1994

ANNALS OF THE NEW YORK ACADEMY OF SCIENCES

Volume 697

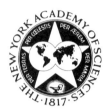

EDITORIAL STAFF

Executive Editor
BILL BOLAND

Managing Editor
JUSTINE CULLINAN

Associate Editor
MARION GARABEDIAN

The New York Academy of Sciences
2 East 63rd Street
New York, New York 10021

CORTICOTROPIN-RELEASING FACTOR AND CYTOKINES: ROLE IN THE STRESS RESPONSE

HANS SELYE SYMPOSIUM ON NEUROENDOCRINOLOGY AND STRESS

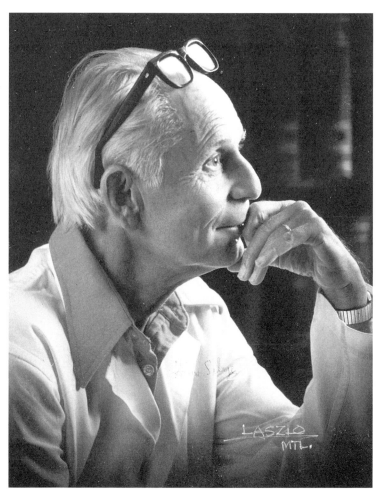

HANS SELYE

Dedicated to Dr. Hans Selye in commemoration of the tenth anniversary of his passing in October 1982.

ANNALS OF THE NEW YORK ACADEMY OF SCIENCES
Volume 697

CORTICOTROPIN-RELEASING FACTOR AND CYTOKINES: ROLE IN THE STRESS RESPONSE

HANS SELYE SYMPOSIUM ON NEUROENDOCRINOLOGY AND STRESS

Edited by Yvette Taché and Catherine Rivier

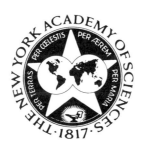

The New York Academy of Sciences
New York, New York
1993

The photograph on the front cover shows The Salk Institute for Biological Studies, La Jolla, California and is reproduced through their courtesy.

Library of Congress Cataloging-in-Publication Data

Hans Selye Symposium on Neuroendocrinology and Stress (3rd : 1992 : Montréal, Québec.
    Corticotropin-releasing factor and cytokines : role in the stress response / Hans Selye Symposium on Neuroendocrinology and Stress ; edited by Yvette Taché and Catherine Rivier.
        p. cm. — (Annals of the New York Academy of Sciences; ISSN 0077-8923 ; v. 697)
    Includes bibliographical references and index.
    ISBN 0-89766-815-4 — ISBN 0-89766-816-2 (paper : alk. paper)
        1. Corticotropin releasing factor—Physiological effect—Congresses.   2. Cytokines—Physiological effect—Congresses.   3. Stress (Physiology)—Congresses.   4. Neuroendocrinology—Congresses.   I. Taché, Yvette.   II. Rivier, Catherine, 1943—   III. Title.   IV. Series.
        [DNLM: 1. Corticotropin-Releasing Factor—physiology—congresses.   2. Cytokines—physiology—congresses.   3. Stress—physiopathology—congresses.   4. Stress—veterinary—congresses.   5. Gastrointestinal System—physiology—congresses.   W1 AN626YL v.697 1993 / QT 162.S8 H249c 1992]
    Q11.N5   vol. 697
    [QR572.C62]
    500 s—dc20
    [616.9'8]
    DNLM/DLC
    for Library of Congress   93-35701
                                                                                                            CIP

SP
Printed in the United States of America
ISBN 0-89766-815-4 (cloth)
ISBN 0-89766-816-2 (paper)
ISSN 0077-8923

ANNALS OF THE NEW YORK ACADEMY OF SCIENCES

Volume 697
October 29, 1993

CORTICOTROPIN-RELEASING FACTOR AND CYTOKINES: ROLE IN THE STRESS RESPONSE[a]

HANS SELYE SYMPOSIUM ON NEUROENDOCRINOLOGY AND STRESS

Editors and Conference Organizers
YVETTE TACHÉ AND CATHERINE RIVIER

Advisory Board
BEATRICE TUCHWEBER, LOUISE DREVET-SELYE, AND SANDOR SZABO

CONTENTS

[a]This volume contains papers presented at the Hans Selye Symposia on Neuroendocrinology and Stress entitled CRF and Cytokines: Role in Stress Response, which was sponsored by the Hans Selye Foundation and held in Montreal, Quebec, Canada on October 11–14, 1992.

Financial assistance was received from:
- FONDS DE LA RECHERCHE EN SANTE DU QUEBEC
- HANS SELYE FOUNDATION
- JOUVEINAL RESEARCH INSTITUTE

Preface

YVETTE TACHÉ

CURE/Digestive Disease Center
V. A. Wadsworth Medical Center, and
Department of Medicine and Brain Research Institute
University of California at Los Angeles
Los Angeles, California 90073

CATHERINE RIVIER

The Clayton Foundation Laboratories for Peptide Biology
The Salk Institute
La Jolla, California 92037

This volume contains the proceedings of the Third Hans Selye Symposium on Neuroendocrinology and Stress, which was devoted to cytokines and the role played by corticotropin-releasing factor (CRF) in mediating the stress response. The meeting was held in Montreal, Canada, on October 11–14, 1992 and commemorates the tenth anniversary of the passing of Hans Selye in Montreal in October 1982.

In 1981, Drs. W. Vale, J. Spiess, C. Rivier, and J. Rivier reported in *Science* the first characterization from ovine hypothalami of a 41-residue peptide that stimulates the secretion of corticotropin and β-endorphin. In subsequent years, CRF became known as a key chemical messenger in the response to stress. The 1992 multidisciplinary conference was the first attempt to address the role of CRF and cytokines in mediating some of the biological responses to stress. Specific topics covered in this volume encompass CRF gene expression, new knowledge on CRF-binding protein, receptor characterization and distribution, influence on endocrine, autonomic, gastrointestinal, and immune functions and behavior. The localization of CRF and CRF receptors in the central nervous system and the potency of the peptide and its antagonist to influence behavior and physiological processes have further emphasized the physiological role played by CRF, particularly as it relates to the chemical coding of stress. The ability of cytokines to stimulate CRF pathways further emphasizes the interactions between activation of immune function and stress. Finally, another aspect of stress covered in this volume is how stress is manifested in domestic animals and its implications. The editors are exceedingly grateful to all the contributors for their thorough articles.

The compilation of these important advances on CRF and cytokines makes this volume an important reference source for understanding the underlying mechanisms mediating the stress response.

The Hans Selye Foundation, established in 1980 by Hans Selye to promote research and education on stress, was the main sponsor of the symposium. The conference would not have taken place without the support of Drs. Beatriz Tuchweber, Louise Drevet-Selye, and Sandor Szabo, members of the standing committee of the Hans Selye Foundation; the dedication of the conference administrator, Joyce Fried; and the help of the local organizing committee, Drs. M. Salas Prato, S. St. Pierre, and B. Tuchweber. We would also like to acknowledge the financial support of the Fonds de la Recherche en Santé du Québec, and Dr. J. L. Junien (Jouveinal Research Institute, France). Last, but not least, Bill M. Boland and Marion Garabedian of the Editorial Department of the New York Academy of Sciences are to be acknowledged for seeing this volume through publication.

Corticotropin-Releasing Factor–Binding Protein

A Putative Peripheral and Central Modulator of the CRF Family of Neuropeptides[a]

DOMINIC P. BEHAN, ELLEN POTTER, STEVE SUTTON,
WOLFGANG FISCHER, PHILIP J. LOWRY,[b]
AND WYLIE W. VALE

Clayton Foundation Laboratories for Peptide Biology
The Salk Institute
La Jolla, San Diego, California 92037

[b]*Department of Biochemistry and Physiology*
Reading University
Reading RG6 2AJ, England

We and others have recently reported the existence of a binding protein for corticotropin-releasing factor (CRF) in human plasma which inhibits the ACTH-releasing activity of the peptide in an *in vitro* pituitary bioassay.[1–6] In order to characterize this putative CRF modulator, we subsequently purified the protein from human plasma by repeated affinity chromatography followed by gel filtration.[7] A 12-million-fold purification resulted in one major band of 37 kDa after SDS PAGE that was estimated to be 95% pure. The protein was tracked throughout the purification by exploiting its ability to inhibit binding of an hCRF antibody to an hCRF-radiolabeled peptide. The purified protein maintained all the characteristics of the crude human plasma protein in that it bound human CRF with high affinity, had a low affinity for the ovine peptide, and gave a dose-dependent inhibition of CRF-induced ACTH secretion *in vitro.*[6] After SDS PAGE and electrophoretic transfer onto nitrocellulose, the band corresponding to the pure protein was excised and subjected to trypsinization. Fragments were then separated by reverse phase HPLC and individually sequenced by Edmann degradation. Amino acid sequence information, obtained for seven tryptic fragments, was then used to develop degenerate cDNA probes for amplification in the polymerase chain reaction (PCR). A 377-bp CRF-binding protein (BP) PCR fragment, amplified from a human liver lambda gt11 cDNA library, was subsequently labeled and used to clone full-length CRF-BP cDNA sequences from human liver and rat brain cDNA libraries, respectively.[8] Both the human and rat cDNA clones, 1.8 and 1.85 kb, respectively, predicted mature proteins of 322 amino acids with each containing one putative N-glycosylation site (FIG. 1), which was in good agreement with Suda *et al.* who reported an increase in electrophoretic mobility of the protein after N-glycanase treatment.[9] Both the human and rat recombinant binding proteins, expressed transiently in COS cells, hindered binding of an hCRF antibody to radiolabeled

[a]This work is supported by NIH grant DK26741 and by the Foundation for Medical Research. D. B. is supported by a fellowship from the Adler Foundation. W. W. V. is an FMR Senior Investigator.

1

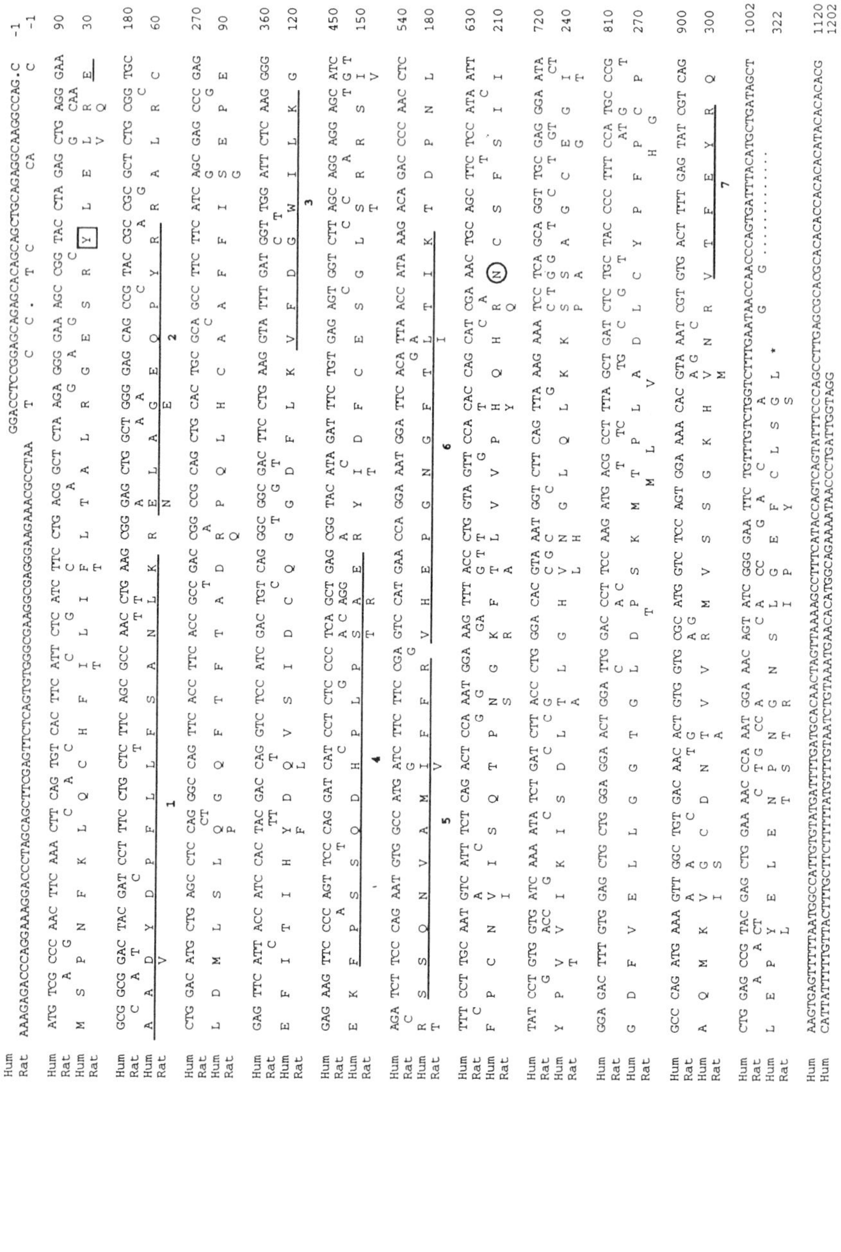

FIGURE 1.

hCRF and dose dependently inhibited CRF-induced ACTH secretion from rat anterior pituitary cells *in vitro*.[8]

The full-length cDNA predicted the presence of 11 cysteines in the CRF-BP precursor, 10 of which remain in the mature molecule after proteolytic cleavage of the signal peptide. Through the sequencing analysis of tryptic fragments of purified recombinant hCRF-BP and examination of mixed sequences before and after reduction, we determined that at least one major form of the recombinant protein has 10 disulfide bonds which are sequentially bonded in tandem pairs.[10] Furthermore, examination of the hCRF-BP gene revealed the presence of six introns and seven exons such that three of the five disulfide loops are encoded by exons 5, 6, and 7. Exons 3 and 4 provide the four cysteines that form the first and second disulfide loops in the sequence with three of the cysteines coming from exon 3 and one from exon 4. Because exons often encode domains within proteins,[11] it is possible that the disulfide loops form functional domains within the mature CRF-BP. Furthermore, this multi-intronic/exonic structure may provide a template for alternate splicing of the CRF-BP primary mRNA transcript resulting in the expression of a different molecule(s) from the same gene by a reorganization of the disulfide loop domains.

We previously reported that CRF-BP is expressed in primate brain and in human liver.[8] However, the protein is not expressed in rat liver which probably explains the lack of a CRF-BP in rat blood. We were, therefore, interested in characterizing promoter elements for this gene that may complement the tissue distribution of the protein. Primer extension analyses revealed the transcriptional initiation site to be 32 bp downstream from a consensus TATA box, which suggested that 900 bp of an extreme 5′ sequence was a putative promoter. Within this extreme 5′ sequence we located transcription elements specific for two liver-specific enhancer proteins, LFA1 and LFB1 at −135 and −598 bp, respectively.[12] These factors may be important in the regulating of blood CRF-BP levels in humans inasmuch as we previously reported the liver to be the most likely source of the circulating protein in normal human plasma.[8] The immune type enhancer elements, NF-kappa B, a transcription factor known to regulate the immunoglobulins and interleukins,[13] and INF-1, a transcription factor known to regulate the interferon gene,[14] were also identified at −305 and −677 bp. This was of particular interest because many genes from the IgG family have exons encoding disulfide-bonded loops[15] and thus bear structural homology to the CRF-BP gene. Finally, a number of estrogen receptor half-sites were located at positions −749, −695, and −273 bp.[16]

The functions of the CRF-binding protein remain to be established. CRF originating from a number of tissues including the brain, spinal cord, adrenal, lung,

←──

FIGURE 1. Diagram of the complete cDNA and predicted amino acid sequences for the human and rat CRF-binding proteins. The first methionine having a Kozak consensus sequence is marked at position +1. The underlined amino acid sequences are those determined for the tryptic fragments. N-terminal sequence analysis revealed the presence of two species: [Y,E] [L,A] [L,D] Y [E,D] [A,P] [A,F], which was attributed to partial proteolytic processing at Arg 29. The most extreme N-terminal amino acid was therefore deduced to be Tyr 25 which is shown by the box. One putative N-glycosylation site was found which is identified by the circle. There are three corrections to the previously published human CRF-BP cDNA sequence,[8] which are summarized as follows: First, there is a transposition of nt 141 and 142 which changes CG to GC and alters the amino acid sequence from DV to EL; second, nt 743 and 744 have been transposed such that AG should be GA which changes the amino acid sequence to G; and third, a C and an A present at positions −29 and −30, respectively, have been deleted.

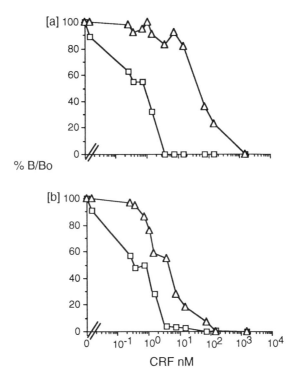

FIGURE 2. Diagram of competitive binding curves for the NP-40 solubilized rat (**a**) and sheep (**b**) membrane CRF-BP. Solubilized membranes were incubated with [125I]rCRF and competed with a range of cold rCRF (*squares*) and/or oCRF (*triangles*) concentrations. Membranes were solubilized with 0.16% NP-40 and diluted in assay buffer (phosphate buffered saline containing EDTA, sodium azide, 0.25% BSA, 0.01% triton X-100). [125I]rCRF was then added and the reaction was incubated for 30 minutes at 25 °C. Bound [125I]CRF was then detected by the addition of a human CRF-BP antibody (5144; 1:1000) followed by a further 30-minute incubation at room temperature. The complex was then finally precipitated by the addition of 200 μL of a preprecipitated sheep antirabbit second antibody mixture. The tubes were then centrifuged (4 °C; 3000 × g) for 15 minutes and the pellets were counted in a gamma counter.

liver,[17] stomach, duodenum,[18] pancreas,[19] joints, inflammatory sites,[20] and placenta[21] may be secreted into the blood and be neutralized by the plasma binding protein.

Many workers have reported the existence of elevated CRF levels in late gestational maternal human plasma which reach a peak in the third trimester and return to normal levels after parturition.[21–24] One function of the protein may be to bind placental-derived CRF and thus modulate the pituitary ACTH-releasing activity of the peptide during late pregnancy when CRF levels are substantially elevated. We have recently found that binding protein levels, as measured by radioimmunoassay, decrease during the third trimester of human pregnancy when CRF levels are inversely increasing.[25] It is possible, therefore, that ligand binding triggers tissue- and/or cell-specific clearance of the complex.

CRF and/or CRF receptors have been identified on splenic lymphocytes and macrophages,[26,27] the adrenal gland,[28] and in a number of neural tissues,[29] suggesting that the peptide can regulate the activity of the immune and autonomic nervous system at peripheral as well as central levels. In support of this, CRF has been shown to regulate a variety of immune responses both directly at the tissue/cell site[20,27,30] and indirectly, presumably via increased glucocorticoid secretion.[31] Thus, in humans, it is likely that both locally produced and circulating CRF-BP can influence the HPA axis and immune system by modulating activity of the peptide at both pituitary and nonpituitary site(s) either by neutralization of the neuropeptide or specific tissue targeting of the bound complex.

Recently, by immunohistochemistry and *in situ* hybridization techniques, we also found CRF-binding protein to be expressed in pituitary corticotropes and centrally in various areas of rat brain including the cerebral cortex, the subcortical limbic system and sensory relays associated with the auditory, olfactory, vestibular, and trigeminal systems.[32]

In its localization to pituitary corticotropes and cortical structures in the central nervous system, CRF-BP shares some regional overlap with CRF receptor binding sites.[29,33] However, other areas of the brain that have been reported to contain a high density of CRF receptors, such as the basal ganglia, thalamus, and cerebellum, appear to express little or no CRF-BP.

Using a CRF-BP ligand immunoradiometric assay (LIRMA) we were able to identify a specific CRF-binding activity in purified plasma membrane fractions prepared from brain and pituitary tissue. In this assay a rabbit CRF-BP antibody raised to the purified recombinant human CRF-BP (5144) and a high-affinity radiolabeled CRF ligand are used. Thus, the radiolabeled CRF binds to the binding protein in the presence of bound CRF-BP antibody, and the whole complex is then

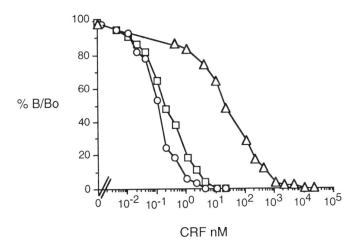

FIGURE 3. Diagram showing competitive binding of hCRF (*squares*), carp urotensin (*circles*), and sauvagine (*triangles*) to the human recombinant CRF-binding protein. Media from CHO cells harboring a stable integrate of the hCRF-BP cDNA were used as a source of the recombinant protein. Respective K_d values for hCRF, carp urotensin, and sauvagine were 0.166, 0.052, and 16.9 nM, respectively. The assay was performed essentially as described in FIGURE 2, except no NP-40 was used. Antisera raised to the recombinant human CRF-BP (5144; 1:1000 initial dilution) was used to detect CRF-BP, and bound complexes were subsequently precipitated by the addition of 200 μL of preprecipitated sheep antirabbit second antibody.

precipitated with a preprecipitated sheep antirabbit second antibody. By use of this assay system, the solubilized rat brain CRF-BP gave K_d values for human and ovine CRF of 0.65 nM and 108 nM, respectively (FIG. 2a). In contrast, however, the CRF-BP solubilized from sheep brain bound ovine CRF with high affinity (K_d hCRF = 0.15 nM; K_d oCRF = 1.75 nM; FIG. 2b), but retained a tenfold higher affinity for the human peptide (FIG. 2b). This suggests that the ovine binding protein has evolved to bind and thus regulate its own oCRF. However, the high affinity maintained for hCRF suggests that ovine CRF-BP may also bind a mammalian CRF homolog that more closely resembles the human peptide in structure.

We also recently demonstrated that the human recombinant binding protein binds urotensins and sauvagine (K_d carp urotensin = 0.052 nM; K_d sauvagine = 16.9 nM), which implies that CRF may not be the sole ligand for the this protein (FIG. 3).

The mechanism of membrane association is yet to be elucidated but the multi-intronic/exonic structure of the CRF-BP gene may provide the potential for alternate splicing and/or posttranslational processing from a larger precursor. Indeed, posttranslational modifications resulting in the addition of fatty acid chains in the form of palmitate,[34] myristate,[34] farnesyl,[35] geranylgeranyl,[36] and phosphatidylinositol groups[37] have resulted in the attachment of a variety of proteins to plasma membranes. Furthermore, other primary sequence characteristics of proteins that lack classical transmembrane domains have resulted in membrane anchorage. One example is the amphiphilic helix which is thought to be responsible for anchoring carboxypeptidase E to the plasma membrane via its C-terminus.[38] It is therefore possible that CRF-BP has similar hydrophobic properties that change the physiochemical characteristics of the protein and result in membrane anchorage. Alternatively, it is possible that a membrane receptor specifically binds CRF-BP at the membrane surface.

The observation of membrane association raises the question of whether CRF-BP participates in any receptor-mediated signal transduction event in addition to its possible role in limiting the action and distribution of the neuropeptide.

REFERENCES

1. LINTON, E. A. & P. J. LOWRY. 1986. A large molecular weight carrier for CRF-41 in human plasma (abstract). J. Endocrinol. **111** (Suppl.)
2. ORTH, D. N. & C. D. MOUNT. 1987. Specific high affinity binding protein for human corticotropin-releasing hormone in normal human plasma. Biochem. Biophys. Res. Commun. **143:** 411–417.
3. LINTON, E. A., C. D. A. WOLFE, D. P. BEHAN & P. J. LOWRY. 1988. A specific carrier substance for human corticotropin releasing factor in late gestational maternal plasma which could mask the ACTH-releasing activity. Clin. Endocrinol. **28:** 315–324.
4. SUDA, T., M. IWASHITA, F. TOZAWA, T. USHIYAMA, N. TAMORI, T. SUMITOMO, Y. NAKAGAMI, H. DEMURA & K. SHIZUM. 1988. Characterization of CRH binding protein in human plasma by chemical cross-linking and its binding during pregnancy. J. Clin. Endocrinol. & Metab. **67:** 1278–1283.
5. ELLIS, M. J., J. H. LIVESEY & R. A. DONALD. 1988. Circulating plasma corticotropin-releasing factor-like immunoreactivity. J. Endocrinol. **117:** 299–307.
6. LINTON, E. A., D. P. BEHAN, P. W. SAPHIER & P. J. LOWRY. 1989. Corticotropin-releasing hormone binding protein: Reduction in the ACTH-releasing activity of placental but not hypothalamic CRH. J. Clin. Endocrinol. & Metab. **70:** 1574–1580.
7. BEHAN, D. P., E. A. LINTON & P. J. LOWRY. 1989. Isolation of the human plasma corticotropin-releasing factor binding protein. J. Clin. Endocrinol. & Metab. **70:** 1574–1580.
8. POTTER, E., D. P. BEHAN, W. H. FISHER, E. A. LINTON, P. J. LOWRY & W. VALE. 1991.

Cloning and characterization of the cDNAs for the human and rat corticotropin-releasing factor binding proteins. Nature **349:** 423–426.

9. SUDA, T., T. SUMITOMO, F. TOZAWA, T. USHIYAMA & H. DEMURA. 1989. CRF-binding protein is a glycoprotein. Biochem. Biophys. Res. Commun. **165:** 703–707.

10. FISCHER, W. H., D. P. BEHAN, E. POTTER, M. PARK, P. J. LOWRY & W. VALE. 1991. Assignment of disulphide bonds in corticotropin releasing factor binding protein. 5th Symposium of the Protein Society, June 22–26, Baltimore, Maryland.

11. GILBERT, W. 1978. Why genes in pieces. Nature **271:** 501.

12. HARDON, E. M., M. FRAIN, G. PAONESSA & R. CORTESES. 1988. Two distinct factors interact with the promoter regions of several liver-specific genes. EMBO J. **7:** 1711–1719.

13. LENARDO, J. M. & D. BALTIMORE. 1989. NF-kB: A pleotrophic mediator of inducible and tissue-specific gene control. Cell **58:** 227–229.

14. FUJITA, T., H. SHIBUYA, H. HOTTA, K. YAMANISHI & T. TANIGUCHI. 1987. Interferon-B gene regulation: Tandemly repeated sequences of a synthetic 6bp oligomer function as a virus-inducible enhancer. Cell **49:** 357–367.

15. BARCLAY, N. A., P. JOHNSON, G. W. McCAUGHAN & A. F. WILLIAMS. 1988. Immunoglobulin-related structures associated with vertebrate cell surfaces. *In* The T-cell Receptors. Plenum. New York, NY.: 53–85.

16. VACCARO, M., A. PAWLAK & J. P. JOST. 1990. Positive and negative regulatory elements of chicken vitellogenin II gene characterized by in vitro transcription competition assays in a homologous system. Proc. Natl. Acad. Sci. USA **87:** 3047–3051.

17. SUDA, T., N. TOMORI, F. YAJIMA, T. SUMITOMO, Y. NAKAGAMI, T. USHIYAMA, H. DEMURA & K. SHIZUME. 1985. Immunoreactive corticotropin-releasing factor in human plasma. J. Clin. Invest. **76:** 2026–2029.

18. NIEUWENHUYSEN KRUSEMAN, A. C., E. A. LINTON, J. F. ACKLAND, G. M. BESSER & P. J. LOWRY. 1984. Heterogeneous immunocytochemical reactivities of O-CRF-like material in the human hypothalamus, pituitary and G.I. tract. Neuroendocrinology **38:** 212–216.

19. PETRUSZ, P., I. MERCHANTHALLER, J. L. MADERDRUT, S. VIGH & A. V. SCHALLY. 1983. Corticotrophin-releasing factor-like immunoreactivity in the vertebrate endocrine pancreas. Proc. Natl. Acad. Sci. USA **80:** 1721.

20. CROFFORD, L., H. SANA, R. WIDLER & G. P. CHROUSOS. 1992. Proinflammatory actions of immune CRH: Detection of peptide and mRNA in the periphery (abstract). Ninth International Congress of Endocrinology. Nice.

21. SASAKI, A., A. S. LIOTTA, M. M. LUCKEY, A. N. MARGIORIS, T. SUDA & D. KRIEGER. 1984. Immunoreactive corticotropin-releasing factor is present in human maternal plasma during the third trimester of pregnancy. J. Clin. Endocrinol. & Metab. **59:** 812–814.

22. CAMPBELL, E. A., E. A. LINTON, C. D. A. WOLFE, P. R. SCRAGGS, M. T. JONES & P. J. LOWRY. 1987. Plasma corticotropin releasing hormone concentrations during pregnancy and parturition. J. Clin. Endocrinol. & Metab. **64:** 1054–1059.

23. LINTON, E. A., C. MACLEAN, A. NIEUNENHUYSEN, F. J. TILDERS, E. A. VAN DER VEEN & P. J. LOWRY. 1987. Direct measurement of human plasma corticotropin-releasing factor by "two-site" immunoradiometric assay. J. Clin. Endocrinol. & Metab. **64:** 1047–1053.

24. GOLAND, R. D., S. L. WARDLAW, R. I. STARK, JR., L. S. B. BROWN & A. G. FRANTZ. 1986. High levels of corticotropin-releasing hormone immunoreactivity in maternal and fetal plasma during pregnancy. J. Clin. Endocrinol. & Metab. **63:** 1199–1203.

25. LINTON, E. A., A. V. PERKINS, R. J. WOODS, F. EBEN, C. D. A. WOLFE, D. P. BEHAN, E. POTTER, W. W. VALE & P. J. LOWRY. 1992. Corticotropin releasing hormone-binding protein [CRH-BP]: Plasma levels decrease during the third trimester of normal human pregnancy. J. Clin. Endocrinol. & Metab. In press.

26. WEBSTER, E. L. & E. B. DESOUZA. 1988. Corticotropin-releasing factor receptors in mouse spleen: Identification, autoradiographic localization, and regulation by divalent cations and guanine nucleotides. Endocrinology **122:** 609–617.

27. McGILLIS, J. P., A. PARK, P. RUBIN-FLETTER, C. TURCK, M. F. DALLMAN & D. G. PAYAN. 1989. Stimulation of rat B-lymphocyte proliferation by corticotropin-releasing factor. J. Neurosci. Res. **23:** 346–352.

28. DAVE, R. J., L. E. EIDEN & R. L. ESKAY. 1985. Corticotropin-releasing factor binding to

peripheral tissue and activation of the adenylate cyclase-adenosine $3',5'$-monophosphate system. Endocrinology **116:** 2152–2159.

29. AGUILERA, G., M. C. MILLAN, R. L. HAUGER & K. J. CATT. 1987. Corticotropin-releasing factor receptors: Distribution and regulation in brain, pituitary, and peripheral tissues. Ann. N.Y. Acad. Sci. **512:** 48.

30. KIANG, J. G. & E. T. WEI. 1987. Corticotropin-releasing factor inhibits thermal injury. J. Pharmacol. Exp. Ther. **243:** 517.

31. IRWIN, M. R., W. VALE & K. T. BRITTON. 1987. Central corticotropin-releasing factor suppresses natural killer cytotoxicity. Brain Behav. Immun. **1:** 81.

32. POTTER, E., D. P. BEHAN, E. A. LINTON, P. J. LOWRY, P. E. SAWCHENKO & W. VALE. 1992. The central distribution of a CRF-binding protein predicts multiple sites and modes of interaction with CRF. Submitted to Proc. Natl. Acad. Sci. USA.

33. DESOUZA, E. B., T. R. INSEL, M. H. PERRIN, J. RIVIER, W. W. VALE & M. J. KUHAR. 1985. Differential regulation of corticotropin-releasing factor receptors in anterior and intermediate lobes of pituitary and in brain following adrenalectomy in rats. Neurosci. Lett. **56:** 121–128.

34. GRAND, R. J. A. 1989. Acylation of viral and eukaryotic proteins. Biochem. J. **258:** 625–638.

35. HANCOCK, J. F., A. I. MAGEE, J. E. CHIDS & C. J. MARSHALL. 1989. All ras proteins are polyisoprenylated but only some are palmitoylated. Cell **57:** 1167–1177.

36. SEABRA, M. C., M. S. BROWN, C. A. SLAUGHTER, T. C. SUDHOF & J. L. GOLDSTEIN. 1992. Purification of component A of Rab geranylgeranyl transferase: Possible identity with chorioderemia gene product. Cell **70:** 1049–1057.

37. LOW, M. 1989. Glycosyl-phosphatidylinositol: A versatile anchor for cell surface proteins. FASEB J. **3:** 1600–1608.

38. FRICKER, L. D., B. DAS & R. HOGUE ANGELETTI. 1990. Identification of a pH-dependent membrane anchor of carboxypeptidase E (EC 3.4.17.10). J. Biol. Chem. **265:** 2476–2482.

Corticotropin-Releasing Factor and Interleukin-1 Receptors in the Brain-Endocrine-Immune Axis

Role in Stress Response and Infection

ERROL B. DE SOUZA

Neurocrine Biosciences, Inc.
1020 Prospect Street, Suite 317
La Jolla, California 92037

Recent evidence suggests that the endocrine, immune, and central nervous systems interact and respond to physiological and pharmacological stimuli in a coordinated manner. Although the influence of the brain in regulating endocrine function has long been recognized, the presence of hormones, neurotransmitters, and receptors common to all three systems supports the view that bidirectional communication exists between the neuroendocrine and immune systems and between the immune and central nervous systems. The brain-endocrine-immune responses to stress and infection provide two examples of how the three systems respond in an integrated manner to physiological and pathological stimuli. Two primary candidates involved in coordinating such responses through the brain-endocrine-immune circuitry are corticotropin-releasing factor (CRF) and interleukin-1 (IL-1).

CRF, a 41-amino-acid peptide, plays a pivotal role in integrating the organism's overall response to stress. CRF, derived from the paraventricular nucleus of the hypothalamus, is the major physiological regulator of the basal and stress-induced release of adrenocorticotropic hormone (ACTH), β-endorphin, and other proopiomelanocortin (POMC)-derived peptides from the pituitary gland.[1] CRF is not only localized in the hypothalamus but is found throughout the central nervous system (CNS).[1] In addition to its effects on the pituitary, substantial evidence exists to suggest that CRF functions as a neurotransmitter/neuromodulator in the CNS to produce a wide spectrum of electrophysiological, autonomic, and behavioral effects.[1] Recent evidence also suggests that CRF may have immunomodulatory actions in the periphery.[2] Overall, CRF appears to be one of the crucial CNS neurotransmitters/ neuromodulators that activates and coordinates the endocrine, behavioral, autonomic, and possibly immune responses to stress.

The cytokine IL-1 is one of the key mediators of the immunological and pathological responses to stress, infection, and antigenic challenge.[3,4] In addition, IL-1 has a variety of effects in the brain including induction of fever,[3,4] alteration of slow wave sleep,[5] reduction of food intake,[6] induction of analgesia,[7] induction of acute phase glycoprotein synthesis,[8] stimulation of thermogenesis,[9] inhibition of gastric acid secretion,[10–12] and alteration of neuroendocrine activity. With regard to its neuroendocrine actions, central administration of IL-1 stimulates the hypothalamic-pituitary-adrenocortical axis,[13–15] inhibits the hypothalamic-pituitary-gonadal axis,[16,17] elevates circulating levels of insulin,[18] while inhibiting release of thyroid hormone.[19] In addition to modulating hormone secretion through indirect effects in brain, IL-1 has been shown to have direct actions at target endocrine organs such as the pituitary[20–23] and testis.[16,24–26]

Because the actions of CRF and IL-1 described above are mediated through membrane receptors, a summary of the characteristics and physiological roles of CRF and IL-1 receptors in the brain-endocrine-immune axis will be provided. The pharmacological and biochemical characteristics and localization and modulation of CRF receptors have been described in detail elsewhere.[27-30] Thus, only an overall summary of the characteristics of CRF receptors in the brain-pituitary-immune axis will be included. The focus of this paper will be on IL-1 receptors. Specifically, the general kinetic and pharmacological characteristics will be described, as well as the modulation of IL-1 receptors by endotoxin and CRF treatment in the brain-endocrine-immune axis. The physiological role of IL-1 in modulating CNS and endocrine activities will be described in the context of the distribution of IL-1 receptors in brain, pituitary, and testis.

CRF RECEPTORS IN THE BRAIN-PITUITARY-IMMUNE AXIS

Radioligand binding studies in membrane homogenates and autoradiographic studies in slide-mounted tissue sections have identified, characterized, and localized CRF receptors in the brain-pituitary-immune axis using a variety of iodine-125-labeled analogs of CRF.

Kinetic, Pharmacological, and Biochemical Characteristics

Specific [^{125}I]CRF binding was identified in homogenates of the anterior[31-33] and neurointermediate[33] lobes of the pituitary gland, brain,[34] and spleen[35] and was found to have comparable kinetic and pharmacological characteristics in all the tissues examined (TABLE 1). [^{125}I]CRF binding was saturable, reversible, and on Scatchard analysis demonstrated the presence of a high-affinity binding site with an apparent K_d value of 200–400 pM. The relative density of CRF binding was highest in the anterior and intermediate lobes of the pituitary, with moderate densities present in brain and low but detectable quantities present in spleen. Data from competition studies demonstrated that the CRF binding sites in the four tissues had comparable pharmacology; the specificity and relative potencies of CRF analogs and fragments inhibiting [^{125}I]CRF binding correlated extremely well with their relative intrinsic potencies in stimulating or inhibiting anterior pituitary secretion of ACTH *in vitro*. These data substantiate earlier suggestions from behavioral and biochemical studies that some structural requirements for CRF activity are shared by the brain, pituitary, and splenic receptors.

Chemical affinity cross-linking studies followed by SDS-PAGE and autoradiography demonstrated that the molecular weight of the CRF receptor is higher in peripheral tissues (75,000 Da in pituitary and spleen) than in brain (58,000 Da) (TABLE 1).[36] Enzymatic digestion studies demonstrated that the CRF receptor is a glycoprotein and that the differences observed in the molecular weight are due to the microheterogeneity of the carbohydrate moieties on the receptors in two types of tissues.[37] Furthermore, limited proteolysis revealed that the CRF receptor protein in the brain or periphery contained similar proteolytic enzyme cleavage sites, suggesting that the protein backbone of the receptor is comparable in all tissues.

Second Messengers

Magnesium ions enhance agonist binding to receptors coupled to adenylate cyclase whereas guanine nucleotides selectively decrease the affinity of agonists for their receptors. In anterior and intermediate lobes of the pituitary,[32] in brain,[34] and in spleen,[35] the addition of guanosine 5′-triphosphate (GTP) and related analogs, but not adenosine 5′-triphosphate (ATP), to the incubation medium resulted in dose-dependent inhibition of [125I]CRF binding (TABLE 1). In contrast, magnesium ions appeared obligatory and produced dose-dependent increases in [125I]CRF binding (TABLE 1). On the other hand, monovalent cations such as NaCl had no major effects of [125I]CRF binding. The effects of magnesium chloride and guanine nucleotides on [125I]CRF binding are consistent with previous data demonstrating

TABLE 1. Similarities and Differences in the *in Vitro* Characteristics of Corticotropin-Releasing Factor (CRF) Receptors in Brain, Pituitary, and Spleen

| Characteristic | Brain | Pituitary | | Spleen |
		Anterior	Intermediate	
Affinity (K_d; pM)	200–400	200–400	200–400	200–400
Binding in the presence of divalent cations (e.g., Mg^{2+})	Increased	Increased	Increased	Increased
Binding in the presence of guanine nucleotides (e.g., GTP)	Decreased	Decreased	Decreased	Decreased
Second messenger (stimulation of adenylate cyclase activity)	Yes	Yes	Yes	Yes
Pharmacology comparable to CRF-stimulated ACTH secretion *in vitro*	Yes	Yes	Yes	Yes
Apparent molecular weight (Da)	58,000	75,000	75,000	75,000
Structural composition	Glycoprotein	Glycoprotein	Glycoprotein	Glycoprotein

the ability of these modulators to alter agonist binding to receptors coupled to adenylate cyclase. The second messenger system mediating the effects of CRF in the anterior and intermediate lobes of the pituitary,[1] in brain,[38] and in spleen[39] involves stimulation of cAMP production.

CRF Receptors in the Pituitary

CRF is the primary physiological regulator of POMC-derived peptide secretion from the pituitary gland.[1] Rat, mouse, bovine or porcine pituitary autoradiograms showed specific binding sites for [125I]CRF in anterior and intermediate lobes; no specific binding sites for CRF were apparent in the posterior pituitary.[31,32] Some differences among species were shown in the relative distribution of CRF receptors in the anterior and intermediate lobes. For example, the density of CRF receptors was somewhat higher in the anterior than in the intermediate lobe in the rat whereas the converse was true in the mouse, pig, and cow. The distribution of CRF binding sites resembled the clustering of corticotropes in the anterior lobe and the uniform distribution of opiomelanocortin-producing cells in the intermediate pituitary. In addition, human pituitary autoradiograms showed the presence of a cluster-like distribution of receptors in the anterior lobe.[40] The distribution pattern of receptors within the pituitary further supports the physiological role of endogenous CRF in regulating POMC-derived hormone secretion from the anterior and intermediate lobes of the pituitary.

CRF Receptors in the CNS

The widespread distribution of CRF-containing neurons in the CNS and the direct CNS-mediated effects of CRF on autonomic function, behavior, and neuronal electrical activity suggest that CRF also functions as a bona fide neurotransmitter in brain.[1] CRF receptors were heterogeneously distributed throughout the CNS with highest concentrations present in brain regions involved in cognitive function (cerebral cortex), in limbic areas involved in emotion and stress responses (amygdala, nucleus accumbens, and hippocampus), in olfactory bulb, in cerebellum, and in brain stem regions important in regulating autonomic function (locus coeruleus and nucleus of the solitary tract).[41] In addition, CRF receptors were localized in spinal cord, with the highest concentrations present in the substantia gelatinosa of the dorsal horn.[42] Overall, the pattern of localization of CRF receptors in CNS further substantiates the pivotal role of the neuropeptide in integrating the endocrine, autonomic, and behavioral responses to stress.

CRF Receptors in the Spleen

CRF also plays a significant role in integrating the response of the immune system to physiological, psychological, and immunological stressors.[2] Autoradiographic studies in mouse spleen demonstrated that specific [^{125}I]CRF binding sites were primarily localized to the splenic pulp and marginal zone regions that have high concentrations of macrophages.[35] The absence of specific CRF binding sites in the periarteriole and peripheral follicular white pulp regions of the spleen suggests that neither T nor B lymphocytes have specific high-affinity CRF receptors. The demonstration of CRF-like immunoreactivity in primary sensory afferents and in human peripheral blood lymphocytes provides possible sources of CRF in spleen that could be released by neurosecretion or paracrine secretion from splenic leukocyte populations, respectively. CRF had been shown to regulate the expression of POMC-derived peptides in mouse splenocytes.[43] The demonstration of functional CRF receptors in macrophage-enriched zones of the spleen raises the possibility that CRF may regulate POMC secretion in mouse macrophages through a cAMP-mediated mechanism similar to that demonstrated in the pituitary. Alternatively, Kavelaars et al.[44] have provided evidence that CRF stimulates human peripheral blood monocytes to secrete IL-1, which, in turn, stimulates B lymphocytes to secrete β-endorphin. Thus, IL-1 from macrophages may mediate CRF-induced secretion of POMC-derived peptides from lymphocytes.

IL-1 RECEPTORS IN THE BRAIN-ENDOCRINE-IMMUNE AXIS

Radioligand binding studies in membrane homogenates have identified and characterized IL-1 receptors in mouse brain,[45,46] pituitary,[47,48] testis,[46,49] kidney,[50] AtT-20 mouse pituitary, and EL-4 6.1 mouse thymoma cell lines[47,48] using iodine-125-labeled recombinant human IL-1α ([125I]IL-1α) or recombinant human IL-1 receptor antagonist ([125I]IL-1ra). In addition, receptor autoradiographic[45,46,49] and *in situ* hybridization histochemical studies[51–53] have been utilized to localize IL-1 and IL-1 receptor mRNA, respectively, in slide-mounted tissue sections of brain, pituitary, and testis.

Kinetic and Pharmacological Characteristics

[125I]IL-1α or [125I]IL-1ra binding to membrane homogenates of mouse (C57BL/6) hippocampus, pituitary, testis, spleen, kidney, AtT-20 mouse pituitary tumor cell line, and EL-4 6.1 thymoma cell line had comparable kinetic and pharmacological characteristics. Specific binding of [125I]IL-1α or [125I]IL-1ra (FIG. 1) was temperature dependent, linear with membrane protein concentration, saturable, reversible, and of high affinity (K_d of 20–100 pM). [125I]IL-1α or [125I]IL-1ra (TABLE 2) binding was specifically inhibited by recombinant human IL-1α, recombinant human IL-1β, and a weak analog, recombinant IL-1β+, in parallel with their relative bioactivities in a murine thymocyte costimulation assay (TABLE 2). The pharmacological specificity of the IL-1 binding site in these tissues was further strengthened by the lack of inhibitory activity of peptides such as CRF and tumor necrosis factor-α. The kinetic and pharmacological characteristics of [125I]IL-1α binding in these tissues were comparable to the characteristics of type I IL-1 receptors found in T lymphocytes and fibroblasts.

IL-1 Receptors in the CNS

Overall, both the receptor autoradiographic and *in situ* hybridization histochemical studies demonstrated low densities of IL-1 receptors and type I IL-1 receptor mRNA throughout the forebrain. One exception was the hippocampus in which high levels of type I IL-1 receptor mRNA (FIG. 2) and receptor expression (FIG. 3) were evident in the molecular and granular layers of the dentate gyrus, which contain intrinsic neurons as well as afferent terminal projections. Although these data suggest that IL-1 receptors in brain are localized primarily to neurons, IL-1 has been reported to stimulate eicosanoid production in rat primary culture astrocytes,[54] to be an astroglial growth factor, and to stimulate astroglial proliferation.[55] Quinolinic acid lesions were used to determine whether IL-1 binding sites in the hippocampus were localized to neurons and/or astroglia.[45] The destruction of intrinsic neurons after local injections of quinolinic acid in the hippocampus was associated with the disappearance of [125I]IL-1α binding, indicating that IL-1 receptors were predominantly associated with intrinsic neurons. The expression of IL-1 has recently been detected after microinjection of lipopolysaccharide (LPS) and γ-interferon into rat hippocampus,[56] and perferent path deafferentation,[57] providing an endogenous substrate for IL-1 receptors in this brain area. Furthermore, both hippocampal neurons and glial cells respond to IL-1 in culture by increasing production of nerve growth factor (NGF).[58,59] Intracerebroventricular injection of IL-1 in rats has also been reported to increase NGF mRNA in the hippocampus.[59]

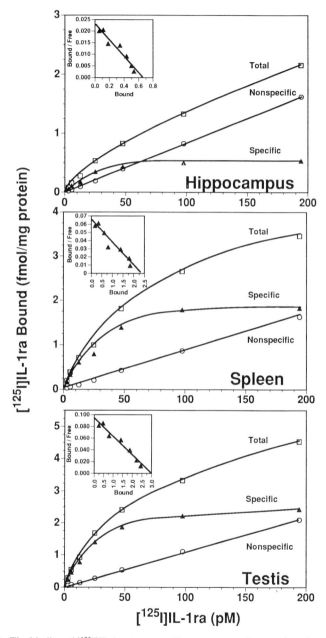

FIGURE 1. The binding of [125I]IL-1ra to mouse hippocampus, spleen, and testis as a function of increasing ligand concentration. Direct plot of data showing the total amount of [125I]IL-1ra bound (Total), binding in the presence of 300 nM IL-1α or β (Nonspecific), and specific (Total minus Nonspecific) binding. The inserted figures demonstrate Scatchard plots of [125I]IL-1ra specific binding. (Takao *et al.*[46] Reproduced, with permission, from the *Journal of Neuroimmunology.*)

TABLE 2. Pharmacological Specificity of $[^{125}I]$IL-1α and $[^{125}I]$IL-1ra Binding to Mouse Tissues

| Peptide | Ki (pM) Hippocampus | | Spleen | Kidney | Testis | | Biological Activity (units/mg) |
	$[^{125}I]$IL-1α	$[^{125}I]$IL-1ra	$[^{125}I]$IL-1ra	$[^{125}I]$IL-1α	$[^{125}I]$IL-1α	$[^{125}I]$IL-1ra	
IL-1α	55 ± 18	70 ± 10	57 ± 9	28 ± 19	14 ± 2	46 ± 8	3.0×10^7
IL-1ra	ND	119 ± 63	104 ± 54	ND	ND	94 ± 49	No activity
IL-1β	76 ± 20	1798 ± 234	3138 ± 1159	53 ± 23	89 ± 6	3672 ± 1317	2.0×10^{7a}
IL-1β+	2940 ± 742	ND	ND	5560 ± 2098	7183 ± 604	ND	1.0×10^6
IL-1βc18	ND	2008 ± 350	2780 ± 919	ND	ND	2732 ± 474	ND
TNF	>100,000	>100,000	>100,000	>100,000	>100,000	>100,000	8.0×10^2
CRF	>100,000	>100,000	>100,000	>100,000	>100,000	>100,000	0.0

NOTE: Peptides at 3–10 concentrations were incubated with approximately 100 pM $[^{125}I]$IL-1α and 40 pM $[^{125}I]$IL-1ra for 120 min at room temperature. All assays were conducted in triplicate in three separate experiments. K_i (inhibitory binding-affinity constant) values were obtained from competition curve data analyzed using the computer program LIGAND.[72] Biological activity data were obtained in a murine thymocyte assay.[73]
[a]IL-1β used in the $[^{125}I]$IL-1ra experiments had lower biological activity than IL-1β used in the $[^{125}I]$IL-1α experiments.
Abbreviations: CRF, rat/human corticotropin-releasing factor; TNF, human recombinant tumor necrosis factor-α; ND, not determined.

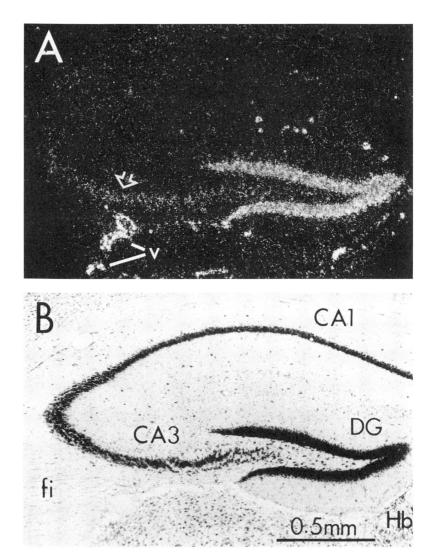

FIGURE 2. Darkfield photomicrograph of an emulsion autoradiogram of a coronal section through the hippocampus after *in situ* hybridization with antisense probe for IL-1 receptor mRNA (**A**). An adjacent Nissl-stained section is shown for reference (**B**). Note the dense autoradiographic signal over granule cells in the dentate gyrus (DG) and, to a lesser extent, over the pyramidal cell layer of the hilus and CA3 region (*arrow*). Note also the dense signal over endothelial cells of postcapillary venules (v). fi, fimbria hippocampus; Hb, medial habenular nucleus (Cunningham *et al.*[51] Reproduced with permission of The Endocrine Society.)

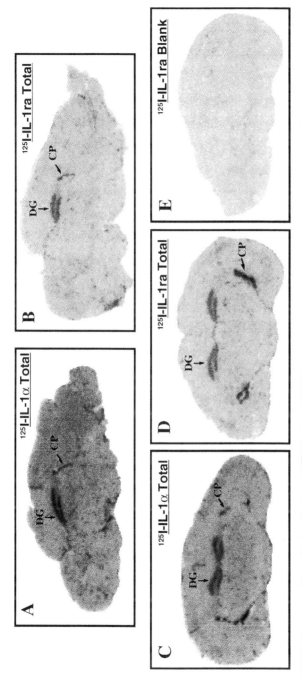

FIGURE 3. Autoradiographic localization of [125I]IL-1α and [125I]IL-1ra in mouse brain cut in sagittal (*top*) and coronal (*bottom*) planes. The images were computer generated using autoradiograms on Hyperfilm. The darker areas in autoradiograms correspond to brain regions displaying higher densities of binding. Note the absence of specific [125I]IL-1ra binding in an adjacent (blank) section **E** coincubated with 100 nM IL-1α. DG, dentate gyrus; CP, choroid plexus. (Takao *et al.*[46] Reproduced, with permission, from the *Journal of Neuroimmunology.*)

Administration of IL-1 alters a variety of functions that are mediated primarily in the hypothalamus. Some of these effects of IL-1 include induction of fever,[3,4] analgesia,[7] and thermogenesis;[9] reduction of food intake[6] and of gastric acid secretion;[11] and alteration of neuroendocrine activity.[13–16] The importance of this brain area in mediating the effects of IL-1 is underscored by immunohistochemical studies identifying neurons positive for IL-1β-like immunoreactivity in the hypothalamus.[60] Very low densities of specific [^{125}I]IL-1α binding sites were detected in homogenate preparations of hypothalamus; however, autoradiographic localization (FIG. 3) and *in situ* hybridization studies demonstrated that the distribution of type I IL-1 binding sites in hypothalamus was unremarkable. There may be several explanations for the apparent discrepancy between the hypothalamic effects of IL-1 and the low densities of receptors in this brain region. Because of the higher endogenous levels of IL-1 and/or IL-1ra in the hypothalamus, the IL-1 receptors may become occupied, resulting in an apparent low level of detectable IL-1 binding sites in this brain area. Alternatively, these effects of IL-1 may be mediated by a subtype of IL-1 receptors in hypothalamus that are not labeled by [^{125}I]IL-1α or [^{125}I]IL-1ra under the conditions used. The effects of IL-1 may also be indirectly mediated through actions of the cytokine on receptors in extrahypothalamic brain areas such as the hippocampus, which, in turn, may influence hypothalamic function.

There was a very high density of IL-1 receptors in the choroid plexus (FIG. 3). The resolution of the autoradiographic technique did not allow the precise localization of IL-1 to a particular component (vasculature, smooth muscle cells, or epithelium) of the choroid plexus. A recent study demonstrated that the choroid plexus was able to present foreign antigen to and stimulate the proliferation of peripheral helper T-lymphocytes.[61] Furthermore, *in vivo,* choroid plexus epithelial cells have access to and are capable of taking up virus-sized particles from the cerebrospinal fluid (CSF).[61] The researchers suggested that the choroid plexus, which constitutes the blood–CSF barrier, may play a role in immunological communication between the CNS and periphery.[61] IL-1-like activity is present in CSF[62,63] and is altered in patients with bacterial meningitis.[63] IL-1 receptors in the choroid plexus may play an important role in the immune and CNS responses to infection.

IL-1 Receptors in the Pituitary

IL-1 receptors[46–48,64] and type I IL-1 receptor mRNA[52] were localized in high densities in the anterior lobe of the mouse pituitary; no specific binding was evident in the intermediate or posterior lobes of the pituitary gland. Within the anterior lobe, there was a homogeneous distribution of IL-1 receptors and mRNA, suggesting a generalized action of the cytokine on hormone synthesis and/or secretion. IL-1 receptors were also detected in high concentrations in AtT-20 mouse pituitary tumor cells. Several groups have shown that IL-1 can directly stimulate ACTH/β-endorphin release in AtT-20 cells,[20,22,23] and ACTH release[21,65] and POMC mRNA production[65] in primary rat pituitary cultures. Although other laboratories were not able to replicate the direct action of IL-1 on pituitary cells,[14,15] IL-1 was found to stimulate pituitary ACTH release by a central action mediated by hypothalamic CRF.[13–15] The controversy of whether IL-1 induces ACTH secretion by a direct stimulation of cells in the pituitary or indirectly via hypothalamic stimulation of CRF remains unresolved.

IL-1 Receptors in the Testis

The autoradiographic localization studies demonstrate a heterogeneous distribution of IL-1 receptors in mouse testis. Low to moderate densities of [^{125}I]IL-1α or [^{125}I]IL-1ra binding sites[46,49] and type I IL-1 receptor mRNA[53] were present in the interstitial areas of the testis. In view of the presence of large amounts of IL-1-like factors in rat testis[66,67] and human testicular cytosolic fluid,[66] it would appear that the IL-1 receptors in the testis may, under physiological conditions, subserve a paracrine function. The functional nature of IL-1 binding sites in testis is further supported by demonstrations that IL-1 inhibited steroidogenesis by cultured Leydig cells[24] and neonatal testicular cells.[25] Further support for a functional role for the IL-1 binding sites in testis come from a study demonstrating that IL-1 stimulated spermatogonial proliferation *in vivo.*[26]

High densities of type I IL-1 receptor mRNA (FIG. 4) and IL-1 receptors were present in both the luminal centers of the epididymis and the lumen of the seminiferous tubules. Moderate densities of binding sites were found in the head, body, and tail of the epididymis. The highest densities of binding sites were found along the luminal borders of the epididymis, with a circumferential pattern of distribution. The role of the very high densities of IL-1 binding sites in the epididymis is, at present, unclear. The detection of IL-1 activity in extracts of epididymal tissue and epididymal sperm[67] provides an endogenous ligand for these binding sites. IL-1 in the epididymis may serve important biological functions involved in the spermatogenic process[26] or, possibly, in the transit of sperm.

Stress, infection, and inflammation are often accompanied by increased IL-1 production and inhibition of reproductive function. In view of the presence of IL-1-like factors[66,67] and IL-1 receptors in testis and the effects of IL-1 to inhibit steroidogenesis,[25,26] it is tempting to speculate on a role for IL-1 at the gonadal level in mediating some of these stress-induced effects on reproductive function. IL-1 may also play a role in modulating reproductive function through actions in the CNS to inhibit GnRH release[16] or its effects to stimulate CRF secretion,[13–15] which, in turn, can inhibit the hypothalamic-pituitary-gonadal axis.[68,69]

In Vivo *Modulation of IL-1 Receptors in Mice after Treatment with Endotoxin*

In an attempt to define the involvement of endogenous IL-1 in the regulation of IL-1 receptors in mouse tissues, we examined [^{125}I]IL-1α binding in hippocampus, pituitary, spleen, kidney, and testis after two intraperitoneal injections of lipopolysaccharide at 0 and 12 h.[50,70] Homogenate binding and autoradiographic studies using a single concentration of radioligand (80–100 pM) demonstrated significant reductions in [^{125}I]IL-1α binding in all the tissues examined at 12 h after the second injection of LPS (FIG. 5). Saturation experiments carried out in testis and kidney demonstrated that the decreases in [^{125}I]IL-1α binding were due to decreases in both the affinity and density of IL-1 receptors. These data provide indirect evidence in support of the contention that LPS treatment increases endogenous IL-1 production which, in turn, down-regulates its receptors. Recently, we have measured IL-1β levels following LPS administration and confirmed that treatment with endotoxin results in increases in IL-1 levels in the various tissues.[70] The effects of IL-1 in brain and in the testis to down-regulate its receptors probably represent paracrine actions of the cytokine because access of circulating cytokine to these tissues may be limited by the blood-brain and blood-testicular barriers, respectively. However, the down-regulation of IL-1 receptors in pituitary, spleen, and kidney may be a consequence of

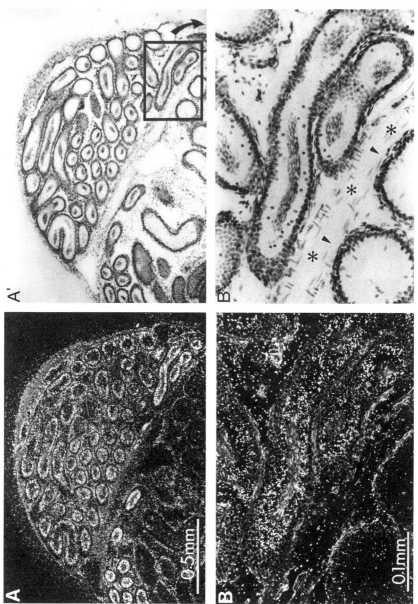

FIGURE 4.

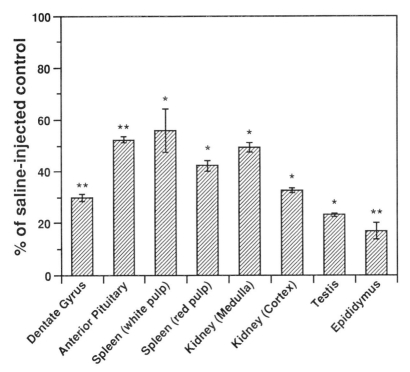

FIGURE 5. Effects of endotoxin treatment on [^{125}I]IL-1α binding in brain, endocrine, and immune tissues using quantitative autoradiography. Mice were injected with lipopolysaccharide (LPS) (30 μg/mouse) at time 0 and 12 h and sacrificed 12 h after the second LPS injection. Data are expressed as a percentage of the mean ± SEM of vehicle-injected controls. Asterisk and double asterisk represent significant differences at $p < 0.05$ and $p < 0.005$, respectively, from saline-injected controls as determined by Student's t test.

increased tissue concentrations of IL-1 as well as the effects of elevated levels of circulating IL-1 in response to treatment with endotoxin. The dramatic compensatory homologous down-regulation of IL-1 receptors in the various tissues following treatment with endotoxin further underscores the importance of the cytokine in regulating brain-endocrine-immune function in response to infection.

FIGURE 4. Low-power (**A**) and high-power (**B**) darkfield photomicrographs of an emulsion autoradiogram of a section through the epididymis after *in situ* hybridization with an antisense probe for type I IL-1 receptor mRNA. Brightfield photomicrographs of the same section counterstained with hematoxylin-eosin are shown for reference (**A′**, **B′**). Note the intense autoradiographic signal over the cells lining the epididymal ducts, denser in the head than the body (*arrowheads*). The head and body of the epididymis are separated in this section by a layer of connective tissue (indicated by *asterisks*). The relatively homogeneous distribution of signal over the entire pseudostratified epithelium of the ducts suggests significant localization to large columnar principal cells, although production by the much smaller basal cells located at the base of the epithelium cannot be excluded. Signal over intraductal sperm cells and over interposed smooth muscle and connective tissue elements (*asterisks*) is comparable to background. (Cunningham *et al.*[53] Reproduced, with permission, from *Neuroendocrinology.*)

In Vitro *Modulation of IL-1 Receptors in Mouse AtT-20 Pituitary Tumor Cells by Treatment with CRF*

In order to further characterize the mechanisms regulating the interactions of IL-1 and CRF, we examined [^{125}I]IL-1α and [^{125}I]CRF binding at 24 h after treatment of AtT-20 cell cultures with rat/human CRF.[71] The treatment of AtT-20 cells for 24 h with CRF produced a dose-dependent increase in [^{125}I]IL-1α binding and a dose-dependent decrease in [^{125}I]CRF binding. The CRF-induced increase in [^{125}I]IL-1α binding appears to be mediated through specific membrane receptors for CRF

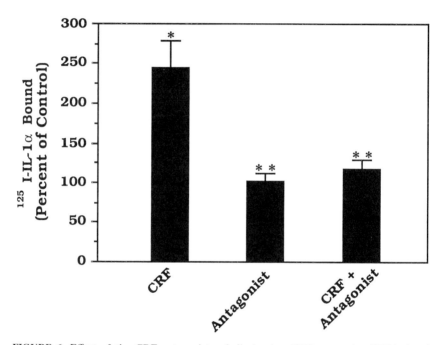

FIGURE 6. Effect of the CRF antagonist, α-helical ovine CRF$_{9-41}$, on the CRF-induced increase in [^{125}I]IL-1α binding to AtT-20 cell membrane homogenates. AtT-20 cells were incubated with vehicle, 10 nM rat/human CRF, 1 mM CRF antagonist, or 10 nM rat/human CRF + 1 mM CRF antagonist for 24 h. Data are expressed as a percentage of vehicle-treated controls. *$p < 0.01$ vs. control; **$p < 0.01$ vs. 10 nM rat/human CRF, as determined by one-way ANOVA and Duncan's Multiple Range Test. (Webster *et al.*[71] Reproduced with permission from the Endocrine Society.)

because the CRF receptor antagonist, α-helical ovine CRF$_{9-41}$, blocked the CRF-induced increase in IL-1 receptors without producing any changes in [^{125}I]IL-1α binding by itself (FIG. 6). [^{125}I]IL-1α saturation assays performed in CRF-treated and control cell cultures indicated that the affinity (K_d) values in the control and CRF-treated cells were similar whereas the density of the receptors in the CRF-treated cultures were significantly higher than in the control-treated group. The increased density of IL-1 receptors after treatment with CRF may involve a variety of mechanisms including increased synthesis of IL-1 receptors, unmasking of cryptic receptors, and/or decrease in internalization of IL-1 receptors. If increased CRF concentrations produce an up-regulation of IL-1 receptors in the anterior pituitary similar to that observed in AtT-20 cells, then one might speculate that IL-1 (which increases in stressful situations) may act at the pituitary level to maintain the elevated plasma ACTH seen following stress.

SUMMARY AND CONCLUSIONS

CRF and IL-1 receptors were identified, characterized, and localized in brain, endocrine, and immune tissues. CRF receptors with comparable kinetic and pharmacological characteristics were localized in the anterior and intermediate lobes of the pituitary, in brain areas involved in mediating stress responses, and in the macrophage-enriched marginal zones of the spleen. The discrete localization of IL-1 receptors in neurons of the hippocampus provides further support for the role of IL-1 as a neurotransmitter/neuromodulator/growth factor in the CNS. The neuroendocrine effects of IL-1 may be mediated through actions of the cytokine in brain. However, given the high densities of IL-1 receptors in the anterior pituitary and testis, direct effects of the cytokine at the pituitary or gonadal levels seem highly likely. Overall, these data support a role for IL-1 and CRF in coordinating and integrating the brain-endocrine-immune responses to physiological, pharmacological, and pathological stimuli.

ACKNOWLEDGMENTS

The work presented in this paper represents the collaborative efforts of numerous colleagues including Drs. Toshihiro Takao, Daniel E. Tracey, Emmett T. Cunningham, Jr., Dimitri E. Grigoriadis, and Elizabeth L. Webster.

REFERENCES

1. DE SOUZA, E. B. & C. B. NEMEROFF, EDS. 1990. Corticotropin-Releasing Factor: Basic and Clinical Studies of a Neuropeptide. CRC Press. Boca Raton, FL.
2. BLALOCK, J. E. 1989. A molecular basis for bidirectional communication between the immune and neuroendocrine systems. Physiol. Rev. **69:** 1–32.
3. DINARELLO, C. A. 1988. Biology of interleukin 1. FASEB J. **2:** 108–115.
4. MIZEL, S. B. 1989. The interleukins. FASEB J. **3:** 2379–2388.
5. KRUEGER, J. M., J. WALTER, C. A. DINARELLO, S. M. WOLFF & L. CHEDID. 1984. Sleep-promoting effects of endogenous pyrogen-(interleukin-1). Am. J. Physiol. **246:** R994–R999.
6. MCCARTHY, D. O., M. J. KLUGER & A. J. VANDER. 1985. Suppression of food intake during infection: Is interleukin-1 involved? Am. J. Clin. Nutrition **42:** 1179–1182.
7. NAKAMURA, H., K. NAKANISHI, A. KITA & T. KADOKAWA. 1988. Interleukin-1 induces analgesia in mice by a central action. Eur. J. Pharmacol. **149:** 49–54.
8. BLATTEIS, C. M., W. S. HUNTER, Q. J. LLANOS, R. A. AHOKAS & T. A. MASHBURN, JR. 1984. Activation of acute-phase responses by intrapreoptic injections of endogenous pyrogen in guinea pigs. Brain Res. Bull. **12:** 689–696.
9. DANSCOMBE, M. J., R. A. LEFEUVRE, B. O. SAGAY, N. J. ROTHWELL & M. J. STOCK. 1989. Pyrogenic and thermogenic effects of interleukin-1 beta in the rat. Am. J. Physiol. **256:** E7–E11.
10. SAPERAS, E., H. YANG, C. RIVIER & Y. TACHÉ. 1990. Central action of recombinant interleukin-1 to inhibit acid secretion in rats. Gastroenterology **99:** 1599–1606.

11. SAPERAS, E., H. YANG & Y. TACHÉ. 1992. Interleukin-1β acts at hypothalamic sites to inhibit gastric acid secretion in rats. Am. J. Physiol. **263:** G414–G418.
12. UEHARA, A., T. OKUMURA, S. KITAMORI, Y. TAKASUGI & M. NAMIKI. 1990. Interleukin-1: A cytokine that has potent antisecretory and anti-ulcer actions via the central nervous system. Biochem. Biophys. Res. Commun. **173:** 585–590.
13. BERKENBOSCH, F., J. VAN OERS, A. DEL REY, F. TILDERS, & H. BESEDOVSKY. 1987. Corticotropin-releasing factor–producing neurons in the rat activated by interleukin-1. Science **238:** 524–526.
14. SAPOLSKY, R., C. RIVIER, G. YAMAMOTO, P. PLOTSKY & W. VALE. 1987. Interleukin-1 stimulates the secretion of hypothalamic corticotropin-releasing factor. Science **238:** 522–524.
15. UEHARA, A., P. E. GOTTSCHALL, R. R. DAHL & A. ARIMURA. 1987. Interleukin-1 stimulates ACTH release by an indirect action which requires endogenous corticotropin-releasing factor. Endocrinology **121:** 1580–1582.
16. RIVIER, C. & W. W. VALE. 1989. In the rat, interleukin-1α acts at the level of the brain and the gonads to interfere with gonadotropin and sex steroid secretion. Endocrinology **124:** 2105–2109.
17. KALRA, P. S., A. SAHU & S. P. KALRA. 1990. Interleukin-1 inhibits the ovarian steroid-induced luteinizing hormone surge and release of hypothalamic luteinizing hormone-releasing hormone in rats. Endocrinology **126:** 2145–2152.
18. CORNELL, R. P. & D. B. SCHWARTZ. 1989. Central administration of interleukin-1 elicits hyperinsulinemia in rats. Am. J. Physiol. **25:** R772–R777.
19. RETTORI, V., J. JURCOVICOVA & S. M. McCANN. 1987. Central action of interleukin-1 in altering the release of TSH, growth hormone, and prolactin in the male rat. J. Neurosci. Res. **18:** 179–183.
20. WOLOSKI, B. M. R. N. J., E. M. SMITH, W. J. MEYER III, G. M. FULLER & J. E. BLALOCK. 1985. Corticotropin-releasing activity of monokines. Science **230:** 1035–1037.
21. BERNTON, E. W., J. E. BEACH, J. W. HOLADAY, R. C. SMALLRIDGE & H. G. FEIN. 1987. Release of multiple hormones by a direct action of interleukin-1 on pituitary cells. Science **238:** 519–521.
22. FAGARASAN, M. O., R. ESKAY & J. AXELROD. 1989. Interleukin-1 potentiates the secretion of β-endorphin induced by secretagogues in a mouse pituitary cell line (AtT-20). Proc. Natl. Acad. Sci. USA **86:** 2070–2073.
23. FUKATA, J., T. USUI, Y. NAITO, Y. NAKAI & H. IMURA. 1989. Effects of recombinant human interleukin-1α, -1β, 2 and 6 on ACTH synthesis and release in the mouse pituitary tumour cell line AtT-20. J. Endocrinol. **122:** 33–39.
24. CALKINS, J. H., M. M. SIGEL, H. R. NANKIN & T. LIN. 1988. Interleukin-1 inhibits Leydig cell steroidogenesis in primary culture. Endocrinology **123:** 1605–1610.
25. FAUSER, B. C. J. M., A. B. GALWAY & A. J. HSUEH. 1989. Inhibitory actions of interleukin-1β on steroidogenesis in primary cultures of neonatal rat testicular cells. Acta Endocrinol. (Copenh.) **120:** 401–408.
26. POLLANEN, P., O. SODER & M. PARVINEN. 1989. Interleukin-1α stimulation of spermatogonial proliferation in vivo. Reprod. Fertil. Develop. **1:** 85–87.
27. DE SOUZA, E. B. & T. R. INSEL. 1990. Corticotropin-releasing factor (CRF) receptors in the rat central nervous system: Autoradiographic localization studies. *In* Corticotropin-Releasing Factor: Basic and Clinical Studies of a Neuropeptide. E. B. De Souza & C. B. Nemeroff, Eds.: 69–90. CRC Press. Boca Raton, FL.
28. DE SOUZA, E. B. & D. E. GRIGORIADIS. 1990. Corticotropin-releasing factor (CRF) receptors in brain: Characterization and regulation. *In* Corticotropin-Releasing Factor: Basic and Clinical Studies of a Neuropeptide. E. B. De Souza & C. B. Nemeroff, Eds.: 115–135. CRC Press. Boca Raton, FL.
29. DE SOUZA, E. B. 1992. Corticotropin-releasing hormone receptors. *In* Handbook of Chemical Neuroanatomy—Neuropeptide Receptors in the CNS, Part III. A. Bjorklund, T. Hokfelt & M. J. Kuhar, Eds.: 145–155. Elsevier. Amsterdam.
30. DE SOUZA, E. B., D. E. GRIGORIADIS & E. L. WEBSTER. 1991. Role of brain, pituitary and spleen corticotropin-releasing factor (CRF) receptors in the stress response. *In* The

Stress of Life, Revisited. 1. Neuroendocrinology of Stress (Methods and Achievements in Experimental Pathology, Vol. 14). G. Jasmin & M. Cantin, Eds.: 23–44. S. Karger. Basel.

31. DE SOUZA, E. B., M. H. PERRIN, J. E. RIVIER, W. W. VALE & M. J. KUHAR. 1984. Corticotropin-releasing factor receptors in rat pituitary gland: Autoradiographic localization. Brain Res. **296:** 202–207.

32. GRIGORIADIS, D. E. & E. B. DE SOUZA. 1989. Corticotropin-releasing factor (CRF) receptors in intermediate lobe of the pituitary: Biochemical characterization and autoradiographic localization. Peptides **10:** 179–188.

33. WYNN, P. C., G. AGUILERA, J. MORELL & K. J. CATT. 1983. Properties and regulation of high-affinity pituitary receptors for corticotropin-releasing factor. Biochem. Biophys. Res. Commun. **110:** 602–608.

34. DE SOUZA, E. B. 1987. Corticotropin-releasing factor receptors in the rat central nervous system: Characterization and regional distribution. J. Neurosci. **7:** 88–100.

35. WEBSTER, E. L. & E. B. DE SOUZA. 1988. Corticotropin-releasing factor receptors in mouse spleen: Identification, autoradiographic localization, and regulation by divalent cations and guanine nucleotides. Endocrinology **122:** 609–617.

36. GRIGORIADIS, D. E. & E. B. DE SOUZA. 1988. The brain corticotropin-releasing factor (CRF) receptor is of lower apparent molecular weight than the CRF receptor in anterior pituitary. J. Biol. Chem. **263:** 10927–10931.

37. GRIGORIADIS, D. E. & E. B. DE SOUZA. 1989. Heterogeneity between brain and pituitary corticotropin-releasing factor (CRF) receptors is due to differential glycosylation. Endocrinology **125:** 1877–1888.

38. BATTAGLIA, G., E. L. WEBSTER & E. B. DE SOUZA. 1987. Characterization of corticotropin-releasing factor receptor-mediated adenylate cyclase activity in the rat central nervous system. Synapse **1:** 572–581.

39. WEBSTER, E. L., G. BATTAGLIA & E. B. DE SOUZA. 1989. Functional corticotropin-releasing factor (CRF) receptors in mouse spleen: Evidence from adenylate cyclase studies. Peptides **10:** 395–401.

40. DE SOUZA, E. B., M. H. PERRIN, P. J. WHITEHOUSE, J. RIVIER, W. W. VALE & M. J. KUHAR. 1985. Corticotropin-releasing factor receptors in human pituitary gland: Autoradiographic localization. Neuroendocrinology **40:** 419–422.

41. DE SOUZA, E. B., T. R. INSEL, M. H. PERRIN, J. RIVIER, W. W. VALE & M. J. KUHAR. 1985. Corticotropin-releasing factor receptors are widely distributed within the rat central nervous system: An autoradiographic study. J. Neurosci. **5:** 3189–3203.

42. BELL, J. A. & E. B. DE SOUZA. 1988. Functional corticotropin-releasing factor (CRF) receptors in the neonatal rat spinal cord: Evidence from autoradiographic and electrophysiological studies. Peptides **9:** 1317–1322.

43. HARBOUR, D. V., E. M. SMITH & J. E. BLALOCK. 1987. Novel processing for proopiomelanocortin in lymphocytes: Endotoxin induction of a new prohormone-cleaving enzyme. J. Neurosci. Res. **18:** 95–100.

44. KAVELAARS, A., R. E. BALLIEUX & C. J. HEIJNEN. 1989. The role of IL-1 in the corticotropin-releasing factor and arginine vasopressin-induced secretion of immunoreactive β-endorphin by human peripheral blood mononuclear cells. J. Immunol. **142:** 2338–2342.

45. TAKAO, T., D. E. TRACEY, W. M. MITCHELL & E. B. DE SOUZA. 1990. Interleukin-1 receptors in mouse brain: Characterization and neuronal localization. Endocrinology **127:** 3070–3078.

46. TAKAO, T., S. G. CULP, R. C. NEWTON & E. B. DE SOUZA. 1992. Type I interleukin-1 receptors in the mouse brain-endocrine-immune axis labelled with [^{125}I]recombinant human interleukin-1 receptor antagonist. J. Neuroimmunol. **41:** 51–60.

47. TRACEY, D. E. & E. B. DE SOUZA. 1988. Identification of interleukin-1 receptors in mouse pituitary cell membranes and AtT-20 pituitary tumor cells. Soc. Neurosci. Abstr. **14:** 1052.

48. DE SOUZA, E. B., E. L. WEBSTER, D. E. GRIGORIADIS & D. E. TRACEY. 1989. Corticotropin-releasing factor (CRF) and interleukin-1 (IL-1) receptors in the brain-pituitary-immune axis. Psychopharmacol. Bull. **25:** 299–305.

49. TAKAO, T., W. M. MITCHELL, D. E. TRACEY & E. B. DE SOUZA. 1990. Identification of interleukin-1 receptors in mouse testis. Endocrinology 127: 251–258.
50. TAKAO, T., W. M. MITCHELL & E. B. DE SOUZA. 1991. Interleukin-1 receptors in mouse kidney: Identification, localization and modulation by lipopolysaccharide treatment. Endocrinology 128: 2618–2624.
51. CUNNINGHAM, E. T., JR., E. WADA, D. B. CARTER, D. E. TRACEY, J. F. BATTEY & E. B. DE SOUZA. 1991. Localization of interleukin-1 receptor messenger RNA in murine hippocampus. Endocrinology 128: 2666–2668.
52. CUNNINGHAM, E. T., JR., E. WADA, D. B. CARTER, D. E. TRACEY, J. F. BATTEY & E. B. DE SOUZA. 1992. In situ histochemical localization of type I interleukin-1 receptor messenger RNA in the central nervous system, pituitary, and adrenal gland of the mouse. J. Neurosci. 12: 1101–1114.
53. CUNNINGHAM, E. T., JR., E. WADA, D. B. CARTER, D. E. TRACEY, J. F. BATTEY & E. B. DE SOUZA. 1992. Distribution of type I interleukin-1 receptor messenger RNA in testis: An in situ histochemical study in the mouse. Neuroendocrinology 56: 94–99.
54. HARTUNG, H-P., B. SCHAFER, K. HEEININGER & K. Y. TOYKA. 1989. Recombinant interleukin-1β stimulates eicosanoid production in rat primary culture astrocytes. Brain Res. 489: 113–119.
55. GIULIAN, D., D. G. YOUNG, J. WOODWARD, D. C. BROWN & L. B. LACHMAN. 1988. Interleukin-1 is an astroglial growth factor in the developing brain. J. Neurosci. 8: 709–714.
56. HIGGINS, G. A. & J. A. OLSCHOWKA. 1991. Induction of interleukin-1β mRNA in adult rat brain. Mol. Brain Res. 9: 143–148.
57. FAGAN, A. M. & F. H. GAGE. 1990. Cholinergic sprouting in the hippocampus: A proposed role for IL-1. Exp. Neurol. 110: 105–120.
58. FRIEDMAN, W. J., L. LARKFORS, C. AYER-LeLIEVRE, T. EBENDAL, L. OLSON & H. PERSSON. 1990. Regulation of β-nerve growth factor expression by inflammatory mediators in hippocampal cultures. J. Neurosci. Res. 27: 374–388.
59. SPRANGER, M., D. LINDHOLM, C. BANDTLOW, R. HEUMANN, H. GRAHN, M. NAHER-NOE & H. THOENEN. 1990. Regulation of nerve growth factor (NGF) synthesis in the rat central nervous system: Comparison between the effects of interleukin-1 and various growth factors in astrocyte cultures and in vivo. Eur. J. Neurosci. 2: 69–76.
60. BREDER, C. D., C. A. DINARELLO & C. B. SAPER. 1988. Interleukin-1 immunoreactive innervation of the human hypothalamus. Science 240: 321–324.
61. NATHANSON, J. A. & L. L. CHUN. 1989. Immunological function of the blood-cerebrospinal fluid barrier. Proc. Natl. Acad. Sci. USA 86: 1684–1688.
62. LUE, F. A., M. BAIL, J. JEPHTHAH-OCHOLA, K. CARAYANNOITIS, R. GORCZYNSKI & H. MOLDOFSKY. 1988. Sleep and cerebrospinal fluid interleukin-1-like activity in the cat. Int. J. Neurosci. 42: 179–183.
63. MUSTAFA, M. M., M. H. LEBEL, O. RAMILO, K. D. OLSEN, J. S. REISCH, B. BEUTLER & G. H. McCRACKEN JR. 1989. Correlation of interleukin-1β and cachectin concentrations in cerebrospinal fluid and outcome from bacterial meningitis. J. Pediatr. 115: 208–213.
64. HAOUR, F., E. BAN, G. MILON, D. BAMAN & G. FILLION. 1990. Brain interleukin-1 receptors: Characterization and modulation after lipopolysaccharide injection. Prog. NeuroEndocrinImmunol. 3: 196–204.
65. BROWN, S. L., L. R. SMITH & J. E. BLALOCK. 1987. Interleukin 1 and interleukin 2 enhance proopiomelanocortin gene expression in pituitary cells. J. Immunol. 139: 3181–3183.
66. KAHN, S. A., O. SODER, V. SYED, K. GUSTAFSSON, M. LINDH & E. M. RITZEN. 1987. The rat testis produces large amounts of an interleukin-1-like factor. Int. J. Androl. 10: 495–502.
67. SYED, V., O. SODER, S. ARVER, M. LINDH, S. KAHN & E. M. RITZEN. 1988. Ontogeny and cellular origin of an interleukin-1-like factor in the reproductive tract of the male rat. Int. J. Androl. 11: 437–447.
68. ONO, N., M. D. LUMPKIN, W. K. SAMSON, J. K. McDONALD & S. M. McCANN. 1984. Intrahypothalamic action of corticotropin-releasing factor (CRF) to inhibit growth hormone and LH release in the rat. Life Sci. 35: 1117–1123.

69. RIVIER, C. & W. W. VALE. 1984. Influence of corticotropin-releasing factor on reproductive functions in the rat. Endocrinology **114**: 914–921.
70. TAKAO, T., S. G. CULP & E. B. DE SOUZA. 1993. Reciprocal modulation of interleukin-1β and interleukin-1 receptors by lipopolysaccharide (endotoxin) treatment in the mouse brain-endocrine-immune axis. Endocrinology **132**: 1497–1504.
71. WEBSTER, E. L., D. E. TRACEY & E. B. DE SOUZA. 1991. Upregulation of interleukin-1 receptors in AtT-20 pituitary tumor cells following treatment with corticotropin-releasing factor. Endocrinology **129**: 2796–2798.
72. MUNSON, P. J. & D. RODBARD. 1980. LIGAND: A versatile computerized approach for characterization of ligand-binding systems. Anal. Biochem. **297**: 220–229.
73. GERY, I., R. K. GERSHON & B. H. WAKSMAN. 1972. Potentiation of the T-lymphocyte response to mitogens. I. The responding cell. J. Exp. Med. **136**: 128–135.

CRF mRNA in Normal
and Stress Conditions

STAFFORD L. LIGHTMAN,[a,b] MICHAEL S. HARBUZ,[a,b]
RICHARD A. KNIGHT,[c] AND HARDIAL S. CHOWDREY[a,b]

[a] Neuroendocrinology Unit
Charing Cross and Westminster Medical School
Charing Cross Hospital
Fulham Palace Road
London W6 8RF, United Kingdom

[c] Department of Cystic Fibrosis
National Heart and Lung Institute
Brompton Hospital
Manresa Road
London SW3 6LR, United Kingdom

Corticotropin-releasing factor (CRF) is a key player in the regulation of mammalian homeostasis and in particular in the regulation of the hypothalamo-pituitary-adrenal (HPA) axis. All the classic regulatory mechanisms of HPA activity seem, at first sight, to involve appropriate changes in the prevalence of CRF mRNA transcripts.

Normal Conditions

Under normal laboratory conditions rats show diurnal changes in ACTH secretion. This also occurs in the absence of circulating corticosteroids after adrenalectomy or during constant steroid levels following a combination of adrenalectomy and corticosterone pellet replacement,[1] suggesting that CRF neurons in the hypothalamic paraventricular nucleus (PVN) respond to afferent neural regulation. CRF mRNA also shows diurnal changes, although it is unclear to what extent these are neurally activated or a response to changes in circulating corticosteroids.[2]

CRF neurons clearly show major responses to changes in corticosteroid feedback. Jingami *et al.*[3] first showed the increase in CRF mRNA after adrenalectomy, which could be reversed by the administration of dexamethasone. Both Swanson and Simmons[4] and we ourselves[5] have shown this inhibition of CRF mRNA by circulating corticosteroids to be concentration dependent. Local administration of glucocorticoid also reduces CRF mRNAs, suggesting that local glucocorticoid receptors in the PVN are responsible for at least part of this inhibitory feedback effect. Evidence also exists, however, for extrahypothalamic involvement via transsynaptic mechanisms.[6,7] The hippocampus is clearly involved in the extrahypothalamic corticosteroid feedback, and destruction of the hippocampal input to the PVN results in increased levels of CRF mRNA[8] and CRF in portal blood.[9]

[b] Present address: Department of Medicine, University of Bristol, Bristol Royal Infirmary, Marlborough Street, Bristol BS2 8HW, U.K.

Acute Stress

Activation of the HPA is part of the normal physiological response to stress. In response to stress, c-fos mRNA in the medial parvocellular PVN neurons rapidly responds by 15 minutes, peaking at 30 minutes, and falling to control levels by 90 minutes.[10] CRF mRNA levels are seen to increase later at 120–180 minutes after stress. We have characterized this CRF mRNA response to a wide variety of physical stressors including footshock, intraperitoneal (i.p.) hypertonic saline, and naloxone-precipitated opiate withdrawal, as well as to the "psychological" stressors including swimming and immobilization.[11–13] Although all these stressors result in increased CRF mRNA, preproenkephalin mRNA which coexists with CRF[14,15] only increased in response to the physical stressors, implying differential activation of afferent PVN pathways by different stressors. Arginine-vasopressin (AVP) mRNA also increases in response to stress,[11] but it is very difficult to quantitate it separately from the adjacent and intermingling magnocellular vasopressin neurons.

Because stress rapidly increases ACTH and corticosterone, all changes in CRF mRNA occur despite a concurrent increase in corticosteroid feedback. We therefore investigated the interrelationship between the level of corticosteroid feedback and the response of CRF mRNA to stressful stimuli. Quite remarkably we found that the CRF mRNA response to stress remains intact at all levels of corticosterone concentration in the blood. Thus, although adrenalectomy results in a considerable increase in CRF mRNA, a superimposed stress in an adrenalectomized animal results in a further increase in CRF mRNA of similar magnitude to that found in a sham-operated animal.[16] Similarly, if we administer exogenous corticosteroids, even in very high doses that cause a marked suppression of basal CRF mRNA levels, a superimposed stress will still result in an increase in CRF mRNA.[16,17] It is therefore clear that the transsynaptic activation of the CRF-containing neurons of the paraventricular nucleus is not dependent on the presence or absence of activated glucocorticoid receptors and presumably activates second messenger systems independent of those affected by glucocorticoid.

Repeated Stress

Good evidence now exists for stress-induced facilitation of ACTH secretion to explain the continuing normal neuroendocrine response to stress despite maintained increases in circulating corticosteroids.[18] There is, however, also evidence that if the same stress is repeated on multiple occasions a process of adaptation can take place so that the responses become smaller and may even disappear. We investigated whether this process happens at the hypothalamic level, and found that there are differences depending on the type of stimulus used. When we gave daily injections of i.p. hypertonic saline a marked and sustained increase in CRF mRNA[16] was observed, whereas daily immobilization stress rapidly resulted in total desensitization and the loss of any CRF mRNA response to the stimulus.[19] The level at which this adaptation takes place clearly needs further experimental investigation.

IMMUNE MEDIATORS OF HPA ACTIVATION

Stressors are known to alter immune function.[20] In recent years the modulatory effects of cytokines and other immunoregulators on the neuroendocrine system have been the subject of considerable interest and have highlighted the bidirectional flow of information between these systems.[21–23]

Interleukin-1 (IL-1) has been shown to release CRF from hypothalamic explants[24] and from fetal hypothalamic cells in culture.[25] In the latter studies their effect could be blocked by both protein kinase C and protein kinase A inhibitors and by the addition of corticosteroids. *In vivo* exogenous IL-1 has been demonstrated to evoke ACTH and/or corticosterone release when administered both peripherally and centrally.[26–28] The essential role of a central and probably hypothalamic activation is evidenced by studies in which these effects could be blocked by deafferentation of the medial basal hypothalamus[29] or immunoneutralization of endogenous CRF.[27,30] Further evidence for the involvement of CRF comes from studies that demonstrated increased CRF turnover,[31] increased CRF release into the hypophy-

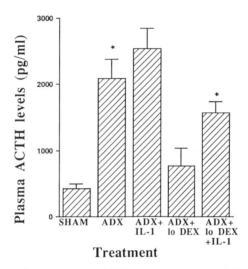

FIGURE 1. The effect of adrenalectomy (ADX) and dexamethasone (lo DEX) replacement on the IL-1β-induced increase in circulating ACTH. *$p < 0.05$ compared with the appropriate control group.

seal portal blood,[27] and increased CRF mRNA in the PVN,[28,32] after administration of IL-1. These effects appear to be predominantly mediated by IL-1β rather than IL-1α.

The mechanism of activation of CRF by IL-1β appears to be distinct from that activated in response to stress because a combination of stress and IL-1β administration results in an additive accumulation of CRF mRNA above that for either stimulus alone.[33] Furthermore, we investigated the interaction of steroid negative feedback on the stimulation of the HPA axis by IL-1β. In adrenalectomized animals IL-1β was unable to elicit an increase in either ACTH (FIG. 1) or CRF mRNA.[33] However, pretreatment of adrenalectomized rats with the synthetic glucocorticoid dexamethasone returned both the ACTH and CRF mRNA responses to IL-1β,[33] even though such pretreatment has been shown to inhibit the ACTH response to stress.[34] These data suggest that the IL-1β-induced activation of the HPA axis may, at least in part, be due to interference with the negative feedback of circulating glucocorticoids at the hypothalamic level.

Although the activation of the HPA axis by IL-1 is well established, the effects of the other cytokines are not as well understood. Corticosteroids are known to reduce IL-1 and IL-2 expression in addition to the well-established negative feedback effects on proopiomelanocortin (POMC) expression in the anterior pituitary. In contrast steroids are known to increase IL-4 expression.[35] We have shown that both IL-1β and IL-2 increase POMC mRNA, whereas IL-4 decreases POMC mRNA in the anterior pituitary.[28,36] Together these findings suggest the possibility of a novel feedback mechanism. Corticosterone acts directly at the pituitary to reduce POMC expression and indirectly via a reduction in IL-1 and IL-2 and an increase in IL-4. The effects of IL-2 and IL-4 do not appear to be mediated through CRF as we have been unable to demonstrate an effect of these cytokines on CRF mRNA in the PVN.[36] However, inasmuch as basal circulating levels of IL-1, IL-2, and IL-4 are undetectable, this mechanism would only become operative in inflammatory situations that activate the production of these cytokines.

ADJUVANT-INDUCED ARTHRITIS AND EXPERIMENTAL ALLERGIC ENCEPHALOMYELITIS

Adjuvant-induced arthritis (AA) is a chronic, immunologically mediated inflammatory disease that has been shown to be T cell dependent. AA can be induced by a single intradermal injection of either ground, heat-killed *Mycobacterium butyricum*[37] or the synthetic adjuvant CP20961,[38] in paraffin oil. Despite the fact that these two adjuvants do not share the same immunogenic determinants, the progress of the disease is remarkably similar. Inflammation becomes apparent approximately 11 days after injection and reaches a peak at 21 days, after which time the acute phase subsides. AA results in a chronic activation of the HPA axis with increased adrenal size, increased POMC mRNA, increased morning ACTH and corticosterone levels, and loss of the normal diurnal rhythm of these hormones.[39] This implies that in this model of chronic inflammatory stress the drive to ACTH secretion is increased, despite the chronic increase in corticosteroid negative feedback from the elevated secretion of corticosterone.

Despite the fact that CRF is the major activator of POMC gene transcription and that CRF mRNA has been demonstrated to be increased after repeated stress,[16] we did not observe an increase in CRF mRNA in the PVN coincident with the development of AA. Indeed the levels in the Piebald-Viral-Glaxo (PVG) rat were found to decrease with increasing severity of disease irrespective of the adjuvant used.[40] There was also a consistent decrease in CRF peptide release into the hypophyseal portal blood. Interestingly, hypophyseal-portal arginine vasopressin release was increased in these animals, suggesting that AVP may be the predominant factor responsible for the activation of the pituitary-adrenal axis in this condition.

Clearly, one candidate that might be responsible for the decrease in CRF mRNA is increased negative feedback due to the increase in plasma corticosterone. However, studies in the adrenalectomized rat have shown that even in the absence of circulating corticosteroids the development of AA is associated with a decrease in CRF mRNA.[41] Other factor(s) clearly must be involved in this seemingly paradoxical response.

The pituitary-adrenal axis is also known to be activated in experimental allergic encephalomyelitis (EAE). EAE is a paralytic disease resulting from an immunological reaction against CNS myelin that has been extensively used as an animal model for multiple sclerosis in humans. In this model the magnitude of the adrenal response not only correlates with disease severity, but is also critical for recovery. We have found that with EAE, as with AA, there is an increase in pituitary POMC mRNA and in plasma corticosterone that are maximal at peak clinical signs. At this time CRF mRNA in the PVN is suppressed suggesting that in EAE, too, the pituitary-adrenal activation is not mediated by CRF. An advantage of the EAE model is that after peak clinical signs full recovery takes place. With recovery the endocrine parameters measured return to normal.

It has recently been suggested that susceptibility to streptococcal cell wall-induced arthritis exhibited by the Lewis strain of rat is due to an inability to mount an appropriate stress response and in particular is a direct result of the nonresponsiveness of CRF mRNA in the PVN.[42] The converse has also been proposed, that is, that

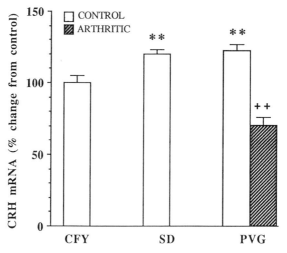

FIGURE 2. CRF mRNA in the parvocellular division of the paraventricular nucleus (pPVN) of CFY, SD, and PVG rat strains. *$p < 0.05$ compared with CFY control group.

the robust stress response as exhibited by the PVG strain of rat is a major factor in the resistance of this strain to EAE.[35] In our studies on AA we used the PVG strain of rat because it is particularly insensitive to encephalopathy. Although PVG and Sprague-Dawley strains of rat, used extensively in stress studies, have a robust corticosterone and CRF mRNA response to acute stress, both strains are sensitive to AA. Clearly, the regulation of CRF mRNA in the PVN is not the only factor responsible for susceptibility to inflammatory stress. Interestingly, basal CRF mRNA levels in both the PVG and Sprague-Dawley strains are significantly greater than levels seen in the resistant CFY strain (FIG. 2). Also of interest is the loss of both corticosterone and CRF mRNA responses to acute stress after the development of arthritis.[41]

MECHANISMS OF ADJUVANT-INDUCED ARTHRITIS LEADING TO ACTIVATION OF HPA AXIS

It has been known for many years that AA is immunologically mediated.[43] For example, leukocyte migration inhibition—a marker of T cell activation—can be detected in response to BCG as early as four days after injection of adjuvant, although, interestingly, the response develops later in rats with sciatic denervation and those in which the pain stimulus has therefore been removed.[44] T cell proliferation to both BCG and to components of inflamed joints such as collagen type II and proteoglycans has also been demonstrated.[44–46] A T cell clone derived from the draining lymph nodes of Lewis rats with AA has been shown to react both with *M. tuberculosis* and proteoglycan,[46] suggesting that antigens of *M. tuberculosis* may cross-react with normal joint components. T cell lines and clones from animals with AA can transfer the disease to irradiated but not to nonirradiated syngeneic rats, and can protect the recipients from active induction of AA.[47] Antibodies to collagen type II have also been described.[45]

It is not surprising, therefore, that soluble inflammatory mediators are increased in animals with AA. The levels of circulating IL-1[48] and IL-6[49] and tumor necrosis factor-α (TNF-α)[48] are raised and the accumulation of IL-1β mRNA in both spleen and thymus is also increased.[50] In adrenalectomized (ADX) rats with AA, splenic IL-1β mRNA is still further increased, in parallel with the heightened severity of the disease in animals with AA.[50] IL-1[51] and IL-6[52] have also been detected in the pituitary, but although we found an increase in pituitary IL-6 mRNA in animals with AA, we were unable to demonstrate increases in pituitary IL-1.[53] Pituitary IL-1β mRNA has, however, been shown to be increased in rats given lipopolysaccharide.[51]

The inflammatory cytokines form a chemical cascade in which, for example, IL-1 and prostaglandin E2 induce the synthesis of IL-6 in inflammatory cells,[54,55] and the serum levels of IL-1 and prostaglandin E2 are also raised in animals with AA.[48] In addition, it has recently been recognized that at least some inflammatory mediators have effects on the HPA axis. For example, both IL-1β and IL-6 increase circulating ACTH.[21,28,56] As discussed previously, the effect of IL-1 is probably exerted at the hypothalamic level, because it increases hypothalamic CRF mRNA[32] and the concentration of CRF in portal blood,[27] and its effects on ACTH are inhibited by anti-CRF antiserum.[57]

We have been interested in the extent to which inflammatory mediators are involved in the neuroendocrine changes found in AA. We approached this question in two ways: first, by comparing the effects of the immunosuppressant cyclosporine A (CsA) on the disease, the inflammatory mediators, and the neuroendocrine system, and, second, by studying the effects of adoptive transfer of spleen cells from animals with AA on the neuroendocrine system, with and without challenge of the recipients with adjuvant.

Cyclosporine A Studies

Continuous administration of CsA from day −3 to day 14 inhibited the development of AA and reduced the concomitant activation of the HPA axis.[53] CsA has also been shown to inhibit the HPA axis under both basal and stimulated (cold stress) conditions.[58] When added to fresh pituitary cell cultures *in vitro*, CsA reduced POMC and IL-6 mRNAs accumulation, and significantly reduced the increase in POMC mRNA expression produced by exogenous CRF.[53] Although CsA suppresses immune responses by reducing the production of IL-1[59] and IL-2[60] and the expression of IL-2 receptors,[61] it is possible that the effects of CsA on the HPA axis in rats with AA were mediated by these direct actions on the pituitary rather than by inhibition of inflammatory mediator expression.

In a separate series of experiments rats were given CsA discontinuously for different periods during the development of the arthritis.[39] Although the immunosuppressant produced a reduction in the degree of elevation of circulating ACTH and corticosterone at all time intervals tested, this effect was most pronounced when the drug was given in the period immediately prior to sacrifice. Cessation of CsA therapy for six or more days before sacrifice would allow the resumption of inflammation, with the possibility of inflammatory mediators being able to resume activation of the HPA axis. Giving CsA right up to the time of decapitation would, conversely, abrogate immune mediator production at the time of sacrifice. These data are therefore consistent with inflammatory mediators being activators of the HPA axis *in vivo*.

Adoptive Transfer Studies

In order to test whether products of activated immune cells directly activate the HPA axis, spleen cells from 14-day-old Sprague-Dawley rats with AA were transferred intraperitoneally to normal syngeneic nonirradiated recipients. On days 1 and 3 after the transfer, pituitary POMC mRNA accumulation and circulating ACTH levels had increased.[62] By day 7, both mRNA and peptide had returned to control levels and remained so up to 14 days after transfer. Rats that received transfer of nonimmune spleen cells showed no change at any time point in pituitary POMC mRNA or circulating ACTH. None of the animals developed AA during the 14-day observation period.

Although inflammatory cells can produce ACTH, it has been reported that mouse spleen cell-derived ACTH contains only the first 25 amino acids.[63] If the same truncated molecule is produced by rat spleen cells, it will lack the C-terminal residues recognized by the antiserum used in the radioimmunoassay. Consequently, the increased ACTH is likely to be derived from the increased pituitary POMC transcription, rather than being an immunological product.

In a second set of experiments, nonirradiated rats received nonimmune and immune cells as described above. Again, none of the recipients developed any clinical signs of AA up to 21 days after the transfer. On day 21 after transfer, both groups were challenged with adjuvant. In the nonimmune recipients, classic AA developed within 14 days of adjuvant administration. However, in the rats that had received immune spleen cells 21 days prior to the adjuvant, no signs of AA developed.

Both pituitary POMC mRNA accumulation and circulating ACTH were increased in nonimmune and immune adjuvant injected groups, irrespective of the development of AA. POMC mRNA and peptide were, however, slightly lower in the immune-protected animals. This demonstrates that the HPA activation seen in arthritic animals does not arise solely from the discomfort and immobility of the disease, but at least in part has an immunological basis. The increased pituitary POMC mRNA and circulating ACTH in the immune-protected, nonarthritic animals are presumably a result of inflammatory mediator production by the secondary immune response induced in these animals by adjuvant challenge.

The precise molecular mechanism of these effects is unknown. In addition to producing interleukins, some of which can activate the HPA axis, inflammatory cells can also express mRNAs and produce peptides related to the hypothalamic releasing hormones.[64,65] Although inflammatory CRF is biochemically distinct from the hypothalamic hormone, it functions effectively in increasing POMC mRNA accumulation in both dispersed pituitary cells and in lymphocytes. Acute administration of IL-1 also increases circulating ACTH, although its action is mediated by increased transcription and release of hypothalamic CRF.[27,32] In rats with AA, however, hypothalamic CRF mRNA and CRF peptide in the portal circulation are reduced,[40] suggesting either that chronic IL-1 may have different effects than those resulting from the acute administration of this cytokine or that in AA, IL-1 is not the major mediator of the immune-neuroendocrine interaction.

These data suggest that neuroendocrine changes are a general accompaniment of chronic inflammation. Evidence exists that neuroendocrine responses in immunological disorders play a role in the susceptibility of individual strains of animals to the development of those disorders. A better understanding of the mechanisms of the immune-neuroendocrine dialogue may improve our ability to manage inflammatory disease in man.

ACKNOWLEDGMENTS

In this review we summarized our current understanding of the mechanisms responsible for the activation of CRF mRNA transcription in response to various stressors. We acknowledge Antonio Chover-Gonzalez, a visiting research fellow from the University of Cadiz, and doctoral students Anastasis Stephanou and Nicholas J. Sarlis for their invaluable contributions to this work.

REFERENCES

1. DALLMAN, M. F., S. F. AKANA, N. LEVIN, *et al.* 1989. Corticosterone (B) replacement in adrenalectomized rats: Insight into the regulation of ACTH secretion. *In* The Control of the Hypothalamo-Pituitary-Adrenocortical Axis. F. C. Rose, Ed. International Universities Press. Madison, CT.
2. WATTS, A. G. & L. W. SWANSON. 1989. Diurnal variations in the content of preprocorticotropin-releasing hormone messenger ribonucleic acids in the hypothalamic paraventricular nucleus of rats of both sexes as measured by in situ hybridization. Endocrinology **125:** 1734–1738.
3. JINGAMI, H., S. MATSUKURA, S. NUMA & H. IMURA. 1985. Effects of adrenalectomy and dexamethasone administration on the level of prepro-corticotropin-releasing factor messenger ribonucleic acid (mRNA) in the hypothalamus and adrenocorticotropin/b lipotropin precursor mRNA in the pituitary in rats. Endocrinology **117:** 1314–1320.
4. SWANSON, L. W. & D. M. SIMMONS. 1989. Differential steroid hormone and neural influences on peptide mRNA levels in CRH cells of the paraventricular nucleus: A hybridization histochemical study in the rat. **285:** 413–435.
5. LIGHTMAN, S. L., M. S. HARBUZ & W. S. I. YOUNG. 1992. Regulation of hypothalamic CRF mRNA. *In* Stress, Neuroendocrine and Molecular Approaches. R. Kvetnansky, R. McCarty & J. Axelrod, Eds. Gordon and Breach, New York, NY.
6. DALLMAN, M. F., N. LEVIN, C. S. CASCIO, S. F. AKANA, L. JACOBSEN & R. W. KUHN. 1989. Pharmacological evidence that the inhibition of diurnal adrenocorticotropin secretion by corticosteroids is mediated via type I corticosterone preferring receptors. Endocrinology **124:** 2844–2850.
7. HERMAN, J. P., S. J. WIEGAND & S. J. WATSON. 1990. Regulation of basal corticotropin-releasing hormone and arginine vasopressin messenger ribonucleic acid expression in the paraventricular nucleus: Effects of selective hypothalamic deafferentations. Endocrinology **127:** 2408–2417.

8. HERMAN, J. P., M. K. H. SHAFER, E. A. YOUNG, et al. 1989. Evidence for hippocampal regulation of neuroendocrine neurons of the hypothalamo-pituitary-adrenocortical axis. J. Neurosci. **9:** 3072–3082.

9. SAPOLSKY, R. M., M. P. ARMANINE, S. W. SUTTON & P. M. PLOTSKY. 1989. Elevation of hypophysial portal concentrations of adrenocorticotropin secretagogues after fornix transection. Endocrinology **125:** 2881–2887.

10. IMAKI, T., T. SHIBASAKI, M. HOTTA & H. DEMARA. 1992. Early induction of c-fos precedes increased expression of corticotrophin-releasing factor messenger ribonucleic acid in the paraventricular nucleus after immobilisation stress. Endocrinology **131:** 240–246.

11. LIGHTMAN, S. L. & W. S. YOUNG III. 1988. Corticotrophin-releasing factor, vasopressin and proopiomelanocortin mRNA responses to stress and opiates in the rat. J. Physiol. **403:** 511–523.

12. HARBUZ, M. S. & S. L. LIGHTMAN. 1989. Responses of hypothalamic and pituitary mRNA to physical and psychological stress in the rat. J. Endocrinol. **122:** 705–711.

13. HARBUZ, M. S., J. A. RUSSELL, B. E. H. SUMNER, M. KAWATA & S. L. LIGHTMAN. 1991. Rapid changes in the content of proenkephalin A and corticotrophin releasing hormone mRNAs in the paraventricular nucleus during morphine withdrawal in urethane-anaesthetized rats. Mol. Brain Res. **9:** 285–291.

14. HOKFELT, T., J. FAHRENKRUG, K. TATEMOTO, V. MUTT, S. WERNER, A. L. HULTING, L. TERENIUS & K. J. CHANG. 1983. The PHI (PHI-27)/corticotropin-releasing factor/enkephalin immunoreactive hypothalamic neuron: Possible morphological basis for integrated control of prolactin, corticotropin, and growth hormone secretion. Proc. Natl. Acad. Sci. USA **80:** 895–898.

15. HISANO, S., Y. TSURUO, S. KATOH, S. DAIKOKU, N. YANAIHARAN & T. SHIBASAKI. 1987. Intragranular colocalization of arginine vasopressin and methionine-enkephalin-octapeptide in CRF-axons in the median eminence. Cell Tissue Res. **249:** 497–507.

16. LIGHTMAN, S. L. & W. S. YOUNG III. 1989. Influence of steroids on the hypothalamic corticotropin-releasing factor and preproenkephalin mRNA responses to stress. Proc. Natl. Acad. Sci. USA **86:** 4306–4310.

17. HARBUZ, M. S., S. A. NICHOLSON, B. GILLHAM & S. L. LIGHTMAN. 1990. Stress responsiveness of hypothalamic corticotrophin-releasing factor and pituitary proopiomelanocortin mRNAs following high dose glucocorticoid treatment and withdrawal in the rat. J. Endocrinol. **127:** 407–415.

18. AKANA, S. F., M. F. DALLMAN, M. J. BRADBURY, K. A. SCRIBNER, A. M. STRACK & C. D. WALKER. 1992. Feedback and facilitation in the adrenocortical system: Unmasking facilitation by partial inhibition of the glucocorticoid response to prior stress. Endocrinology **131:** 57–68.

19. LIGHTMAN, S. L. & M. S. HARBUZ. 1992. Expression of corticotropin-releasing factor mRNA in response to stress. In CIBA Foundation Symposium: 173–187. Wiley. Chichester.

20. KHANSARI, D. N., A. J. MURGO & R. E. FAITH. 1990. Effects of stress on the immune system. Immunol. Today **11:** 170–175.

21. DUNN, A. J. 1990. Interleukin 1 as a stimulator of hormone secretion. Prog. NeuroEndo-crinImmunol. **3:** 26–29.

22. ROTHWELL, N. J. 1991. Functions and mechanisms of interleukin 1 in the brain. Trends Pharmacol. Sci. **12:** 430–436.

23. HARBUZ, M. S. & S. L. LIGHTMAN. 1992. Stress and the hypothalamo-pituitary-adrenal axis: Acute, chronic and immunological activation. J. Endocrinol. **134:** 327–339.

24. TSAGARAKIS, S., G. GILLIES, L. H. REES, M. BESSER & A. GROSSMAN. 1989. Interleukin-1 directly stimulates the release of corticotrophin releasing factor from rat hypothalamus. Neuroendocrinology **49:** 98–101.

25. HU, S. B., L. A. TANAHILL & S. L. LIGHTMAN. 1992. Interleukin-1β (IL-1β) induces corticotropin releasing factor-41 release from cultured hypothalamic cells through protein kinase C and cAMP dependent protein kinase pathways. J. Neuroimmunol. **40:** 49–56.

26. BESEDOVSKY, H., A. DEL REY, E. SORKIN & C. A. DINARELLO. 1986. Immunoregulatory feedback between interleukin-1 and glucocorticoid hormones. Science **233:** 652–654.

27. SAPOLSKY, R., C. RIVIER, G. YAMAMOTO, P. PLOTSKY & W. VALE. 1987. Interleukin-1 stimulates the secretion of hypothalamic corticotropin-releasing factor. Science **238:** 522–524.

28. HARBUZ, M. S., A. STEPHANOU, N. SARLIS & S. L. LIGHTMAN. 1992. The effects of recombinant interleukin (IL)-1α, IL-1β or IL-6 on hypothalamo-pituitary-adrenal axis activation. J. Endocrinol. **133:** 349–355.

29. OVADIA, H., O. ABRAMSKY, V. BARAK, N. CONFORTI, D. SAPHIER & J. WIEDENFELD. 1989. Effect of interleukin-1 on adrenocortical activity in intact and hypothalamic deafferentated male rats. Exp. Brain Res. **76:** 246–249.

30. BERKENBOSCH, F., J. VAN OERS, A. DEL REY, F. TILDERS & H. BESEDOVSKY. 1987. Corticotropin-releasing factor-producing neurons in the rat activated by interleukin-1. Science **238:** 524–526.

31. BERKENBOSCH, F., D. E. C. DE GOEIJ, A. DEL REY & H. O. BESEDOVSKY. 1989. Neuroendocrine, sympathetic and metabolic responses induced by interleukin-1. Neuroendocrinology **50:** 570–576.

32. SUDA, T., F. TOZAWA, T. USHIYAMA, T. SUMITOMO, M. YAMADA & H. DEMURA. 1990. Interleukin-1 stimulates corticotropin releasing factor gene expression in the rat hypothalamus. Endocrinology **126:** 1223–1229.

33. CHOVER-GONZALEZ, A. J., M. S. HARBUZ & S. L. LIGHTMAN. Effect of adrenalectomy and stress on interleukin-1β mediated activation of hypothalamic corticotropin releasing factor mRNA. J. Neuroimmunol. In press.

34. WEIDENFELD, J., O. ABRAMSKY & H. OVADIA. 1989. Effect of interleukin-1 on ACTH and corticosterone secretion in dexamethasone and adrenalectomized pretreated male rats. Neuroendocrinology **50:** 650–654.

35. MASON, D. 1991. Genetic variation in the stress response: Susceptibility to experimental allergic encephalomyelitis and implications for human inflammatory disease. Immunol. Today **12:** 57–60.

36. HARBUZ, M. S., A. STEPHANOU, R. A. KNIGHT, A. J. CHOVER-GONZALEZ & L. L. S. Action of interleukin-2 and interleukin-4 on CRF mRNA in the hypothalamus and POMC mRNA in the anterior pituitary. Brain Behav. Immun. In press.

37. PEARSON, C. M. 1956. Development of arthritis, periarthritis and periostitis in rats given adjuvant. Proc. Soc. Exp. Biol. Med. **91:** 95–103.

38. CHANG, Y.-H., C. M. PEARSON & C. ABE. 1980. Adjuvant polyarthritis. IV. Induction by a synthetic adjuvant: Immunologic, histopathologic, and other studies. Arthritis Rheum. **23:** 62–71.

39. SARLIS, N. J., A. STEPHANOU, H. S. CHOWDREY, R. A. KNIGHT & S. L. LIGHTMAN. 1992. Pituitary-adrenal axis and anterior pituitary prolactin and growth hormone mRNA responses of adjuvant-arthritic rats to cyclosporine A are dependent upon its time of administration. Prog. NeuroEndocrinImmunol. **5:** 141–150.

40. HARBUZ, M. S., R. G. REES, D. ECKLAND, D. S. JESSOP, D. BREWERTON & S. L. LIGHTMAN. 1992. Paradoxical responses of hypothalamic corticotropin releasing factor (CRF) messenger ribonucleic acid (mRNA) and CRF-41 peptide and adenohypophysial proopiomelanocortin mRNA during chronic inflammatory stress. Endocrinology **130:** 1394–1399.

41. HARBUZ, M. S., R. G. REES & S. L. LIGHTMAN. Hypothalamo-pituitary responses to acute stress and changes in circulating glucocorticoids during chronic adjuvant-induced arthritis in the rat. Am. J. Physiol. In press.

42. STERNBERG, E. M., W. S. I. YOUNG, R. BERNARDINI *et al.* 1989. A central nervous system defect in biosynthesis of corticotropin-releasing hormone is associated with susceptibility to streptococcal cell wall-induced arthritis in Lewis rats. Proc. Natl. Acad. Sci. USA **86:** 4771–4775.

43. PEARSON, C. M. & F. D. WOOD. 1963. Mycobacteria wax D subfractions in induction of adjuvant induced arthritis. Int. Arch. Allergy **35:** 456–464.

44. BERRY, H., D. A. WILLOUGHBY & J. P. GIROUD. 1973. Evidence for an endogenous antigen in the adjuvant arthritic rat. J. Pathol. **111:** 229–238.

45. TRENTHAM, D. E., W. J. MCCUNE, P. SUSMAN & J. R. DAVID. 1980. Autoimmunity to collagen in adjuvant arthritis of rats. J. Clin. Invest. **66:** 1109–1117.

46. VAN EDEN, W., J. HOLOSCHITZ, Z. NEVO, A. FRENKEL, A. KLAJMAN & I. R. COHEN. 1985. Arthritis induced by a T-lymphocyte clone that responds to *Mycobacterium tuberculosis* and to cartilage proteoglycans. Proc. Natl. Acad. Sci. USA **82**: 5117–5120.

47. HOLOSCHITZ, J., A. MATITIAU & I. R. COHEN. 1984. Arthritis induced in rats by cloned T lymphocytes responsive to bacteria but not to collagen type II. J. Clin. Invest. **73**: 211–215.

48. SHINMEI, M., K. MASUDA, T. KIKUSHI & Y. SHINOMURA. 1989. Interleukin 1, tumour necrosis factor and interleukin 6 as mediators of cartilage destruction. Semin. Arthritis Rheum. **18 (Suppl. 1)**: 27–31.

49. LEISTEN, J. C., W. A. GAARDE & W. SCHOLZ. 1990. Interleukin 6 serum levels correlate with footpad swelling in adjuvant-induced arthritic Lewis rats treated with cyclosporin A or indomethacin. Clin. Immunol. Immunopathol. **56**: 108–114.

50. STEPHANOU, A., N. J. SARLIS, R. A. KNIGHT, H. S. CHOWDREY & S. L. LIGHTMAN. 1992. Response of pituitary and spleen pro-opiomelanocortin mRNA, and spleen and thymus interleukin-1β mRNA to adjuvant arthritis in the rat. J. Neuroimmunol. **37**: 59–63.

51. KOENIG, J. J., W. SNOW, B. D. CLARK, *et al.* 1990. Intrinsic pituitary interleukin-1β is induced by bacterial lipopolysaccharide. Endocrinology **126**: 3053–3058.

52. CARMELIET, P., H. VANKELEKOM, J. VAN DAMME, A. BILLIAU & C. DENEF. 1991. Release of interleukin-6 from anterior pituitary cell aggregates: Developmental pattern and modulation by glucocorticoids and forskolin. Neuroendocrinology **53**: 29–34.

53. STEPHANOU, A., N. J. SARLIS, R. A. KNIGHT, S. L. LIGHTMAN & H. S. CHOWDREY. Effects of cyclosporine A on the hypothalamic-pituitary-adrenal axis and anterior pituitary interleukin-6 mRNA expression during chronic inflammatory stress in the rat. J. Neuroimmunol. In press.

54. ZHANG, Y., J.-X. LIN & J. VILCEK. 1988. Synthesis of interleukin 6 (interferon β2–B cell stimulating factor) in human fibroblasts is supported by an increase in intracellular cyclic AMP. J. Biol. Chem. **263**: 6177–6180.

55. WALTHER, Z., L. T. MAY & P. B. SEGHAL. 1988. Transcriptional regulation of the interferon β2/B cell differentiation factor BSF2/hepatocyte stimulating factor gene in human fibroblasts by other cytokines. J. Immunol. **140**: 974–978.

56. NAITOH, Y., J. FUKATA, T. TOMINAGA *et al.* 1988. Interleukin-6 stimulates the secretion of adrenocorticotropic hormone in conscious, freely moving rats. Biochem. Biophys. Res. Commun. **155**: 1459–1463.

57. UEHARA, A., P. E. GOTTSCHALL, R. P. DAHL & A. ARIMURA. 1987. Interleukin-1 stimulates ACTH release by an indirect action which requires endogenous corticotropin-releasing factor. Endocrinology **121**: 1580–1582.

58. HIRANO, T., K. YAMADA & K. OKA. 1988. Effects of cyclosporine on adrenocortical stress response of Wistar rats. Res. Commun. Chem. Pathol. Pharmacol. **60**: 3–5.

59. BUNJES, D., C. HARDT, M. ROLLINGHOFF & H. WAGNER. 1981. Cyclosporin A mediates immunosuppression of primary cytotoxic T cell response by impairing the release of interleukin 1 and interleukin 2. Eur. J. Immunol. **11**: 657–661.

60. ANDRUS, L. & K. J. LAFFERTY. 1982. Inhibition of T-cell activity by cyclosporin A. Scand. J. Immunol. **15**: 449–458.

61. PRINCE, H. E. & J. K. JOHN. 1986. Cyclosporin inhibits the expression of receptors for interleukin 2 and transferrin on mitogen-activated human T lymphocytes. Immunol. Invest. **15**: 463–465.

62. KNIGHT, R. A., A. STEPHANOU, N. J. SARLIS, H. S. CHOWDREY & S. L. LIGHTMAN. Direct stimulation of the pituitary by transfer of activated leucocytes. Submitted.

63. SMITH, E. M., S. F. GALIN, R. D. LEBOEUF, D. H. COPPENHAVER, D. V. HARBOUR & J. E. BLALOCK. 1990. Nucleotide and amino acid sequence of lymphocyte derived corticotropin: Endotoxin induction of a truncated peptide. Proc. Natl. Acad. Sci. USA **87**: 1057–1060.

64. STEPHANOU, A., D. S. JESSOP, R. A. KNIGHT & S. L. LIGHTMAN. 1990. Corticotrophin-releasing factor-like immuno-reactivity and mRNA in human leukocytes. Brain Behav. Immun. **4**: 67–72.

65. STEPHANOU, A., R. A. KNIGHT & S. L. LIGHTMAN. 1991. Production of a growth hormone-releasing hormone-like peptide and its mRNA by human lymphocytes. Neuroendocrinology **53**: 628–633.

Phenotypic Plasticity of CRF Neurons during Stress[a]

F. J. H. TILDERS,[b] E. D. SCHMIDT,
AND D. C. E. DE GOEIJ[c]

Graduate School Neurosciences Amsterdam
Neuroscience Research Institute Free University
Department of Pharmacology, Faculty of Medicine
1081 BT Amsterdam, the Netherlands

Since the original report on the existence of somatostatin immunoreactivity in sympathetic ganglia, there have been many examples described of neurons in which a peptide is colocalized with a classical transmitter.[1] These colocalized peptides are produced, packaged in secretory granules, stored in nerve terminals, and secreted upon appropriate stimuli. Therefore, such neurons are considered to be multimessenger neurons. Colocalized messengers are not necessarily secreted concomitantly. In several systems, low-stimulation frequencies have been found to induce preferential release of the neurotransmitter whereas neuropeptide secretion becomes prominent at high-stimulation frequencies.[1,2] Thus, the biochemical composition of the signal that is produced by a multimessenger neuron can vary with the conditions of stimulation. In some systems, these colocalized peptides are known to modulate the response of the target cells of the neurotransmitter. Alternatively, these peptides may act presynaptically to modulate the stimulation-secretion characteristics of the terminals or act at more remote targets.[1–3]

In addition, peptidergic neurons often express more than one peptide gene. A most intriguing example of peptidergic multimessenger neurons is shown by the CRF-producing parvocellular neurons in the paraventricular nucleus of the hypothalamus (PVN) that control ACTH secretion from the anterior pituitary gland. In rats, these neurons have the capacity to express at least eight neuropeptide genes in addition to that of CRF. A considerable proportion of these CRF neurons has been found to coproduce arginine-vasopressin (AVP), neurotensin, enkephalin or the transmitter GABA, whereas other peptides such as angiotensin II, cholecystokinin (CCK), galanin, vasoactive intestinal peptide (VIP/PHI) or thyrotropin releasing hormone (TRH) are less frequently found (FIG. 1). Whether all these peptides are expressed to the same extent under physiological conditions is not fully clear because the high doses of colchicine that are needed to visualize the peptides in the cell bodies can by themselves induce expression of certain neuropeptide genes.[4] By the use of electron microscopic techniques, at least some of the above-mentioned peptides have been detected in CRF-containing nerve terminals of rats not treated with colchicine. For instance, most if not all immunodetectable vasopressin in the external zone of the median eminence (ZEME) of rats was found in CRF-containing nerve terminals.[5,6] In fact, up to 50% of the CRF-containing terminals in this region

[a]This work was supported by the Netherlands Organization for Scientific Research (grant 900-543-101).
[b]Corresponding author.
[c]Present address: Organon International, Oss, the Netherlands.

costore pro-AVP-derived products.[5–10] Further, enkephalin has been detected in a significant proportion of the CRF terminals in the ZEME.[11,12] Thus, at least in the rat, the CRF-producing neurons in the medial parvocellular PVN are heterogenic with respect to the coproduction and costorage of neuropeptides or transmitters (see also ref. 13). Because the substances that are costored with CRF in the nerve terminals can be secreted upon appropriate stimuli, activation of CRF neurons may lead to the release of a bouquet of signaling substances of which the exact composition will depend on the peptide makeup of the CRF neurons involved in the response.

With the exception of AVP, little is known about the physiological significance of the cosecretion of the substances that are costored with CRF. It is conceivable that the secretory products may reach the portal blood and may help to orchestrate the

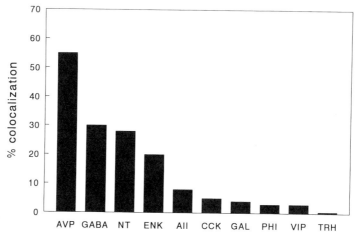

FIGURE 1. Colocalization of neuropeptides and GABA in CRF neurons in the parvocellular part of the paraventricular nucleus of the hypothalamus of rats. The numbers represent estimates of the percentages of CRF neurons coproducing vasopressin,[94] gamma aminobutyric acid,[95] neurotensin,[96] enkephalin,[96] angiotensin II,[95] cholecystokinin,[96] galanin,[96] peptide histidine isoleucine/vasoactive intestinal polypeptide,[96] and thyrotropin.[96]

endocrine response of the anterior pituitary gland. This may involve modulation of the response of the corticotrope cells to CRF[14–21] as well as actions on other endocrine or nonendocrine cell types in the anterior pituitary gland. In addition, these substances may act in the ZEME to modulate the secretion of products from CRF terminals (presynaptic autocrine effects) or act on other nerve terminals or cells in the ZEME (paracrine effects).[22] Strong evidence has been presented to support the view that AVP can be cosecreted with CRF from the nerve terminals in the ZEME into the portal blood and that it plays an important role in the physiological control of ACTH secretion.[16,23–25] Therefore, in the present paper we will focus on the occurrence of AVP in CRF neurons and will briefly discuss the occurrence of phenotypically different CRF neurons, their changes in peptide makeup in response to adrenalectomy or to chronic stress, and the consequences of these changes for the composition of the hypothalamic signal driving ACTH secretion.

QUANTITATIVE IMMUNOCYTOCHEMISTRY

In our studies, we have approached the study of CRF neurons by examining changes in the peptide content of their nerve terminals located in the ZEME. Quantitative information on the CRF content can easily be retrieved from radioimmunological determinations of CRF in median eminence extracts, because the terminals of interest represent the major source of CRF in this brain structure. However, the situation with respect to AVP is different because AVP stored in the CRF terminals represents only a small fraction of the total AVP content of the median eminence. In intact rats, most of the AVP is present in the internal zone of the median eminence in fibers *en passant* that originate from the magnocellular neurons and terminate in the posterior pituitary. Although it cannot be excluded that AVP from these fibers can reach the corticotropes in the anterior pituitary gland, the activity of the magnocellular AVP neurons do not seem to contribute much to the control of ACTH secretion.[26] Therefore, AVP that is involved in the physiological control of ACTH secretion appears to originate primarily from AVP costoring CRF terminals in the ZEME.

In order to detect AVP changes in the ZEME without contamination with AVP from the internal zone, we used the quantitative immunocytochemical approach as described earlier.[27] Briefly, tissue specimens were immersion fixed, embedded together in a cryomold, frozen in nitrogen-cooled isopentane, and sectioned (10 μm) by using a motor-driven cryostat. Thus, each section contains material of each specimen. Adjacent sections were stained for CRF or AVP by using indirect immunofluorescence techniques. In some experiments double-staining procedures were used.[28] For details of the procedures and specificity of the antibodies see references 29 and 30.

The staining intensity was quantitated by the use of a computer-assisted microfluorimeter (Leitz MPV II). In each section, 10 measurements (diameter measuring spot 12.5 μm) were made in the ZEME and six in the area of the arcuate nucleus (background). Of each median eminence specimen, three sections were analyzed between the levels A 4100 and A 4500 according to Koenig and Klippel.[31] After background subtraction, the mean fluorescence intensity was calculated. For interexperimental comparison of the results, hypothalami from a group of normal untreated rats ($n = 6$) were included in each experiment and served as a reference standard. Within these groups, the average variation in CRF and AVP readings in the ZEME was 5% and 10%, respectively.

To validate the results of quantitative immunocytochemical analysis, experiments have been carried out in which groups of rats were subjected to manipulations leading to decreases or increases of CRF stores in the ZEME. The hypothalami of half of each group were processed for quantitative immunocytochemistry, whereas the other half was used for measurements of CRF in hypothalamic extracts by radioimmunoassay. As illustrated in FIGURE 2, both parameters showed a good linear correlation (see also ref. 32). Thus, changes in CRF as determined by quantitative immunocytochemistry can legitimately be interpreted as proportional changes in the amounts of peptide stored in the tissues. By inference, quantitative immunocytochemical data on AVP are likely to reflect proportional changes in actual AVP content.

PEPTIDE DEPLETION RATE—AN INDEX OF SECRETORY ACTIVITY

Our "peptide turnover" approach[27] is based on the view that the amount of peptide stored in the nerve terminals reflects the net balance between the rate of supply of newly formed material and the rate of release of the peptide. Thus, changes in peptide stores in the terminals may reflect changes in either parameter and can therefore not been interpreted unequivocally. We postulated that if we could prevent the supply of newly formed material, the secretion rate would determine the rate of depletion of the peptide stores in the terminals. Intracisternal administration of a low nontoxic dose (5 μg/rat) of colchicine leads to a transient (6–8 h) blockade of fast axonal transport of peptides in hypothalamic neurons, with minor interference

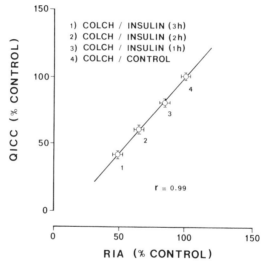

FIGURE 2. Correlation between changes in CRF as measured by radioimmunoassay (RIA) and by quantitative immunocytochemistry (QICC) in the external zone of the median eminence. Four groups of rats ($n = 14$) were subjected to different treatments. Of each group, eight were processed for RIA and six were processed for QICC. Data refer to means and SEM. For details see reference 34.

with the activity of neuroendocrine control mechanisms.[27,32–35] Colchicine or saline (10 μl) is injected into the cisterna magna under light ether anesthesia, and animals are sacrificed 5 or 6 hours later.[27] The injection procedure itself induced transient ACTH, alpha-MSH, corticosterone, and prolactin responses that disappeared within 60 minutes. At the nontoxic dose used in these experiments, colchicine did not affect hormone secretion up to 5 hours after administration[27] and did not interfere with stress-induced ACTH secretion.[9] In addition, we found that this low dose of colchicine did not affect CRF and AVP in the ZEME of intact rats under resting conditions when the activity of the hypothalamic-pituitary-adrenal (HPA) axis is low, but did reduce CRF and/or AVP during conditions of high HPA activity. By using this approach, information can be obtained on stimulus-induced CRF and AVP secretion from the ZEME in a freely moving awake animal. Although the method has many applications, its use is limited to conditions that lead to release of a significant proportion (> 10–20%) of the peptide stores. Therefore, it cannot be used to study the hypothalamic responses to short and/or mild stressors such as ether or novel environment.

CHANGES IN PEPTIDE MAKEUP AFTER ADRENALECTOMY

In the mid-1970s, several groups reported that adrenalectomy of rats leads to increased AVP immunostaining in the ZEME that could be prevented by daily administration of dexamethasone.[36] In adrenalectomized (ADX) rats, as in intact controls, AVP immunoreactivity in the ZEME was found to be localized in CRF containing terminals.[8,12] In contrast to intact animals in which less than half of the CRF terminals contain AVP (see above), in ADX rats, the vast majority ($> 90\%$) of the CRF terminals costore AVP.[6,8] Apparently, ADX causes those CRF neurons that normally do not produce and store AVP, to switch to the AVP coproducing mode. This is supported by the results of immunocytochemical staining of the cell bodies showing a high degree of CRF and AVP colocalization in the parvocellular PVN of ADX rats.[37] These studies further disclosed that the rate of synthesis of both AVP and CRF in these neurons is enhanced after adrenalectomy,[38–42] which is in accordance with large increments in the levels of pro-AVP and pro-CRF mRNA in this part of the PVN.[43–46] Inasmuch as elevated concentrations of CRF and AVP occur in the portal blood of ADX animals,[47–50] enhanced production of these peptides appears to be associated with increased secretion rates of both peptides (see also refs. 27 and 51).

The enhanced secretion of CRF drives, at least partly, the ACTH hypersecretion in ADX rats. Peripheral administration of a CRF antiserum or of a CRF-receptor antagonist caused a prompt drop in the high plasma ACTH levels in such animals,[52–54] whereas these substances did not affect resting ACTH levels in intact animals.[53,55] In view of this, we were struck by the finding that the CRF content of the median eminence as measured by quantitative immunocytochemistry or by RIA in rats adrenalectomized one week previously was similar to that of intact controls.[27] In some but not all strains (and substrains) of rats, this situation can be maintained for at least four weeks after ADX.[51] Because the amount of peptide stored in the nerve terminals reflects the balance between supply of newly synthesized material and release, it is conceivable that the slightest imbalance between these two processes will result in a gradual increase or decrease of the peptide stores. Accordingly, the discordant data reported on ADX-induced changes in CRF stores in the median eminence[38,48,50,56,57] may reflect only slight imbalances between these two processes, which are both strongly accelerated by the absence of circulating glucocorticoids.

In contrast to its variable effects on CRF stores, ADX always leads to a progressive accumulation of AVP in the ZEME that can be detected from the first day onwards.[51] This increase in AVP is at least partly caused by a prompt increase in the fraction of the CRF neurons coproducing AVP and, consequently, an increase of the fraction of CRF terminals costoring AVP.[8,58] Nearly complete colocalization of CRF and AVP has been observed in the ZEME as early as three days after adrenalectomy.[8] Thus, adrenalectomy induces a fast and nearly complete transition of the CRF motor neurons from the AVP nonproducing phenotype to the AVP coproducing phenotype. In addition to an increase in the numbers of AVP coproducing CRF neurons, AVP synthesis per neuron also increases as illustrated by a progressive increase of AVP immunoreactivity and of pro-AVP mRNA in CRF neurons.[40,44,59] Within the CRF nerve terminals, adrenalectomy induced marked changes with respect to the peptide content of their secretory granules as indicated by double-label immunocytochemistry. Electron microscopy studies on intact rats revealed that most of the granules were positive for CRF or for both CRF and AVP, whereas very few were only AVP positive. In contrast, these AVP-positive/CRF-negative granules represent a large population of the secretory granules in CRF terminals of ADX rats,[6] indicating that secretory granules appear that store predominantly (or even exclusively) AVP. The consequences of these changes in peptide makeup for the composition of the signal produced by the CRF neurons in ADX rats will be discussed below.

All of the above-mentioned ADX-induced changes in CRF neurons can be prevented or reversed by the administration of corticosterone or dexamethasone.[8,44,59–62] A wealth of information indicates that the CRF neurons in the PVN are sensitive to glucocorticoid feedback and that in normal intact rats, mRNA expression and, to a larger extent, the synthesis of AVP and CRF are tonically suppressed by the circulating corticosterone.[62–64] Although this may also be true for the synthesis of angiotensin II and CCK in the parvocellular PVN,[13,65,66] other peptides that can be expressed in CRF neurons (e.g., enkephalin, neurotensin) are not affected by adrenalectomy.[44,63] The exact mechanism by which glucocorticoids suppress CRF synthesis is not known as the CRF gene does not appear to exhibit a glucocorticoid-responsive element. Such an element is present on the AVP gene but *in vitro* studies have shown that glucocorticoids can enhance or inhibit AVP gene transcription *in vitro* depending on the conditions used.[67]

CHANGES IN PEPTIDE MAKEUP DURING CHRONIC STRESS

If glucocorticoids indeed play a dominant role in suppressing AVP and CRF synthesis under physiological situations, one would anticipate that conditions leading to elevated corticosteroid levels (e.g., stress) will exert a suppressive action on CRF and AVP gene transcription and translation. Although indications for such an action have been found,[68] until recently available information indicated that chronic stress did not reduce but rather increased CRF mRNA in the PVN.[69–72] However, in some chronic stress paradigms, unchanged[70,72] or decreased message levels have been found.[73] After a single exposure of rats to a strong stressor, a fast increase in CRF mRNA was recorded,[70,74] which disappeared within 24 hours (S. L. Lightman, personal communication). This short-term increase in message possibly relates to a short-term increase in CRF biosynthesis, which is necessary to substitute for the losses of CRF in the nerve terminals caused by secretion. Indeed, a single exposure to a strong stressor (e.g., immobilization) causes a fast decline in CRF and AVP stores in the ZEME (1–3 h),[9] but these stores were replenished to their prestress levels within 24 hours (Tilders *et al.,* unpublished observations).

In contrast to the remarkable stability of the CRF and AVP stores as measured one day after a single stress experience, repeated or chronic stress leads to characteristic changes of the peptide stores in the ZEME 24 hours after the last challenge. For instance, after 3–4 weeks of "chronic psychosocial stress" induced by housing male rats in a hierachically controlled colony, the CRF content in the ZEME of the subordinate males had not changed, but their AVP content had increased to 160–190% of that of the controls who were housed in pairs. Because their subordinate status correlated with the AVP content in the ZEME, the intensity of the stress experienced by the animal appears to be an important determinant for the increase in AVP in the ZEME.[75] In most chronic stress models, animals are exposed intermittently to one (or a variety of) aversive stimulus. We selected two stimuli to which rats do not respond with marked habituation or sensitization of the ACTH responses. One consists of repeated administration once daily of a hypoglycemic dose of insulin,[34,76] which results in a progressive increase of AVP in the ZEME to 160% after 11 days. According to our observations in rats exposed to chronic psychosocial stress, intermittent hypoglycemia did not result in elevated CRF stores but rather in a transient reduction of this peptide in the ZEME.[75,76] In addition, repeated exposure to immobilization once daily did not affect the CRF content but resulted in a progressive increase (> twofold after 16 days) in AVP stored in the ZEME.[9] Irrespective of the reported differences in the fraction of CRF terminals costoring AVP in normal untreated rats, which may relate to differences in methodology, rat strains or prior history of animals,[7,9,10] repeated immobilization was found to increase twofold the numbers of double-labeled terminals in the ZEME.[9,10] At the level of the CRF cell bodies in the PVN, both message and peptide levels are enhanced after repeated immobilization,[10,28] but the increases of AVP peptide and message appear stronger than those of CRF. Furthermore, by using double-label immunocytochemistry, the numbers of AVP coproducing CRF neurons in the PVN showed a two- to threefold increase[28] which is in harmony with the observed changes in the ZEME of repeatedly stressed rats. Taken together, these observations indicate that chronic stress drives the CRF neurons from the non-AVP-producing to the AVP-coproducing phenotype.

Chronic stress-induced changes in CRF neurons need time to develop. We only observed significant changes in chronic stress paradigms that lasted for more than five days. An obvious conclusion is that the number of repetitions or the duration of the aversive situation is an important parameter for the development of these adaptive changes in CRF neurons. However, it is not clear whether this is indeed the case. Recently, we found that such changes can also be observed two weeks after a single period (2 h) of hypoglycemia (de Goeij, unpublished observations) or after exposure of rats to a single period (15 min) of electric footshocks.[77] Accordingly, we cannot exclude the possibility that it is the time elapsed since the first stress encounter, rather than the number of repetitions or duration of the stressful period, that determines these changes. Future studies are needed to clarify this point.

It is intriguing that the phenotypic changes in CRF neurons that occur in ADX animals and that can be prevented by the administration of glucocorticoids can also be observed during conditions of chronic stress (TABLE 1). Apparently, the glucocorticoid status of the animal is not the crucial factor for this aspect of phenotypic plasticity of CRF neurons. A common aspect of ADX and chronic stress is that both conditions are associated with secretory hyperactivity of the CRF neurons in the PVN. Accordingly, we hypothesized that the expression, production, and storage of AVP is an intrinsic property expressed by activated CRF neurons.[9] If this hypothesis is correct, the amount of AVP stored in the ZEME and the fraction of CRF neurons coproducing AVP might be used as a postmortem index of the antemortem activity of these CRF neurons. In support of this hypothesis, we recently found that AVP expression in parvocellular CRF neurons in the PVN of the human hypothalamus increases with aging,[78] a condition that appears to be associated with hyperactivity of the HPA axis.[79]

SIGNIFICANCE OF CHANGES IN PEPTIDE MAKEUP
FOR THE COMPOSITION OF THE SIGNAL

Based on a series of elegant studies, Whitnall[80] hypothesized that only the AVP-storing population of CRF neurons can respond to stressors with the secretion of their contents into the portal blood. By inference, the non-AVP-storing CRF neurons represent a "dormant" population of cells. According to this hypothesis, AVP coproduction is not a consequence of prior hyperactivity, but rather reflects a phenotype of CRF neurons that is selectively involved in the stress response. Assuming that in normal unstressed rats, AVP present in the ZEME is localized in up to 50% of the CRF-containing terminals, and that CRF and AVP stored in these terminals are secreted concomitantly (see below), any stress-induced depletion of the CRF stores in the ZEME should be accompanied by the disappearance of at least a twofold higher fraction of the AVP stores. This is clearly not the case. Although several stressors including hypoglycemia,[76] immobilization,[9] and histamine (unpublished observations) diminish the CRF and AVP stores in the ZEME, other stimuli (e.g., interleukin-1) result in a selective depletion of CRF,[35,81] whereas social interactions can lead to a selective fall in AVP without detectable effects on the CRF stores.[75] In addition, we reported that the stress-induced declines of the AVP and

TABLE 1. Effects of Adrenalectomy and Chronic or Repeated Stress on CRF-Producing Neurons in the Rat[a]

	Adrenalectomy	Chronic Stress
External zone of the median eminence		
AVP content (QICC)	↑	↑
CRH content (ICC, RIA)	↓ → ↑	→
% AVP costoring CRF terminals	↑	↑
% AVP positive secretory granules	↑	↑
Secretion AVP	↑	↑
Secretion CRF	↑	→
Signal ratio AVP/CRF	↑	↑
Parvocellular part PVN		
AVP staining (cell numbers)	↑	↑
CRF staining (cell numbers)	↑	↑
AVP/CRF colocalization (cell numbers)	↑	↑
AVP mRNA	↑	↑
CRF mRNA	↑	↑

[a]Note that both conditions induce increasing numbers of CRF neurons to transcribe and translate the AVP gene and to store AVP in the terminals. Furthermore, both conditions shift the composition of the hypothalamic signal towards increased AVP/CRF ratio.

CRF stores in the ZEME often follow different time courses.[32] Accordingly, the secretion of CRF and of AVP from the nerve terminals in the ZEME appear to be two independently controlled processes.

This is in accord with a wealth of information indicating that the ACTH responses to certain stressors are very dependent on AVP, whereas those to other stimuli are not or are to a much lesser extent.[23,82,83] Although the exact neuronal origin of the AVP found in portal blood is still disputed, the results of such studies support the notion that AVP contributes to the signal for ACTH secretion during certain conditions but not during others.[16] Therefore, it seems most likely that both phenotypes of CRF neurons (non-AVP producing and AVP coproducing) can participate in the stress response and that their specific contribution to the hypothalamic signal driving ACTH secretion varies with the nature, intensity, and duration of the stressor. This view implies that the two phenotypes of CRF neurons may have different afferent inputs and/or express different receptors for neuronal and/or humoral signaling substances. Therefore, it would be most interesting to know whether the transition from one phenotype to the other is associated with changes in the responsiveness to specific humoral or neuronal signals. At least one observation supports this possibility. Although discordant results have been reported,[84] under the conditions used in our studies,[35,81] interleukin-1 appears to selectively activate the non-AVP producing phenotype of CRF neurons. However, after adrenalectomy when this phenotype disappears (see above) interleukin-1 loses its capacity to stimulate ACTH secretion[85] (Berkenbosch, unpublished observations). We feel that such peptide makeup associated change in responsiveness of CRF neurons may not only occur after adrenalectomy but also after chronic or repeated stress.

Another explanation for the finding that AVP and CRF secretion from the ZEME are independently controlled may be that colocalized peptides are not necessarily secreted concomitantly and in the same ratio as found in the terminal. To study whether this may be the case, we analyzed AVP and CRF secretion in ADX rats, because in these animals the CRF terminals in the ZEME show a high degree of homogeneity in the sense that they are almost all of the AVP costoring phenotype. Thus, we postulated that major discordances between the secretion rates of CRF and AVP point toward preferential secretion of one peptide over the other. Indeed, in long-term (4 wk), but not in short-term (1 wk) in ADX rats, the chance of AVP being secreted was approximately twice as high as that of CRF.[51] Although alternative explanations can be given, the possibility can no longer be excluded that the composition of the signal produced by a multimessenger CRF neuron may vary with its stimulation conditions as has been demonstrated for amine-peptide–containing neurons (see introduction). Recently it became clear that one of the prerequisites for differential release, namely, heterogeneity of the secretory granules, appears to be met. Although CRF can be colocalized with AVP and enkephalin in the same secretory granules,[5,12] our observations (FIG. 3) and those of others[6,10] involving double-label immunocytochemistry show a marked heterogeneity in the labeling intensity of different secretory granules within CRF nerve terminals that are likely to be related to differences in their peptide content.

Only limited information is available on the consequences of chronic stress–induced increases in the AVP load of the ZEME on the composition of the signal driving ACTH secretion. In our studies on the effects of repeated stress on hypoglycemia-induced activation of CRF neurons, CRF secretion remained unchanged or even decreased, whereas the amounts of AVP that were secreted progressively increased to approximately 150% after 11 days as the duration of the chronic stress increased.[76] Similar changes have been found in the signal produced by CRF neurons of ADX rats. Also in this condition, the progressive increase in AVP content of the ZEME is accompanied by a progressive increase in the AVP/CRF ratio of the signal produced by these neurons. Thus both during chronic stress and after adrenalectomy, the hypothalamic signal produced by the CRF neurons gradually changes from a CRF-dominated signal to a more AVP-dominated signal. This is in accordance with *in vitro* studies demonstrating enhanced AVP secretion from hypothalami of chronically stressed and ADX rats.[56,86,87]

SIGNIFICANCE OF CHANGES IN PEPTIDE SIGNAL FOR PITUITARY FUNCTION

Let us briefly consider the physiological impact of an increase of the AVP/CRF ratio of the signal produced by the CRF neurons of animals exposed to chronic stress. Because of the synergistic actions of AVP and CRF on ACTH secretion from

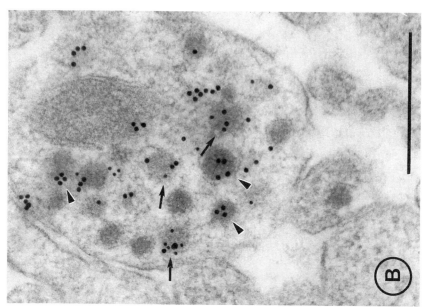

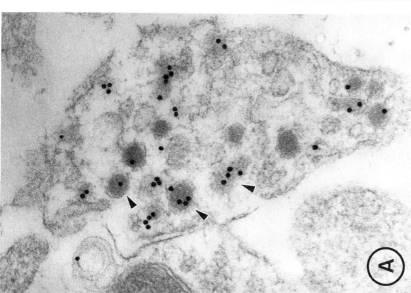

FIGURE 3. Electron micrographs of phenotypically different CRF terminals in the external zone of the median eminence of an intact rat. **Panel A** shows a terminal containing secretory granules labeled only for CRF (15 nm gold, *arrowheads*), whereas the terminal shown in **panel B** contains granules labeled for CRF and/or AVP-neurophysin (10 nm gold particles, *arrows*). Images obtained after postembedding immunogold double-labeling for CRF (antiserum 5 Bo, supplied by F. Berkenbosch) and for AVP-neurophysin (monoclonal PS41, kindly supplied by H. Gainer). Note the heterogeneity in labeling density between granules. Bar = 500 nm.

the corticotropes, it can be anticipated that in the presence of increased AVP levels, the same amounts of CRF provoke exaggerated ACTH responses. This by itself will result in an increased power of these CRF neurons. This increased power may relate to the ACTH hyperresponsiveness often observed when repeatedly stressed rats are exposed to an unfamiliar stimulus. In contrast, repeated exposure to the same stimulus may result in habituation of the ACTH response, a phenomenon that is at least partly controlled by suprahypothalamic mechanisms, and that can occur in animals with high as well as with low AVP levels in the ZEME.

The increased AVP/CRF ratio of the hypothalamic response to repeated (12 times) hypoglycemia was not associated with increased ACTH responses.[76] This suggests a gradual loss of the responsiveness of corticotrope cells to either or both of these hypothalamic signals. Accordingly, chronic stress is known to result in down-regulation of CRF receptors of corticotropes and in a concomitant reduction of their responsiveness to CRF.[88,89] Although CRF alone can down-regulate CRF receptors *in vivo* and *in vitro*, AVP has been reported to facilitate this phenomenon.[90–93] In contrast to the stress-induced loss of pituitary responsiveness to CRF, the ACTH releasing activity of AVP was not attenuated in chronically stressed rats.[88] These observations point toward an interesting parallel between the shift in the composition of the hypothalamic signal (more AVP dominated) and the change in pituitary responsiveness to these signals. Thus, on the one hand, AVP facilitates CRF receptor down-regulation making ACTH secretion more AVP driven, whereas, on the other hand, AVP continues to potentiate the crippled CRF signal.[88]

Although the biological significance of these changes remains to be elucidated, it should be noted that CRF- and AVP-induced ACTH secretion differ strongly with respect to their sensitivity to glucocorticoids. That is, CRF-induced ACTH secretion is more sensitive to the suppressive action of glucocorticoids than is AVP-induced ACTH secretion.[17] Accordingly, it can be anticipated that the prolonged ACTH responses as observed in chronically stressed animals may, at least in part, be related to changes in the composition of the hypothalamic signal driving ACTH secretion.

CONCLUSIONS

CRF neurons that project to the ZEME are multimessenger neurons that have the capacity to produce various substances along with CRF. In normal rats less than 50% of these neurons are of the AVP-coproducing phenotype, whereas the remaining CRF neurons are of the non-AVP producing phenotype. These neurons show a remarkable form of neuronal plasticity, namely, that during chronic stress and after adrenalectomy AVP production is switched on in previously non-AVP producing neurons. Under both conditions, the increase in AVP gene expression and AVP synthesis is associated with increased numbers of AVP plus CRF storing terminals and an overall increase of the AVP/CRF ratio of the peptide stores in the ZEME. In addition, these phenotypic changes in CRF neurons induced by chronic stress and adrenalectomy are associated with an increase of the AVP/CRF ratio of the signal produced by these neurons. This change in the hypothalamic signal may have major repercussions for the functioning of the HPA axis during chronic stress and stress-related disorders.

ACKNOWLEDGMENT

We thank Mr. H. Nordsiek for producing the figures.

REFERENCES

1. HÖKFELT, T., B. EVERITT, B. MEISTER, T. MELANDER, M. SCHALLING, O. JOHANSSON, J. M. LUNDBERG, A. HULTING, S. WERNER, C. CUELLO, H. HEMMINGS, C. OUIMET, I. WALAAS, P. GREENGARD & M. GOLDSTEIN. 1986. Recent Prog. Horm. Res. **42:** 1–69.
2. STJÄRNE, L. 1989. Rev. Physiol. Biochem. Pharmacol. **112:** 1–138.
3. JAN, Y. N. & L. Y. JAN. 1983. TINS **6:** 320–325.
4. CECCATELLI, S., R. CORTES & T. HÖKFELT. 1991. Mol. Brain Res. **9:** 57–69.
5. WHITNALL, M. H., E. MEZEY & H. GAINER. 1985. Nature **317:** 248–250.
6. BERTINI, L. T. & J. Z. KISS. 1991. Neuroscience **42:** 237–244.
7. WHITNALL, M. H., D. SMYTH & H. GAINER. 1987. Neuroendocrinology **45:** 420–424.
8. WHITNALL, M. H., S. KEY & H. GAINER. 1987. Endocrinology **120:** 2180–2182.
9. DE GOEIJ, D. C. E., R. KVETNANSKY, M. H. WHITNALL, D. JEZOVA, F. BERKENBOSCH & F. J. H. TILDERS. 1991. Neuroendocrinology **53:** 150–159.
10. BARTANUSZ, V., D. JEZOVA, L. T. BERTINI, F. J. H. TILDERS, J. AUBRY & J. Z. KISS. 1993. Endocrinology **132:** 895–902.
11. HISANO, S., S. DAIKOKU, N. YANAIHARA & T. SHIBASAKI. 1986. Brain Res. **370:** 321–326.
12. HISANO, S., Y. TSURUO, S. KATOH, S. DAIKOKU, N. YANAIHARA & T. SHIBASAKI. 1987. Cell Tissue Res. **249:** 497–507.
13. SWANSON, L. W. 1991. Prog. Brain Res. **87:** 181–200.
14. GILLIES, G. E., E. A. LINTON & P. J. LOWRY. 1982. Nature **299:** 355–357.
15. VALE, W., J. VAUGHAN, M. SMITH, G. YAMAMOTO, J. RIVIER & C. RIVIER. 1983. Endocrinology **113:** 1121–1131.
16. ANTONI, F. A. 1986. Endocr. Rev. **7:** 351–378.
17. OKI, Y., T. W. PEATMAN, Z. C. QU & D. N. ORTH. 1991. Endocrinology **128:** 1589–1596.
18. SPINEDI, E. & A. NEGRO VILAR. 1983. Neuroendocrinology **37:** 446–453.
19. REISINE, T. & R. JENSEN. 1986. J. Pharmacol. Exp. Ther. **236:** 621–626.
20. HOOI, S. C., D. M. MAITER, J. B. MARTIN & J. L. KOENIG. 1990. Endocrinology **127:** 2281–2289.
21. TILDERS, F. J. H., K. TATEMOTO & F. BERKENBOSCH. 1984. Endocrinology **115:** 1633–1635.
22. GAMBACCIANI, M., S. S. YEN & D. D. RASMUSSEN. 1986. Neuroendocrinology **43:** 533–536.
23. RIVIER, C. & W. VALE. 1983. Nature **305:** 325–327.
24. RIVIER, C. & W. VALE. 1983. Endocrinology **113:** 939–942.
25. LINTON, E. A., F. J. H. TILDERS, S. HODGKINSON, F. BERKENBOSCH, I. VERMES & P. J. LOWRY. 1985. Endocrinology **116:** 966–970.
26. AGUILERA, G., S. L. LIGHTMAN & A. KISS. 1993. Endocrinology **132:** 241–248.
27. BERKENBOSCH, F. & F. J. H. TILDERS. 1988. Brain Res. **442:** 312–320.
28. DE GOEIJ, D. C. E., D. JEZOVA & F. J. H. TILDERS. 1992. Brain Res. **577:** 165–168.
29. BERKENBOSCH, F., E. A. LINTON & F. J. H. TILDERS. 1986. Neuroendocrinology **44:** 338–346.
30. VAN DER SLUIS, P. J., C. W. POOL & A. A. SLUITER. 1988. Electrophoresis **9:** 654–661.
31. KOENIG, J. F. R. & R. A. KLIPPEL. 1963. The Rat Brain. A Stereotactic Atlas of the Forebrain and Lower Parts of the Brainstem. Williams & Wilkins. Baltimore, MD.
32. TILDERS, F. J. H., D. C. E. DE GOEIJ & F. BERKENBOSCH. 1989. Turnover of corticotropin releasing factor and vasopressin in the median eminence and control of pituitary-adrenal activity. *In* The Control of the Hypothalamo-Pituitary-Adrenal Axis. F. C. Rose, Ed.: 7–24. International University Press. Madison, WI.
33. PARISH, D. C., E. M. RODRIQUEZ, S. D. BIRKETT & B. T. PICKERING. 1981. Cell Tissue Res. **220:** 809–827.
34. BERKENBOSCH, F., D. C. E. DE GOEIJ & F. J. H. TILDERS. 1989. Endocrinology **125:** 28–34.
35. BERKENBOSCH, F., D. C. E. DE GOEIJ, A. D. REY & H. O. BESEDOVSKY. 1989. Neuroendocrinology **50:** 570–576.
36. ZIMMERMAN, E. A., M. A. STILLMAN, L. D. RECHT, J. L. ANTUNES, P. W. CARMEL & P. C. GOLDSMITH. 1977. Ann. N.Y. Acad. Sci. **297:** 405–419.
37. WHITNALL, M. H. 1988. J. Comp. Neurol. **275:** 13–28.
38. BUGNON, C., D. FELLMANN & A. GOUGET. 1983. Neurosci. Lett. **37:** 43–49.
39. TRAMU, G., C. CROIX & A. PILLEZ. 1983. Neuroendocrinology **37:** 467–469.

40. KISS, J. Z., E. MEZEY & L. SKIRBOLL. 1984. Proc. Natl. Acad. Sci. USA **81:** 1854–1858.
41. SAWCHENKO, P. E., L. W. SWANSON & W. W. VALE. 1984. Proc. Natl. Acad. Sci. USA **81:** 1883–1887.
42. ALONSO, G., A. SZAFARCZYK & I. ASSENMACHER. 1986. Exp. Brain Res. **61:** 497–505.
43. FRIM, D. M., B. G. ROBINSON, K. B. PASIEKA & J. A. MAJZOUB. 1990. Am. J. Physiol. **258:** E686–E692.
44. SWANSON, L. W. & D. M. SIMMONS. 1989. J. Comp. Neurol. **285:** 413–435.
45. YOUNG, W. S., E. MEZEY & R. E. SIEGEL. 1986. Neurosci. Lett. **70:** 198–203.
46. YOUNG, W. S., E. MEZEY & R. E. SIEGEL. 1986. Mol. Brain Res. **1:** 231–241.
47. ECKLAND, D. J. A., K. TODD & S. L. LIGHTMAN. 1988. J. Endocrinol. **117:** 27–34.
48. FINK, G., I. C. ROBINSON & L. A. TANNAHILL. 1988. J. Physiol. (Lond.) **401:** 329–345.
49. KOENIG, J. I., H. Y. MELTZER, G. D. DEVANE & G. A. GUDELSKY. 1986. Endocrinology **118:** 2534–2539.
50. PLOTSKY, P. M. & P. E. SAWCHENKO. 1987. Endocrinology **120:** 1361–1369.
51. DE GOEIJ, D. C. E., F. BERKENBOSCH & F. J. H. TILDERS. 1993. J. Neuroendocrinol.
52. CONTE-DEVOLX, B., M. REY, F. BOUDOURESQUE, P. GIRAUD, E. CASTANAS, Y. MILLET, J. L. CODACCIONI & C. OLIVER. 1983. Peptides **4:** 301–304.
53. RIVIER, C., J. RIVIER & W. VALE. 1982. Science **218:** 377–379.
54. RIVIER, J., C. RIVIER & W. VALE. 1984. Science **224:** 889–891.
55. VAN OERS, J. W. A. M. & F. J. H. TILDERS. 1991. Endocrinology **128:** 496–503.
56. SPINEDI, E., M. GIACOMINI, M. C. JACQUIER & R. C. GAILLARD. 1991. Neuroendocrinology **53:** 160–170.
57. SUDA, T., N. TOMORI, F. TOZAWA, T. MOURI, H. DEMURA & K. SHIZUME. 1983. Endocrinology **113:** 1182–1184.
58. KISS, J. C. & L. T. BERTINI. 1992. Brain Res. **597:** 353–357.
59. KOVACS, K., J. Z. KISS & G. B. MAKARA. 1986. Neuroendocrinology **44:** 229–234.
60. JINGAMI, H., S. MATSUKURA, S. NUMA & H. IMURA. 1985. Endocrinology **117:** 1314–1320.
61. KOVACS, K. J. & E. MEZEY. 1987. Neuroendocrinology **46:** 365–368.
62. SAWCHENKO, P. E. 1987. Brain Res. **403:** 213–223.
63. SAWCHENKO, P. E. 1987. J. Neurosci. **7:** 1093–1106.
64. HERMAN, J. P., M. K. SCHAFER, R. C. THOMPSON & S. J. WATSON. 1992. Mol. Endocrinol. **6:** 1061–1069.
65. LIND, R. W., L. W. SWANSON, T. O. BRUHN & D. GANTEN. 1985. Brain Res. **338:** 81–89.
66. MEZEY, E., T. D. REISINE, L. SKIRBOLL, M. BEINFELD & J. Z. KISS. 1986. Proc. Natl. Acad. Sci. USA **83:** 3510–3512.
67. VERBEECK, M. A. E., W. SUTANO & J. P. H. BURBACH. 1991. Mol. Endocrinol. **5:** 795–801.
68. SAWCHENKO, P. E., T. IMAKI & W. VALE. 1992. Co-localization of neuroactive substances in the endocrine hypothalamus. *In* Functional anatomy of the neuroendocrine hypothalamus. J. Chadwick & J. Marsh, Eds.: 16–42. John Wiley & Sons. Chichester.
69. LIGHTMAN, S. L. & W. S. YOUNG. 1988. J. Physiol. (Lond.) **403:** 511–523.
70. HARBUZ, M. S. & S. L. LIGHTMAN. 1989. J. Endocrinol. **122:** 705–711.
71. HERMAN, J. P., K. H. SCHAFER, C. D. SLADEK, R. DAY, E. A. YOUNG, H. AKIL & S. J. WATSON. 1989. Brain Res. **501:** 235–246.
72. IMAKI, T., J. L. NAHAN, C. RIVIER, P. E. SAWCHENKO & W. VALE. 1991. J. Neurosci. **11:** 585–599.
73. HARBUZ, M. S., R. G. REES, D. ECKLAND, D. S. JESSOP, D. BREWERTON & S. L. LIGHTMAN. 1992. Endocrinology **130:** 1394–1400.
74. IMAKI, T., T. SHIBASAKI, M. HOTTA & H. DEMURA. 1992. Endocrinology **131:** 240–246.
75. DE GOEIJ, D. C. E., H. DIJKSTRA & F. J. H. TILDERS. 1992. Endocrinology **131:** 847–853.
76. DE GOEIJ, D. C. E., R. BINNEKADE & F. J. H. TILDERS. 1992. Am. J. Physiol. **263:** E394–E399.
77. VAN DIJKEN, H. H., D. C. E. DE GOEIJ, W. SUTANTO, J. MOS, E. R. DE KLOET & F. J. H. TILDERS. 1993. Neuroendocrinology. In press.
78. RAADSHEER, F. C., A. A. SLUITER, RAVID, F. J. H. TILDERS & D. F. SWAAB. 1993. Brain Res. In press.
79. DODT, C., J. DITTMANN, J. HRUBY, E. SPATH SCHWALBE, J. BORN, R. SCHUTTLER & H. L. FEHM. 1991. J. Clin. Endocrinol. Metab. **72:** 272–276.

80. WHITNALL, M. H. 1989. Neuroendocrinology **50:** 702–707.
81. BERKENBOSCH, F., J. W. A. M. VAN OERS, A. DEL REY, F. J. H. TILDERS & H. BESEDOVSKY. 1987. Science **238:** 524–526.
82. VAN OERS, J. W. A. M., D. JEZOVA, R. KVETNANSKY & F. J. H. TILDERS. 1993. Submitted.
83. RIVIER, C. 1991. Neuroendocrine mechanisms of anterior pituitary regulation in the rat exposed to stress. *In* Stress. Neurobiology and Neuroendocrinology. M. R. Brown, G. F. Koop & C. Rivier, Eds.: 119–136. Marcel Dekker. New York, NY.
84. WHITNALL, M. H., R. S. PERLSTEIN, E. H. MOUGEY & R. NETA. 1992. Endocrinology **131:** 37–44.
85. WEIDENFELD, J., O. ABRAMSKY & H. OVADIA. 1989. Neuroendocrinology **50:** 650–654.
86. HOLMES, M. C., F. A. ANTONI, K. J. CATT & G. AGUILERA. 1986. Neuroendocrinology **43:** 245–251.
87. AGUILERA, G., A. KISS, R. L. HAUGER & Y. TIZABI. 1992. Regulation of the hypothalamic-pituitary-adrenal axis during stress: Role of neuropeptides and neurotransmitters. *In* Stress: Neuroendocrine and Molecular Approaches. R. Kvetnansky, R. McCarty & J. Axelrod, Eds.: 365–383. Gordon & Breach Science Publishers. New York, NY.
88. HAUGER, R. L., M. A. MILLAN, M. LORANG, J. P. HARWOOD & G. AGUILERA. 1988. Endocrinology **123:** 396–405.
89. HAUGER, R. L., M. LORANG, M. IRWIN & G. AGUILERA. 1990. Brain Res. **532:** 34–40.
90. TIZABI, Y. & G. AGUILERA. 1992. Neuroendocrinology **56:** 611–618.
91. HOFFMAN, A. R., G. CEDA & T. D. REISINE. 1985. J. Neurosci. **5:** 234–242.
92. RIVIER, C. & W. VALE. 1983. Endocrinology **113:** 1422–1426.
93. WYNN, P. C., J. P. HARWOOD, K. J. CATT & G. AGUILERA. 1988. Endocrinology **122:** 351–358.
94. WHITNALL, M. H. & H. GAINER. 1988. Neuroendocrinology **47:** 176–180.
95. MEISTER, B., T. HOKFELT, M. GEFFARD & W. OERTEL. 1988. Neuroendocrinology **48:** 516–526.
96. CECCATELLI, S., M. ERIKSSON & T. HOKFELT. 1989. Neuroendocrinology **49:** 309–323.

Amygdaloid CRF Pathways

Role in Autonomic, Neuroendocrine, and Behavioral Responses to Stress

T. S. GRAY

Department of Cell Biology, Neurobiology and Anatomy
Loyola Stritch School of Medicine
2160 South First Avenue
Maywood, Illinois 60153

A wealth of evidence suggests that the amygdala is a focal region for mediating the biological response to stress. Activation of the amygdala produces a constellation of changes that strikingly resemble the stress response. Damage to the amygdala will usually alter one or more of the neuroendocrine, autonomic or behavioral measures of the stress response. Anatomical studies have demonstrated relatively direct routes by which the amygdala can modulate neuroendocrine, autonomic, and behavioral systems. The neurotransmitters that are crucial for the mediation of the stress response are located in the neuronal pathways that connect the amygdala with other parts of the brain.

Corticotropin-releasing factor (CRF) is one of the most important hormones and putative neurotransmitters involved in the expression of the various components of the stress response. Central administration of CRF produces behavioral and visceral effects that resemble stimulation of the amygdala. The amygdala contains an abundance of CRF cell bodies, terminals, and receptors. These observations have prompted numerous studies that have attempted to further define the role of CRF in amygdaloid functions. The purpose of this paper is to review these studies and speculate on the function of the various CRF pathways related to the amygdala.

AMYGDALA, CRF, AND STRESS

Numerous studies have demonstrated the importance of the amygdala in the expression of autonomic, neuroendocrine, and behavioral changes that occur in response to fearful or aversive stimuli. Destruction of the amygdala markedly reduces various measures of fear or anxiety. It has been known since the classical work of Kluver and Bucy[1] that lesions involving the amygdala greatly reduce emotional responsiveness. Lesion studies indicate that the central amygdaloid nucleus (CeA) is particularly important for mediation of responses associated with conditioned or learned stressors. Bilateral ablation of the CeA impedes or blocks a variety of behavioral, autonomic, and neuroendocrine responses to learned stress. These responses include alterations in heart rate, blood pressure, defecation, and secretion of corticosterone in several animal species.[2–6] The visceral responses to the physical stressor alone are usually unaffected by amygdaloid lesions. These data suggest that the amygdala regulates responses to stimuli that signal an impending threat. Additional data indicate that the CeA is part of the neural circuitry mediating anxiety. Electrical stimulation of the amygdala in conscious human subjects elicits fully integrated experiences of fear and anxiety.[7,8] The perceptions of fear following amygdaloid stimulation are strikingly realistic and are usually associated with memories of the subject's past. Stimulation-induced fear is accompanied by increases in heart rate and blood pressure, pupillary dilatation, sweating, and distressed facial expressions. Similar responses have been observed after electrical or chemical stimulation of the amygdala (mainly the CeA) in conscious animals.[6,9–11] Overall the data strongly suggest that during stressful and anxious situations the CeA is activated.

Some recent studies have provided more direct evidence on the role of the CRF neurons in amygdaloid functions. After immobilization stress, neurons in the central nucleus express high levels of the early-immediate gene c-fos.[12,13] The protein product of the c-fos gene has proved to be a useful marker for detecting changes in neuronal activity. Specifically, immobilization stress induces increased c-fos expression in central nucleus neurons in the rat. As many as 100 c-fos immunoreactive neurons per section were detected using immunocytochemistry in the central nucleus after two or more hours of immobilization. When these sections were stained for CRF immunoreactivity, it was discovered that most of the CRF neurons also expressed the c-fos protein. This data provides evidence that amygdaloid CRF neurons are activated during immobilization stress. Glucocorticoid receptors have also been located with CRF cell bodies of the CeA.[14] This suggests that adrenal steroid feedback could also modulate amygdaloid CRF-containing neurons. However, these effects were seen in other peptide-expressing neurons of the CeA. Neurotensin, enkephalin, and somatostatin immunoreactive neurons also contained c-fos staining after immobilization stress and glucocorticoid receptor immunoreactivity.[13–15]

Another interesting study examined the effects of intracerebroventricular injections of CRF upon c-fos expression in the forebrain.[16] Neurons in the CeA exhibited elevated c-fos expression. Other areas expressing Fos protein increases included the bed nucleus of the stria terminalis, paraventricular nucleus, and ventrolateral septum. In addition to its autonomic and neuroendocrine actions, central injections of CRF enhance rat responses to acoustic startle.[17] This enhancement of the acoustic startle response can be blocked by bilateral lesions of the CeA.[18] Ablation of the hypothalamic paraventricular nucleus had no effect upon CRF facilitation of the acoustic startle response.

Finally, central injections of the CRF antagonist, alpha-helical CRF_{9-41}, reduce emotionality in socially defeated rats.[19] Changes in emotionality are reflected in altered behavioral response to a dominant rat. Intra-amygdaloid administration of the CRF antagonist also significantly reduced the behavioral posturing normally observed in this conflict paradigm. Overall these experiments provide strong data supporting an important role for CRF neurons and their receptors in functions mediated by the amygdala.

AMYGDALA, CRF, AND ANATOMICAL SUBSTRATES

CRF immunoreactive cell bodies and terminals are located throughout the amygdala.[20,21] The central amygdaloid nucleus contains an especially large number of CRF cell bodies and terminals. It is estimated that 1750 CRF neurons are located per side in the central nucleus.[22] Because this nucleus is the source of most of the amygdaloid cells that project to brain stem, it is not surprising that it is the origin of numerous CRF pathways. Recently, colocalization of CRF and neurotensin in the CeA was demonstrated.[23] This finding is not surprising in light of the observation that neurotensin cells in the CeA completely overlap the CRF cell distribution and project to the same regions outside of the amygdala. CRF-containing cells in the central amygdala project to the bed nucleus of the stria terminalis, lateral hypothalamus, mesencephalic reticular formation, midbrain central gray, lateral and medial parabrachial nuclei, mesencephalic nucleus of the trigeminal nerve, and the dorsal vagal complex (i.e., nucleus of the solitary tract and motor nucleus of the vagus).[24-26] In addition, anterograde tracing studies have demonstrated that the CeA and one of its main targets, the bed nucleus of the stria terminalis, innervate CRF neurons in the paraventricular hypothalamic nucleus and lateral hypothalamus.[26-29] Both nuclei also project to vasopressin and oxytocin cells in the paraventricular nucleus.[27,30,31] The CeA and bed nucleus of the stria terminalis also innervate dopaminergic neurons in the substantia nigra/A8 cell group region, serotonergic neurons in the dorsal raphe nucleus, noradrenergic neurons in the locus coeruleus, and both adrenergic and noradrenergic cells in the nucleus of the solitary tract.[32-34] An additional amygdaloid extrinsically projecting CRF pathway originates in the corticomedial nucleus, which innervates the ventromedial hypothalamus.[24] Although CRF cell bodies are heavily distributed in the CeA, CRF-receptor binding studies indicate heaviest binding in the lateral/basolateral amygdaloid complex.[35] These amygdaloid

TABLE 1. Probable Projections of Amygdaloid CRF Neurons: Different Types of Cells Innervated and Their Locations

Source	Location
Hypothalamus	
CRF	Paraventricular and lateral hypothalamus
Vasopressin	Paraventricular nucleus
Oxytocin	Paraventricular nucleus
Midbrain	
Dopamine	Substantia nigra/A8 region
Serotonin	Dorsal raphe nucleus
Pons/Medulla	
Adrenaline	Nucleus of solitary tract
Noradrenaline	Nucleus of solitary tract

nuclei project heavily into the CeA.[36] Recently, studies have demonstrated a dense distribution of CRF-binding protein and its mRNA in the CeA.[37] This protein is thought to bind to CRF and neutralize its biological activity.

Thus, anatomical pathway tracing studies of CRF amygdaloid connections suggest a complex organization involving (1) amygdaloid projections to CRF neurons of different regions related to autonomic and neuroendocrine functions and (2) CRF innervation of monoaminergic cells that project back to the forebrain possibly affecting widespread populations of cells (see TABLE 1 for summary). The function of the various amygdaloid projections may be to activate regions of the brain that initiate or modify components of the defense or stress response. For example, bilateral lesions of the CeA block freezing and cardiovascular response to threatening stimuli.[38] Lesions of the central gray block the freezing response, but not the cardiovascular response. Destruction of the lateral hypothalamus blocks the cardiovascular response, but not the freezing response. This would suggest that different targets of the CeA may mediate these two responses.

If CRF-expressing neurons in the amygdala are activated during stress, it is of interest to determine what type of terminals innervate these cells. The central amygdaloid nucleus contains an abundance of neuropeptide as well as monoaminergic terminals. Recent studies have indicated that CRF immunoreactive neurons are innervated by a heterogeneous population of nerve terminals (see TABLE 2 for summary). CRF neurons are densely innervated by calcitonin gene-related peptide (CGRP) containing terminals.[39,40] The CGRP terminals originate from the parabrachial nucleus.[41,42] Inasmuch as substance P coexists with CGRP in neurons that project to the CeA, it is likely that they also form synaptic contacts on CRF cells.[43] More recently, it has been demonstrated that amygdaloid CRF neurons are innervated by CRF terminals.[40,44] A dense plexus of CRF terminals are found in the region of CRF neurons of the CeA. Some of the CRF terminals formed synaptic contacts with CRF dendrites and perikarya.[22] The source of these terminals is from cell bodies located in the lateral hypothalamus, dorsal raphe, and intrinsic CRF cells in the CeA. In addition to CRF terminals, a dense plexus of many other different types of

TABLE 2. Inputs of Amygdaloid CRF Neurons: A List of Putative Neurotransmitters and Their Sources

Source	Neurotransmitter
Hypothalamus	CRF
	Dynorphin
Midbrain	CRF
	Cholecystokinin
	Dopamine
	Dynorphin
	Serotonin
	Vasoactive intestinal polypeptide
Pons/Medulla	Calcitonin gene-related peptide
	Substance P
	Neurotensin
	Noradrenaline
	Adrenaline
Unknown	Angiotensin II
	Atrial natriuretic peptide
	Bombesin
	Thyrotropin-releasing hormone

peptidergic terminals overlap the distribution of the CRF neurons in the CeA.[45] It is likely that CRF neurons are also innervated by one or more of the following peptidergic terminal types: enkephalin, substance P, cholecystokinin, angiotensin II, vasoactive intestinal polypeptide, atrial natriuretic peptide, and thyrotropin-releasing hormone. Dopaminergic, noradrenergic, and serotonergic terminals are distributed in the regions where amygdaloid CRF neurons are located (for a review see ref. 46). Noradrenergic terminals originate from the nucleus of the solitary tract and the locus coeruleus. Dopaminergic terminals arise from the substantia nigra region. Serotonergic terminals arise from neurons located in the dorsal raphe nucleus, but their distribution within the CeA is relatively sparse compared to dopaminergic and noradrenergic terminals. A final potential modulator of CRF cells in the CeA is gamma amino butyric acid (GABA)-containing cells. These cells are located adjacent to CRF neurons in the CeA and also express enkephalin.[47] Thus, amygdaloid CRF neuronal activity can be modulated by inputs from (1) extrinsic and intrinsic CRF terminals, (2) extrinsic and intrinsic peptidergic and GABA-containing terminals, and (3) various extrinsic monoaminergic cell groups.

The expected function of inputs to amygdaloid CRF neurons would be to increase or decrease their activity. CGRP and thyrotropin-releasing hormone have intra-amygdaloid actions that resemble the stress response. Both produce increases in heart rate, blood pressure, and plasma catecholamines.[48,49] Bilateral lesions of the CeA significantly reduce the ACTH/corticosterone response to immobilization stress.[2,4] Immobilization stress results in increased noradrenergic activity in the CeA suggesting a facilitating role for noradrenaline.[50] Dopaminergic activity in the CeA decreased during immobilization stress indicating an inhibitory role for this monoamine. Serotonergic activity in the amygdala increased during immobilization stress.[2]

SUMMARY

The results of numerous studies have provided compelling evidence that CRF plays an important function in the amygdala. Stimulation of the amygdala produces physiological changes similar those observed after central injections of CRF. Central injections of CRF activate neurons in the amygdala as measured by increases in c-fos protein expression. Destruction of cells or injections of CRF antagonist in the amygdala can attenuate some of the central effects of CRF. The amygdala is the origin of major CRF-containing pathways in the brain. Amygdaloid CRF neurons project to widespread regions of the basal forebrain and brain stem. These amygdaloid pathways mainly arise from the central amygdaloid nucleus where there are a large number of CRF immunoreactive neuronal perikarya. Glucocorticoid and CRF-binding protein are located in cells of the central amygdaloid nucleus. CRF neurons in the central nucleus send their axons to the bed nucleus of the stria terminalis, lateral hypothalamus, midbrain central gray, raphe nuclei, parabrachial region, and the nucleus of the solitary tract. Tract tracing studies have suggested that amygdaloid CRF neurons also innervate CRF neurons in some of these regions and, furthermore, that CRF neurons in some of these areas project back to the CRF neurons in the amygdala. Thus, the amygdala is part of a network of brain nuclei interconnected by CRF pathways. In addition, amygdaloid CRF neurons may project directly to dopaminergic, noradrenergic, and serotonergic neurons, which have widespread projections throughout the neuroaxis. Thus, amygdaloid CRF neurons could participate in an intrinsic CRF brain circuitry and activate the more classical neurotransmitter systems in the brain. These may form the anatomical and biochemical substrates for amygdaloid-mediated responses to stress.

REFERENCES

1. KLUVER, H. & P. C. BUCY. 1939. Preliminary analysis of functions of the temporal lobe in monkeys. Arch. Neurol. Psychiatry **42:** 979–1000.
2. BEAULIEU, S., T. DiPAOLO & N. BARDEN. 1986. Control of ACTH secretion by the central nucleus of the amygdala: Implication of the serotonergic system and its relevance to the glucocorticoid delayed feedback mechanism. Neuroendocrinology **44:** 247–254.
3. SANANES, C. B. & B. A. CAMPBELL. 1989. Role of the central nucleus of the amygdala in olfactory heart rat conditioning. Behav. Neurosci. **103:** 519–525.
4. VAN DE KAR, L. D., R. A. PIECHOWSKI, P. A. RITTENHOUSE & T. S. GRAY. 1991. Amygdaloid lesions: Differential effect on conditioned stress and immobilization-

induced increases in corticosterone and renin secretion. Neuroendocrinology **54:** 89–95.

5. VANDERWOLF, C. H., M. E. KELLY, P. KRAEMER & A. STREATHER. 1988. Are emotion and motivation localized in the limbic system and nucleus accumbens? Behav. Brain Res. **27:** 45–58.

6. IWATA, J., K. CHIDA & J. E. LEDOUX. 1987. Cardiovascular responses elicited by stimulation of neurons in the central nucleus of amygdala in awake, but not anesthetized rats, resemble conditioned emotional responses. Brain Res. **418:** 183–188.

7. CHAPMAN, W. P., H. R. SCHROEDER, G. GEYER, M. A. B. BRAZIER, C. FAGER, J. L. POPPEN, H. C. SOLOMON & P. I. YAKOVLEV. 1954. Physiological evidence concerning importance of the amygdaloid nuclear region in the integration of circulatory function and emotion in man. Science **120:** 949–950.

8. GLOOR, P. 1986. Role of the human limbic system in perception, memory, and affect: Lessons from temporal lobe epilepsy. *In* The Limbic System: Functional Organization and Clinical Disorders. B. K. Doane & K. E. Livingston, Eds.: 159–169. Raven Press. New York, NY.

9. STOCK, G., U. RUPPRECHT, H. STUMPF & K. H. SCHLOR. 1981. Cardiovascular changes during arousal elicited by stimulation of amygdala, hypothalamus and locus coeruleus. J. Auton. Nerv. Syst. **3:** 503–510.

10. GALENO, T. M. & M. J. BRODY. 1983. Hemodynamic responses to amygdaloid stimulation in spontaneously hypertensive rats. Am. J. Physiol. **245:** R281–286.

11. KAADA, B. R. 1951. Somato-motor, autonomic and electrocorticographic responses to electrical stimulation of rhinencephalic and other structures in primates, cat and dog: A study of responses from the limbic, subcallosal, orbito-insular, piriform and temporal cortex, and amygdala. Acta Physiol. Scand. **24(S.83):** 1–285.

12. HONKANIEMI, J., T. KAINU, S. CECCATELLI, L. RECHARDT, T. HOKFELT & M. PELTO-HUIKKO. 1992. Fos and jun in rat central amygdaloid nucleus and paraventricular nucleus after stress. Neuroreport **3:** 849–852.

13. HONKANIEMI, J. 1992. Colocalization of peptide- and tyrosine hydroxylase-like immunoreactivities with Fos-immunoreactive neurons in rat central amygdaloid nucleus after immobilization stress. Brain Res. **598:** 107–113.

14. HONKANIEMI, J., K. FUXE, L. RECHARDT, J. KOISTINAHO, J. ISOLA, J. A. GUSTAFSSON, S. OKRET & M. PELTO-HUIKKO. 1992. Colocalization of Fos-corticoid and glucocorticoid receptor-like immunoreactivities in the rat amygdaloid complex after immobilization stress. J. Neuroendocrinol. **4:** 547–555.

15. HONKANIEMI, J., M. PELTO-HUIKKO, L. RECHARDT, J. ISOLA, A. LAMMI, K. FUXE, J. A. GUSTAFSSON, A. C. WIKSTROM & T. HOKFELT. 1992. Colocalization of peptide and glucocorticoid receptor immunoreactivities in rat central amygdaloid nucleus. Neuroendocrinology **55:** 451–459.

16. ARNOLD, F. J. L., M. D. BUENO, H. SHIERS, D. C. HANCOCK, G. I. EVAN & J. HERBERT. 1992. Expression of c-fos in regions of the basal limbic forebrain following intracerebroventricular corticotropin-releasing factor in unstressed or stressed male rats. Neuroscience **51:** 377–390.

17. LIANG, K. C., K. R. MELIA, M. J. D. MISERENDINO, W. A. FALLS, S. CAMPEAU & M. DAVIS. 1992. Corticotropin-releaasing factor—long-lasting facilitation of the acoustic startle reflex. J. Neurosci. **12:** 2303–2312.

18. LIANG, K. C., K. R. MELIA, S. CAMPEAU, W. A. FALLS, M. J. D. MISERENDINO & M. DAVIS. 1992. Lesions of the central nucleus of the amygdala, but not the paraventricular nucleus of the hypothalamus, block the excitatory effects of corticotropin-releasing factor on the acoustic startle reflex. J. Neurosci. **12:** 2313–2320.

19. HEINRICHS, S. C., E. M. PICH, K. A. MICZEK, K. T. BRITTON & G. F. KOOB. 1992. Corticotropin-releasing factor antagonist reduces emotionality in socially defeated rats via direct neurotropic action. Brain Res. **581:** 190–197.

20. SWANSON, L. W., P. E. SAWCHENKO, J. RIVIER & W. W. VALE. 1983. Organization of ovine corticotropin-releasing factor immunoreactive cells and fibers in the rat brain: An immunohistochemical study. Neuroendocrinology **36:** 165–186.

21. SAKANAKA, M., T. SHIBASAKI & K. LEDERIS. 1987. Corticotropin releasing factor-like

immunoreactivity in the rat brain as revealed by a modified cobalt-glucose oxidase-diaminobenzidine method. J. Comp. Neurol. **260:** 256–298.

22. GRAY, T. S. 1990. The organization and possible function of amygdaloid corticotropin-releasing factor pathways. *In* Corticotropin-Releasing Factor: Basic and Clinical Studies of a Neuropeptide. E. B. De Souza & C. B. Nemeroff, Eds.: 53–68. CRC Press, Inc. Boca Raton, FL.

23. SHIMADA, S., S. INAGAKI, Y. KUBOTA, N. OGAWA, T. SHIBASAKI & H. TAKAGI. 1989. Coexistence of peptides (corticotropin releasing factor/neurotensin and substance P/somatostatin) in the bed nucleus of the stria terminalis and central amygdaloid nucleus of the rat. Neuroscience **30:** 377–383.

24. SAKANAKA, M., T. SHIBASAKI & K. LEDERIS. 1986. Distribution and efferent projections of corticotropin-releasing factor-like immunoreactivity in the rat amygdaloid complex. Brain Res. **382:** 213–238.

25. GRAY, T. S. 1991. Limbic pathways and neurotransmitters as mediators of autonomic and neuroendocrine responses to stress: The amygdala. *In* Stress: Neurobiology and Neuroendocrinology. M. R. Brown, G. F. Koob & C. Rivier, Eds.: 73–89. Marcel Dekker, Inc. New York, NY.

26. GRAY, T. S. & D. J. MAGNUSON. 1992. Peptide immunoreactive neurons in the amygdala and the bed nucleus of the stria terminalis project to the midbrain central gray in the rat. Peptides **13:** 451–460.

27. MAGNUSON, D. J. & T. S. GRAY. 1988. Amygdala directly innervates parvocellular paraventricular hypothalamic CRF, vasopressin and oxytocin containing cells. Soc. Neurosci. Abstr. **14:** 1288.

28. GRAY, T. S., M. E. CARNEY & D. J. MAGNUSON. 1989. Direct projections form the central amygdaloid nucleus to the hypothalamic paraventricular nucleus: Possible role in stress-induced ACTH release. Neuroendocrinology **50:** 433–446.

29. MAGNUSON, D. J. & T. S. GRAY. 1991. Amygdala directly innervates CRF neurons in the lateral hypothalamus. Soc. Neurosci. Abstr. **17:** 472.

30. GRAY, T. S. & D. J. MAGNUSON. 1992. Bed nucleus of stria terminalis directly innervates CRF neurons in the lateral hypothalamus. Soc. Neurosci. Abstr. **18:** 1415.

31. MAGNUSON, D. J. & T. S. GRAY. 1989. Bed nucleus of the stria terminalis directly innervates parvocellular paraventricular hypothalamic CRF, vasopressin and oxytocin containing cells. Soc. Neurosci. Abstr. **15:** 135.

32. MAGNUSON, D. J. & T. S. GRAY. 1990. Central nucleus of the amygdala and bed nucleus of the stria terminalis projections to serotonin or tyrosine hydroxylase immunoreactive cells in the dorsal and median raphe nuclei in the rat. Soc. Neurosci. Abstr. **16:** 121.

33. WALLACE, D. M., D. J. MAGNUSON & T. S. GRAY. 1992. Organization of amygdaloid projections to brainstem dopaminergic, noradrenergic, and adrenergic cell groups in the rat. Brain Res. Bull. **28:** 447–454.

34. WALLACE, D. M., D. J. MAGNUSON & T. S. GRAY. 1989. The amygdalo-brainstem pathway: Selective innervation of dopaminergic, noradrenergic and adrenergic cells in the rat. Neurosci. Lett. **97:** 252–258.

35. DE SOUZA, E. B. 1987. Corticotropin-releasing factor receptors in the rat central nervous system: Characterization and regional distribution. J. Neurosci. **7:** 88–100.

36. KRETTEK, J. E. & J. L. PRICE. 1978. A description of the amygdaloid complex in the rat and cat with observations on intra-amygdaloid connections. J. Comp. Neurol. **178:** 255–280.

37. POTTER, E., D. P. BEHAN, E. A. LINTON, P. J. LOWRY, P. E. SAWCHENKO & W. W. VALE. 1992. The central distribution of a corticotropin-releasing factor (CRF)-binding protein predicts multiple sites and modes of interaction with CRF. Proc. Natl. Acad. Sci. USA **89:** 4192–4196.

38. LEDOUX, J. E., J. IWATA, P. CICCHETTI & D. J. RIES. 1988. Different projections of the central amygdaloid nucleus mediate autonomic and behavioral correlates of conditioned fear. J. Neurosci. **8:** 2517–2529.

39. SHIMADA, S., S. INAGAKI, Y. KUBOTA, S. KITO, H. FUNAKI & H. TAKAGI. 1989. Light and electron microscopic studies of calcitonin gene-related peptide-like immunoreactive terminals in the central nucleus of the amygdala and the bed nucleus of the stria terminalis of the rat. Exp. Brain Res. **77:** 217–220.

40. HARRIGAN, E., D. J. MAGNUSON & T. S. GRAY. 1991. Amygdaloid CRF neurons are innervated by CGRP neurons. Soc. Neurosci. Abstr. **17:** 471.
41. SCHWABER, J. S., C. STERNINI, N. C. BRECHA, W. T. ROGERS & J. P. CARD. 1988. Neurons containing calcitonin gene-related peptide in the parabrachial nucleus project to the central nucleus of the amygdala. J. Comp. Neurol. **270:** 416–426.
42. SHIMADA, S., S. SHIOSAKA, P. C. EMSON, C. J. HILLYARD, S. GIRGIST, I. MACINTYRE & M. TOHYAMA. 1985. Calcitonin gene-related peptidergic projection from the parabrachial area to the forebrain and diencephalon in the rat: An immunohistochemical analysis. Neuroscience **16:** 607–616.
43. YAMANO, M., C. J. HILLYARD, S. GIRGIS, I. MACINTYRE, P. C. EMSON & M. TOHYAMA. 1988. Presence of a substance P-like immunoreactive neurone system from the parabrachial area to the central amygdaloid nucleus of the rat with reference to coexistence with calcitonin gene-related peptide. Brain Res. **451:** 179–188.
44. URYU, K., T. OKUMURA, T. SHIBASAKI & M. SAKANAKA. 1992. Fine structure and possible origins of nerve fibers with corticotropin-releasing factor-like immunoreactivity in the rat central amygdaloid nucleus. Brain Res. **577:** 175–179.
45. GRAY, T. S. 1989. Autonomic neuropeptide connections of the amygdala. *In* Neuropeptides and Stress: Hans Selye Symposium on Neuroendocrinology and Stress. Y. Taché, J. E. Morley & M. R. Brown, Eds.: 92–106. Springer-Verlag. New York, NY.
46. FALLON, J. H. & P. CIOFI. 1992. Distribution of monoamines within the amygdala. *In* The Amygdala: Neurobiological Aspects of Emotion, Memory, and Mental Dysfunction. J. P. Aggleton, Ed.: 97–114. Wiley-Liss, Inc. New York, NY.
47. OERTEL, W. H., G. RIETHMULLER, E. MUGNAINI, D. E. SCHMECHEL, A. WEINDL, C. GRAMSCH & A. HERZ. 1983. Opioid peptide-like immunoreactivity localized in GABAergic neurons of rat neostriatum and central amygdaloid nucleus. Life Sci. **33:** 73–76.
48. BROWN, M. R. & T. S. GRAY. 1988. Peptide injections into the amygdala of conscious rats: Effects on blood pressure, heart rate and plasma catecholamines. Regul. Pept. **21:** 95–106.
49. NGUYEN, K. Q., M. A. SILLS & D. M. JACOBOWITZ. 1986. Cardiovascular effects produced by microinjection of calcitonin gene-related peptide into the rat central amygdaloid nucleus. Peptides **7:** 337–339.
50. BEAULIEU, S., T. DI PAOLO, J. COTE & N. BARDEN. 1987. Participation of the central amygdaloid nucleus in the response of adrenocorticotropin (ACTH) secretion to immobilization stress: Opposing roles of the noradrenergic and dopaminergic systems. Neuroendocrinology **45:** 37–46.

The Psychoendocrinology of Stress[a]

SEYMOUR LEVINE

Laboratory of Developmental Psychobiology
Building 7-930T
Department of Psychiatry and Behavioral Sciences
Stanford University School of Medicine
Stanford, California 94305

Over a decade ago we published a paper[1] in which we hypothesized that the response of the hypothalamic-pituitary-adrenal system (HPA) is a reflection of changes in the level of arousal. We had attempted to develop a psychoendocrine model of the control of HPA activity and to demonstrate that the response of the HPA system represents a component of a unified theory of arousal. Based primarily on the work of D. E. Berlyne, the major stimulators of arousal were hypothesized to be novelty, uncertainty, and conflict. These have been labeled as collative factors because it is necessary to compare stimulus similarities and differences between stimulus elements (novelty), or between simultaneously evoked expectations (uncertainty) or responses (conflict). Thus, the basic cognitive mechanism responsible for eliciting or reducing arousal was one of comparison. In general, the data appeared to support the notion that comparator operations can determine the pituitary-adrenal response to a variety of environmental events. The response to novelty, for example, which appears to be pervasive and species independent, requires a comparison between the existing stimulus patterns and the features of the stimuli that can be retrieved from the long-term memory stores. The greater the discrepancy between the existing stimulus patterns and the prior experience with specific features of the environment the greater the adrenocortical response.

In recent years we have described another class of psychological events that appear to have profound influences on the response of the HPA system. Although there are numerous factors that determine the magnitude of the endocrine responses to stress and, in fact, determine whether or not a response will be elicited, one important variable appears to be the presence of familiar social partners and biologically significant social relationships. An extensive literature now exists that points to the importance of social relationships in determining an individual's ability to cope with stress (coping is defined here as any behavior, cognitive process, or other environmental event that results in a reduction or elimination of the secretion of adrenal glucocorticoid).

In our laboratory we have been studying the influence of psychosocial variables on the response of the HPA axis to stress. This is part of the broader perspective of this laboratory, that is, to emphasize the role of behavior and environment in the regulation of HPA activity. In order to examine the influence of psychosocial factors on physiological processes it was first necessary to find an appropriate animal model in which social behavior was an integral part of the animal's adaptive processes. Although many forms of social organization and social behavior exist among animals, one of the most striking features of adaptation in all primate species appears to be

[a]This research was supported by grants MH-45006 and MH-47573 from the National Institute of Mental Health (NIMH), and U. S. Public Health Service Research Scientist Award MH-19936 from NIMH to S. L.

61

living and interacting in social groups. Hans Kummer has stated, "Primates seem to have only one unusual asset in coping with their environments: a type of society which, through constant associations of young and old animals and through a long life duration, exploits their large brains to produce adults of great experience. One may, therefore, expect to find specific primate adaptations in the way primates do things as social groups."[2] For these reasons we chose as our experimental animal a small South American primate: the squirrel monkey (*Saimiri sciureus*). These monkeys were originally imported from Guyana. However, almost all of the studies we will discuss were based on data collected from animals born in captivity.

ADRENOCORTICAL RESPONSE TO SOCIAL SEPARATION

Our initial studies of social influences on adrenocortical activity were conducted as part of an extensive series of experiments concerned with the psychobiology of squirrel monkey mother–infant relationships. In these studies we first attempted to characterize the effects of temporary disruptions in mother–infant relationships on the activation of the HPA system using the conventional separation paradigm. Our initial observations demonstrated unequivocally that separation of mothers and infants can provoke striking and reproducible elevations in plasma cortisol in both mothers and infants.[3,4] Indeed, mother–infant separations appear to be one of the most reliable activators of adrenocortical activity in these animals; elevations in infant plasma cortisol persist despite numerous episodes of separation and little evidence exists that habituation occurs even after multiple brief separations.[5] In our initial studies, however, we temporarily isolated separated infants in a novel environment. Thus, the infant was exposed to at least two conditions that might activate an adrenocortical response: novelty and maternal loss.

To distinguish between the effects of novelty and maternal loss, in subsequent work we temporarily separated mothers and infants in several different ways.[6,7] In one condition, the infant was separated from its mother and all other members of its social group, and placed in unfamiliar surroundings. In a second condition, the infant was separated from the mother but all other physical and social aspects of the environment remained the same for the infant. A third condition consisted of removing both the mother and the infant from their familiar surroundings and placing them in separate adjacent cages. Thus, in the third condition both members of the mother-infant dyad could see, hear, and smell one another, but could not physically touch one another.

In general, these studies indicate that the infant squirrel monkey's adrenocortical response to social separation is very much dependent upon the type of separation paradigm that is used.[6,7] Although all infants responded to separation with increases in circulating levels of cortisol, the magnitude of these changes appeared to be a function of the degree of social support available during the period of separation (FIG. 1). The most dramatic elevations in plasma levels of cortisol occurred when infants were completely isolated in a novel environment during separation (Total). Infants placed adjacent to their mothers during separation showed a cortisol response that was reduced (Adjacent), in comparison to those of totally isolated infants (Total), but higher than those observed in infants that remained in their home cage with familiar social companions (Home). Thus, when separated infants remained in a familiar social environment that included other mothers and infants, these infants showed minimal signs of behavioral distress and a marked reduction in adrenocortical activity. These findings, together with those from other studies,[3,4,8] clearly indicate that for infant squirrel monkeys, the presence of familiar social companions buffers or ameliorates stress-induced elevations in adrenocortical activity.

SOCIAL SUPPORT AND ADRENOCORTICAL ACTIVITY

That the presence of familiar social companions buffers or ameliorates stress-induced elevations in plasma cortisol is not limited to squirrel monkey mother–infant relationships. We initially obtained evidence suggestive of social buffering in group-housed adult squirrel monkeys that were presented with unfamiliar objects such as moving toys. Although these animals frequently avoided these objects, we did not detect any changes in adrenocortical activity. These data suggested either that the unfamiliar moving toys were not sufficiently intense to elicit an adrenocortical response or that, in the presence of familiar adult companions, social buffering of adrenocortical activity had indeed occurred.

In an attempt to resolve the problem of stimulus intensity, we chose a more salient naturalistic stimulus—visual exposure to a live caged snake. Snakes are

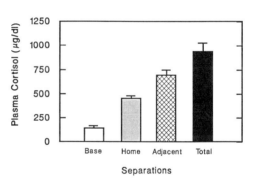

FIGURE 1. Plasma cortisol levels in infant squirrel monkeys (mean ± SEM) 24 hours after separation in different conditions (home, adjacent, and total), as compared with base.

known to provoke strong behavioral reactions in both human and nonhuman primates that do not readily habituate over repeated exposures.[9] Thus, squirrel monkeys were exposed to a live boa constrictor that was presented above their cage. The snake was always confined in a plastic box that prevented direct physical contact between the monkeys and the snake. Nevertheless, all monkeys showed increased levels of vigilance, agitation, and avoidance of the snake when tested individually or as a group. The snake did not elicit an increase in adrenocortical activity, however, when the monkeys were tested together as a group.[9]

Although these results indicate that for adult squirrel monkeys the presence of familiar social companions can buffer the responsiveness of the HPA system to potentially threatening naturalistic stimuli, it should be noted that social buffering appears to occur only when adult squirrel monkeys are living with multiple partners. Surprisingly, when animals are pair-housed, not only do we not see evidence of social buffering, but in some cases the adrenocortical response to the snake is actually exacerbated.[10] Moreover, in the experiments with snakes the monkeys could actively avoid the provocative stimulus by moving to lower perches in the cages, thus exercising some degree of control. Studies of rodents indicate that control is a potent variable ameliorating physiological and somatic responses to stress.[11]

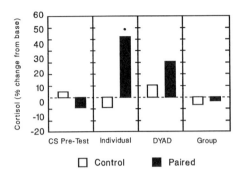

FIGURE 2. Cortisol responses of adult squirrel monkeys to nonreinforced conditioned stimulus (CS) presentations in the home cage before training (CS Pre-test) and after training as a function of social housing condition. The CS Pre-test occurred under individual housing (● differs from control and from zero-percent baseline, $p < 0.05$).

Consequently, in our subsequent attempts to demonstrate social buffering of adrenocortical activity in adult monkeys, we used a different paradigm designed to prevent the monkeys from exercising control.[12] The classical conditioning paradigm used in this study also provided a stressful stimulus that was unequivocally psychological in nature. Adult monkeys were first trained to associate a previously neutral flashing light with a mildly aversive electric shock. To accomplish this, individual monkeys were presented in a test chamber with multiple pairings of the flashing light (conditioned stimulus) and the shock (unconditioned stimulus). After a short training period, all animals were tested in their home cage, and their behavioral and adrenocortical responses were measured after presentation of the flashing light. Animals were tested alone, in pairs, and in a group with six familiar adult companions. When tested alone, exposure to the flashing light (without the shock) produced a dramatic elevation in plasma cortisol levels. In contrast, when the flashing light was presented to animals in the larger social group, no elevations of cortisol were observed (FIG. 2), although a significant increase in behavioral agitation occurred. These findings confirm that in adult squirrel monkeys the adrenocortical response to stressful psychological events can indeed be reduced by the presence of familiar social companions.

CHRONIC ELEVATIONS IN PLASMA CORTISOL IN RESPONSE TO SOCIAL DISRUPTION

Thus far we have discussed some of the beneficial effects of psychosocial factors as regulators of adrenocortical activity of squirrel monkeys. Not all aspects of social life, however, are beneficial. Recent evidence indicates, for example, that chronic disruptions in social relationships can produce prolonged elevations in adrenocortical activity. The formation of new social groups composed of unfamiliar conspecifics, for example, can activate the HPA axis and result in increased levels of circulating cortisol, especially in dominant adult males.[13,14] With the development of stable social relationships, cortisol levels generally return to previously observed levels. However, in instances where social relationships within the group remain unstable and where antagonistic dominance-related behavior persists, cortisol levels may remain elevated for several weeks.[15]

Recently, Rosenblum and Paully[16] discovered that by experimentally altering the effort required to find food, it is also possible to produce chronic disruptions in the social behavior of bonnet macaques. For example, when food is made more difficult to obtain by hiding it in gravel,[17] a marked increase in antagonistic dominance-related behavior occurs. We recently conducted a series of studies using a similar experimental paradigm to evaluate whether social disruption produced by this type of environmental demand chronically elevates plasma cortisol in adult squirrel monkeys.

In these studies,[18] groups of female squirrel monkeys were exposed to either a high demand (HD) or a low demand (LD) condition, based on the effort required to find food. In the HD condition, sufficient food was provided to maintain normal body weights, but food was made more difficult to find by burying it in wood shavings. The LD condition, in contrast, essentially consisted of free feeding. In the first experiment all animals were exposed on alternate two-week blocks to both HD and LD conditions. The results of this experiment indicated a marked change in social behavior during the HD condition. A common affiliative activity in squirrel monkeys is social huddling. In captive groups, adult female squirrel monkeys typically spend considerable amounts of time in affiliative contact huddling with their cagemates.[19] During the HD condition, measures of social contact were markedly reduced, and subsequently remained low throughout the 12-week study. However, no increase in aggressive behavior was evident, nor were other indications of social instability. Nevertheless, one of the most striking findings in this experiment was that plasma cortisol remained elevated during the HD condition, and returned to basal levels during the LD condition.

Based on these preliminary observations, we conducted a second experiment with two groups of adult females exposed to a chronic HD regime and two additional groups of females exposed to a variable demand regime consisting of alternating two-week blocks of HD and LD conditions. Monkeys exposed to the persistent HD condition once again exhibited lower levels of social contact and showed elevations in plasma cortisol levels that persisted for nine weeks. As observed in the first study, behavioral measures and cortisol levels in the variable demand regime tended to reflect the demand condition. During periods of high demand, measures of social contact were relatively low (FIG. 3) and cortisol levels were elevated (FIG. 4); during periods of low demand, behavioral and adrenocortical measures resembled those observed during baseline conditions.

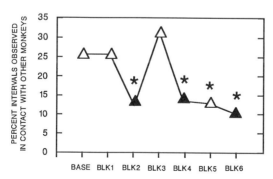

FIGURE 3. Mean percentage of observations when adult female squirrel monkeys were in contact with other adult females during alternating two-week blocks of conditions of low demand (*open triangles*) and of high demand (*solid triangles*) compared to undisturbed base (*$p < 0.05$ in comparison to base).

Recently, we began a series of studies using the foraging-demand paradigm to investigate the effects of environmental demands on the psychobiology of mother–infant relationships. Social groups composed of five mother-infant pairs were examined in three conditions: (1) a chronic HD condition, (2) a chronic LD condition, and (3) a variable demand (VD) regime in which mothers and infants were exposed to alternating HD and LD conditions. In the HD condition, the previously described disruptions in affiliative social contact among adult members of the group were once again detected. Surprisingly, there were no observable indications of behavioral disruption in mother–infant relationships. Infants in the HD condition, however, showed significant reductions in play behavior, a finding that replicates Baldwin's observations of squirrel monkeys in a slightly different experimental setting.[20]

The experimental foraging-demand paradigm also had significant effects on plasma cortisol. In keeping with the previously described studies of adult females, cortisol levels in mothers clearly reflected the demand condition. Mothers in the HD condition (either chronic HD or intermittent HD in the VD regime) showed high levels of cortisol, whereas cortisol levels in mothers in the LD condition (either

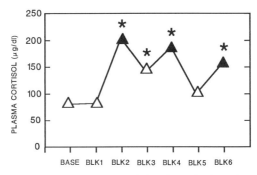

FIGURE 4. Mean plasma cortisol levels of adult female squirrel monkeys during alternating two-week blocks of conditions of low demand (*open triangles*) and of high demand (*solid triangles*) compared to undisturbed base (*$p < 0.05$ in comparison to base).

chronic or intermittent) were not different from those observed previously during baseline conditions. Remarkably, the cortisol responses of infants also closely tracked the demand conditions and resembled those observed in adults.

One possible explanation for this outcome is that the infants responded to some subtle change in their mother's behavior, and their cortisol levels tracked those of their mothers. The correlations between plasma cortisol levels in individual mothers and their infants were highly variable, however, and for only a few mother-infant dyads were these statistically significant. In contrast, the correlations between the group average of the cortisol levels of the mothers and that of the infants were highly significant (HD group $r = 0.72$; VD group $r = 0.78$; LD group $r = 0.60$), indicating that infants may have been responding to changes in the social milieu, rather than to specific changes in their mother's behavior.

An intriguing aspect of research on the HPA system has been the difficulty in producing chronically high levels of any hormone associated with stress. Rose[21] comments that "despite its theoretical importance there are relatively few studies describing endocrine responses to chronic stress." In light of the chronic elevations in plasma cortisol found in our preliminary foraging-demand studies, this experimental paradigm may provide a useful animal model for more extensive studies aimed at understanding the neurobiology of chronic stress.

CONCLUSIONS AND IMPLICATIONS

The body of evidence we presented is another important example of the influence of the behavioral and environmental influences on the HPA system. We demonstrated that throughout a greater part of the life span of the squirrel monkey social factors can both activate and inhibit the activity of this system. We attempted to interpret these findings within the framework of a general theory of stress and coping.[22] However, we must entertain the hypothesis that in a species where social behavior appears to be of extreme significance it is possible that the effects of social factors on HPA activity may have unique and idiosyncratic properties.

These findings do, however, bear on another issue that has plagued the field of stress, namely, our understanding of the afferent limb of the stress cascade. Throughout the history of research in this field numerous attempts have been made to classify the types of stimuli that can activate the HPA system. Among these are distinctions such as "psychological versus physical" and "neurogenic versus systemic."[22] What has been abundantly clear is that different stimuli do not act in identical ways. Recent reports describe different stimulus-dependent patterns in the release of hypothalamic secretagogues.[23] Recently we stated, "The contemporary view of stress can be characterized as an imposition model. . . . This view is fostered in a voluminous number of studies, originating with Selye, in which severely traumatic stimuli were used to elicit a stress response." Our hypothesis is that many situations that activate the HPA axis have the property of representing the absence of critical features in the environment and thus can be viewed as an "omission" model.[24] If we take this perspective, then many of the stimuli that have been classified as psychological or neurogenic represent signals that indicate something is missing or about to disappear. Certainly the loss of social stimuli can be viewed within this framework. However, this hypothesis extends to a wide variety of events, for example, novelty, frustration, conflict, which are characterized by the lack of information or failure of expectancies and where the brain registers this informational discrepancy.

Many suggestions have been made that different neural pathways may exist that are stimulus specific. The anatomical studies by Sawchenko[25] describe at least five different pathways that activate the CRF neuron. Stress-induced feedback or facilitation of the ACTH response is dependent on the type of stimuli used.[26] There is evidence obtained using the developing rat as a model which also indicates that different neural mechanisms are invoked by different stimuli. The infant rodent during the SHRP can elicit an ACTH response to specific stimuli. However, there are many stimuli to which the infant is nonresponsive. One such example is the difference between the infant's response to immune signals and the response to novelty and/or an injection of saline. Exposure to endotoxin[27] and IL-1β (unpublished data) results in a significant increase in ACTH in neonatal rat pups at 6 and 12 days of age, whereas control injections do not. It has been argued that the failure to respond to mild stress is a function of the immaturity of the mechanisms of the limbic system that are involved in processing these stimuli. However, more recent data suggest that the neonates HPA system is quite capable of eliciting a vigorous ACTH response to novelty and/or saline injection, but under normal conditions the neural systems responsible appear to be inhibited by the dam.[28]

We have not attempted to engage in the polemics of "what is stress," but rather to describe a different class of events that involves cognitive processing concerning informational discrepancies and most likely involves limbic system mediation.

REFERENCES

1. HENNESSY, J. W. & S. LEVINE. 1979. Stress, arousal, and the pituitary-adrenal system: A psychoendocrine hypothesis. *In* Progress in Psychobiology and Physiological Psychology. J. M. Sprague & A. N. Epstein, Eds. Vol. **8:** 133–178. Academic Press. New York, NY.
2. KUMMER, H. 1971. Primate Societies: Group Techniques of Ecological Adaptations. Aldine-Atherton. Chicago, IL.
3. MENDOZA, S. P., W. P. SMOTHERMAN, M. T. MINER, J. KAPLAN & S. LEVINE. 1978. Pituitary-adrenal response to separation in mother and infant squirrel monkey. Dev. Psychobiol. **11:** 169–175.
4. LEVINE, S., C. L. COE & W. P. SMOTHERMAN. 1978. Prolonged cortisol elevation in the infant squirrel monkey after reunion with mother. Physiol. & Behav. **20:** 7–10.
5. HENNESSY, M. B. 1986. Multiple, brief maternal separations in the squirrel monkey: Changes in hormonal and behavioral responsiveness. Physiol. & Behav. **36:** 245–250.
6. WIENER, S. G., F. BAYART, K. F. FAULL & S. LEVINE. 1990. Behavioral and physiological responses to maternal separation in squirrel monkeys (*Saimiri sciureus*). Behav. Neurosci. **104:** 108–115.
7. BAYART, F., K. T. HAYASHI, K. F. FAULL, J. D. BARCHAS & S. LEVINE. 1990. Influence of maternal proximity on behavioral and physiological responses to maternal separation in infant rhesus monkeys (*Macaca mulatta*). Behav. Neurosci. **104:** 98–107.
8. WIENER, S. G., E. L. LOWE & S. LEVINE. 1992. Pituitary-adrenal response to weaning in squirrel monkeys. Psychobiology **20:** 65–70.
9. VOGT, J. L., C. L. COE & S. LEVINE. 1981. Behavioral and adrenocorticoid responsiveness of squirrel monkeys to a live snake: Is flight necessarily stressful? Behav. Neurol. Biol. **32:** 391–405.
10. COE, C. L., D. FRANKLIN, E. R. SMITH & S. LEVINE. 1982. Hormonal responses accompanying fear and agitation in the squirrel monkey. Physiol. & Behav. **29:** 1051–1057.
11. WEINBERG, J. & S. LEVINE. 1980. Psychobiology of coping in animals: The effects of predictability. *In* Coping and Health. S. Levine & H. Ursin, Eds.: 39–59. Plenum Press. New York, NY.
12. STANTON, M. E., J. M. PATTERSON & S. LEVINE. 1985. Social influences on conditioned cortisol secretion in the squirrel monkey. Psychoneuroendocrinology **10:** 125–134.
13. MENDOZA, S. P., C. L. COE, E. L. LOWE & S. LEVINE. 1979. The physiological response to group formation in adult male squirrel monkeys. Psychoneuroendocrinology **3:** 221–229.
14. COE, C. L., E. R. SMITH, S. P. MENDOZA & S. LEVINE. 1983. Varying influence of social status on hormone levels in the squirrel monkey. *In* Hormones, Drugs, and Social Behavior. S. Kling & H. D. Steklis, Eds.: 7–32. Spectrum. New York, NY.
15. GONZALEZ, C. A., M. B. HENNESSY & S. LEVINE. 1981. Subspecies differences in hormonal and behavioral responses after group formation in squirrel monkeys. Am. J. Primatol. **1:** 439–452.
16. ROSENBLUM, L. A. & G. S. PAULLY. 1984. The effects of varying environmental demands on maternal and infant behavior. Child Dev. **55:** 305–314.
17. PLIMPTON, E. H., K. B. SWARTZ & L. A. ROSENBLUM. 1981. The effects of foraging demand on social interactions in a laboratory group of bonnet macaques. Int. J. Primatol. **2:** 175–185.
18. LEVINE, S., M. CHAMPOUX & S. G. WIENER. 1991. Social modulation of the stress response. *In* Stress and Related Disorders from Adaptation to Dysfunction. A. R. Genazzani, G. Nappi, F. Petraglia & E. Matignoni, Eds.: 121–128. The Parthenon Publishing Group. NJ.
19. ROSENBLUM, L. A., E. J. LEVY & I. C. KAUFMAN. 1968. Social behaviour of squirrel monkeys and the reaction to strangers. Anim. Behav. **16:** 288–293.

20. BALDWIN, J. D. & J. I. BALDWIN. 1976. Effects of food ecology on social play: A laboratory simulation. Z. Tierpsychol. **40:** 1–14.
21. ROSE, R. M. 1984. Overview of endocrinology of stress. *In* Neuroendocrinology and Psychiatric Disorders. G. M. Brown, S. H. Koslow & S. Reichlin, Eds.: 95–122. Raven Press. New York, NY.
22. KELLER-WOOD, M. E. & M. F. DALLMAN. 1984. Corticosteroid inhibition of ACTH secretion. Endocrine Rev. **5:** 1–24.
23. PLOTSKY, P. M. 1991. Neural coding of stimulus-induced ACTH secretion. *In* Stress, Neurobiology and Neuroendocrinology. M. R. Brown, G. F. Koob & C. Rivier, Eds.: 137–150. Marcel Dekker. New York, NY.
24. LEVINE, S. & H. URSIN. 1991. What is stress? *In* Stress, Neurobiology and Neuroendocrinology. M. R. Brown, G. F. Koob & C. Rivier, Eds.: 3–22. Marcel Dekker. New York, NY.
25. SAWCHENKO, P. E. 1991. The final common path: Issues concerning the organization of central mechanisms controlling corticotrophin secretion. *In* Stress, Neurobiology and Neuroendocrinology. M. R. Brown, G. F. Koob & C. Rivier, Eds.: 55–72. Marcel Dekker. New York, NY.
26. DALLMAN, M. F., S. F. AKANA, K. A. SCRIBNER, M. J. BRADBURY, C. D. WALKER, A. M. STRACK & C. S. CASCIO. 1992. Stress, feedback and facilitation in the hypothalamo-pituitary-adrenal axis. J. Neuroendocrinol. **4:** 517–526.
27. WITEK-JANUSEK, L. 1988. Pituitary-adrenal response to bacterial endotoxin in developing rats. Am. J. Physiol. **255:** E757–E763.
28. SUCHECKI, D., D. MOZAFFARIAN, G. GROSS, P. ROSENFELD & S. LEVINE. 1993. Effects of maternal deprivation on the ACTH stress response in the infant rat. Neuroendocrinology **57:** 204–212.

Individual Differences in the Hypothalamic-Pituitary-Adrenal Stress Response and the Hypothalamic CRF System[a]

MICHAEL J. MEANEY,[b] SEEMA BHATNAGAR,
SYLVIE LAROCQUE, CHERYL McCORMICK,
NOLA SHANKS, SHAKTI SHARMA, JAMES SMYTHE,
VICTOR VIAU, AND PAUL M. PLOTSKY[c]

Developmental Neuroendocrinology Laboratory
Douglas Hospital Research Centre
Departments of Psychiatry, and Neurology and Neurosurgery
McGill University
Montreal, Quebec H4H 1R3, Canada

[c]*Department of Psychiatry and Behavioral Sciences*
Emory University
Atlanta, Georgia 30322

The adrenal glucocorticoids, together with the medullary catecholamines, comprise a frontline of defense for mammalian species under conditions that threaten homeostasis (conditions commonly referred to as stress). These hormones serve as major endocrine regulators of carbohydrate and lipid metabolism, cardiovascular tone, muscle function, immunocompetence, and behavior. The adrenal glucocorticoids represent the end product of the hypothalamic-pituitary-adrenal (HPA) axis. Under most conditions, this axis lies under the dominion of specific peptides secreted by neurons located in paraventricular nucleus (PVN) of the hypothalamus. Most notable among these peptides is corticotropin-releasing factor (CRF). The neurons of the PVN are thus the major target for both the stimulatory effects of neural signals associated with stress and the inhibitory effects associated with glucocorticoid negative-feedback. The nature of the HPA response to stress occurs as a function of the integration of these signals at the level of the CRF neurons in the PVN.

The development of the HPA response is shaped by events occurring early in life. These effects are surprisingly robust and account, at least in part, for the individual differences that occur in neuroendocrine responses to stress. Considerable evidence now exists for the idea that these early environmental factors ultimately affect

[a]This research was supported by grants from the Medical Research Council of Canada (MRCC) to M.J.M. and from the National Institute of Mental Health to P.M.P. M.J.M. is the recipient of an MRCC Scientist career award. N.S., J.S., and C.M.M. are postdoctoral fellows of the Natural Sciences and Engineering Research Council of Canada (NSERC). S.B. is a graduate fellow of the Fonds de la Recherche en Santé du Québec (FRSQ), the Canadian Heart Foundation, and the Medical Research Council of Canada.

[b]Address correspondence to Dr. Michael J. Meaney, Developmental Neuroendocrinology Laboratory, Douglas Hospital Research Centre, 6875 Boul. LaSalle, Montreal, Quebec H4H 1R3, Canada.

activity at the level of the CRF neurons of the PVN, either directly or indirectly via their effects on systems that mediate the inhibitory signals associated with glucocorticoid negative-feedback. These changes persist throughout the life of the animal and are accompanied by altered endocrine responses to stress. Such developmental effects likely represent one way in which early life events can predispose an individual to pathology in later life.

ADRENOCORTICAL RESPONSE TO STRESS

The HPA axis, as described by Selye,[1] is highly responsive to stress. Neural signals associated with stress are transduced into endocrine responses via their effects at the level of the mediobasal hypothalamus. Thus, the secretion of CRF and co-secretagogues such as vasopressin (AVP) from PVN neurons into the portal system of the anterior pituitary during stress causes an increase in the release of adrenocorticotropin (ACTH) into circulation.[2–9] The elevated ACTH levels, in turn, stimulate an increase in the release of adrenal glucocorticoids. The highly catabolic glucocorticoids produce lipolysis, which increases the level of free fatty acids; glycogenolysis, which increases blood glucose levels; and in protein catabolism, which increases amino acid availability as substrates for gluconeogenesis, further increasing blood glucose levels.[10,11] Together, these actions assist the organism under stressful conditions, in part at least, by increasing the availability of energy substrates. The glucocorticoids also suppress immunological responses,[11] protecting against the occurrence of inflammation at a time when mobility may be important to the animal.

However, continued exposure to elevated glucocorticoid levels can present a serious risk for the organism. In addition to a general suppression of anabolic processes, prolonged glucocorticoid exposure can lead to muscle atrophy, decreased sensitivity to insulin and a risk of steroid-induced diabetes, hypertension, hyperlipidemia, hypercholesterolemia, arterial disease, amenorrhea, impotency, and the impairment of growth and tissue repair, as well as immunosuppression.[10,11] Thus, once the stressor is terminated, it is very clearly in the animal's best interest to "turn off" the HPA stress response. The efficacy of this process is determined by the ability of the glucocorticoids to inhibit subsequent ACTH release (i.e., glucocorticoid negative-feedback).

Circulating glucocorticoids feed back onto the pituitary and specific brain regions to inhibit the release of ACTH from the anterior pituitary cells.[12–17] The focus for glucocorticoid negative-feedback inhibition is the population of CRF and CRF/AVP neurons in the parvocellular region of the mediobasal hypothalamus. Thus, glucocorticoids serve to decrease mRNA levels,[18–22] content,[23–25] and release[26] of both CRF and AVP. These effects occur either directly on CRF and CRF/AVP neurons, or via effects on other brain regions. Accordingly, the hypothalamus is not the only relevant brain site for glucocorticoid feedback effects.

In addition to the PVN, considerable evidence exists for the importance of extrahypothalamic regions in the inhibition of CRF synthesis and HPA activity. Most notable among these regions is the hippocampus.[27] In the rat, hippocampal lesions or ablations are associated with elevated corticosterone (B; the principal glucocorticoid in rodents) levels under both basal, stress, and poststress conditions.[28–32] Moreover, hippocampectomized animals show reduced suppression of ACTH after exogenous glucocorticoid administration[28] and increased CRF and AVP mRNA levels in the PVN of the hypothalamus;[24] fornix lesions decrease glucocorticoid inhibition over CRF and AVP release in the portal system.[34] These findings, together with the fact that the hippocampus is rich in corticosteroid receptors,[25] suggest that this structure is involved in the inhibitory influence of glucocorticoids over adrenocortical activity (see refs. 27 and 35 for recent reviews).

Probably the strongest support for the role of the hippocampus in the regulation of HPA activity comes from studies on the role of hippocampal corticosteroid receptor systems. Evidence from a number of models (see refs. 27 and 35–38) suggests that a decrease in hippocampal corticosteroid receptor density is associated with a hypersecretion of B both under basal conditions and following the termination of stress (i.e., less effective negative-feedback). There are decreased levels of hippocampal corticosteroid receptors binding in the aged rat, lactating rats, and immature rats and these animals also hypersecrete B under basal and/or stressful conditions. Perhaps the most impressive evidence comes from studies with the vasopressin-deficient Brattleboro rat.[31] These animals show a deficit in corticosteroid receptors in the hippocampus and pituitary and hypersecrete B following stress. The hippocampal receptor deficit is reversed with vasopressin treatment and, as long as the treatment is continued, receptor levels remain elevated and the animals exhibit normal B secretion following stress.[31]

The uptake of B in rat brain is associated with at least two distinct corticosteroid receptor subtypes.[39–46] The mineralocorticoid (or type I) receptor binds *in vitro* to both B and the mineralocorticoids, aldosterone and RU 26752, with high affinity, and binds the synthetic glucocorticoid, RU 28362, with very low affinity. The greatest concentration of mineralocorticoid receptor sites is found in the hippocampus. The glucocorticoid (or type II) receptor is far more diffusely distributed throughout the brain, binds B, dexamethasone, and RU 28362 with high affinity, and RU 26752 and aldosterone with lower affinity. Although both receptors bind B with high affinity, the K_d of the mineralocorticoid receptor for B (~ 0.5 nM) is lower than that of the glucocorticoid receptor (~ 2.0–5.0 nM[42]).

A physiological consequence of this difference in affinity for B is that these receptors then show different rates of occupancy under basal B levels. A considerable percentage (~ 50–90%) of the mineralocorticoid sites are occupied under basal B levels,[42–45,47] rendering the hippocampal mineralocorticoid receptor relatively insensitive to dynamic variations in B levels. In contrast, the glucocorticoid receptor is more responsive to dynamic changes in B titers, such as those occurring during stress.[42–45,48] Under conditions of basal circulating B, only about 10–15% of the glucocorticoid receptors are occupied. Stress results in a dramatic increase in the hormone-receptor signal, such that immediately after a 20-minute period of restraint about 75–85% of glucocorticoid receptors are occupied. B injections that mimic the steroid levels seen during stress also result in about a 75% occupancy of glucocorticoid receptors. Finally, Sapolsky *et al.*[34] found that the level of glucocorticoid receptor occupancy in the hypothalamus and hippocampus was negatively correlated with portal CRF concentrations. These findings, together with the known negative-feedback efficacy of the synthetic corticoids such as dexamethasone, once thought to selectively bind to the glucocorticoid receptor, suggested that it was this site that mediated the negative-feedback actions of glucocorticoids.

However, Dallman and colleagues[12] have provided evidence for the involvement of both mineralocorticoid and glucocorticoid receptors in the regulation of basal ACTH levels in rats. In subsequent studies hippocampal implants of both the glucocorticoid receptor antagonist, RU 38486, and the mineralocorticoid receptor antagonists, RU 26752 and spironolactone, resulted in elevated levels of plasma ACTH.[49] Moreover, Ratka *et al.*[50] have found that systemic injections of either antagonist resulted in elevated poststress B levels in intact rats. Finally, aldosterone, which acts selectively at mineralocorticoid sites, reduces both basal and stress-induced ACTH secretion.[51] These findings suggest that glucocorticoid negative-feedback almost certainly involves both mineralocorticoid and glucocorticoid receptor sites.

EFFECT OF HANDLING ON THE HPA RESPONSE TO STRESS

Several years ago Ader and Grota,[52] Hess *et al.*,[53] and Levine *et al.*[54–56] described the effects of postnatal "handling" on the development of behavioral and endocrine responses to stress. As adults, handled rats exhibited attenuated fearfulness in novel environments and a less pronounced increase in the secretion of the adrenal glucocorticoids in response to a variety of stressors. These findings clearly demonstrated that the development of rudimentary, adaptive responses to stress could be modified by environmental events. In addition, the handling paradigm provides a marvelous opportunity to examine how subtle variations in the early environment alter the development of specific neurochemical systems, leading to stable individual differences in biological responses to stimuli that threaten homeostasis.

The handling procedure usually involved removing rat pups from their cage, placing the animals together in small containers, and 15–20 minutes later, returning the animals to their cage and their mothers. The manipulation is generally performed daily for the first 21 days of life and the animals are tested as fully mature adults. In response to a wide variety of stimuli, handled (H) rats secrete less B and show a faster return to basal B levels after the termination of stress than do nonhandled (NH) animals.[52–58] The integrated plasma B response to stress (prestress to 120 min poststress) is usually 75–100% higher in the NH rats. These differences are apparent as late as 24–26 months of age,[57] indicating that the handling effect persists over the entire life of the animal. The differences in HPA function are not due to changes in adrenal sensitivity to ACTH or in pituitary sensitivity to CRF.[58,59] Moreover, no differences exist between H and NH animals in the metabolic clearance rate for ACTH and B.[58,59] Rather, the difference lies in the fact that the NH animals show increased secretion of B both during and following stress.

Young adult H and NH animals do not differ in levels of corticosteroid-binding globulin (CBG), the principal plasma binder for B[58,60] or in free B levels.[60] This finding is of considerable importance because brain uptake of B appears to approximate the non-CBG bound (free + albumin-bound) portion of the steroid.[61] Thus, differences in total B are likely predictive of differences in brain uptake of the steroid. Interestingly, the handling effects on HPA function are specific to conditions of stress. Young adult H and NH animals do not differ in basal B levels at any time point over the diurnal cycle.[58,60] This finding also indicates that differences in HPA activity observed during stress cannot be accounted for by differences in prestress, basal glucocorticoid levels.

H and NH animals also differ in plasma ACTH responses to stress. As with B, plasma ACTH levels are higher both during and following stress in NH compared with H animals.[58,62] Generally, the integrated plasma ACTH response (prestress to 60 min poststress) is about 50–100% higher in the NH rats. These findings, along with an earlier report[63] on differences in CRF-like bioactivity between H and NH animals, suggest that the mechanism(s) for differences between H and NH animals is located above the level of the pituitary and may be related to differential sensitivity of CNS negative-feedback processes.

EFFECT OF HANDLING ON HPA NEGATIVE-FEEDBACK PROCESSES

We examined whether the relative hypersecretion of ACTH and B by NH animals might be related to differences in negative-feedback sensitivity to circulating glucocorticoids between H and NH animals. We[58] used a classical negative-feedback paradigm based on the finding that high levels of circulating glucocorticoids feed back onto the brain and/or pituitary to inhibit subsequent HPA activity.[12–14,17] Such delayed, negative-feedback persists for hours following exposure to elevated glucocorticoid levels.[14] H and NH animals were injected with one of five doses of either B or dexamethasone three hours before a 20-minute period of restraint. Both glucocorticoids were more effective in suppressing stress-induced HPA responses in the H animals, that is, the ID_{50} for both B and dexamethasone was 5–10 times lower in the H animals. These data suggest that H animals are indeed more sensitive to the negative-feedback effects of circulating glucocorticoids on HPA activity.

Because this delayed form of negative-feedback is mediated by the binding of B to soluble intracellular receptors, we measured both mineralocorticoid and glucocorticoid receptor sites in selected brain regions and pituitary of young adult H and NH animals.[57,58,60,64–67] The results of these studies demonstrated significant tissue-specific differences in glucocorticoid receptor binding capacity as a function of handling. H animals show increased glucocorticoid receptor binding capacity in the hippocampus, but not in septum, amygdala, hypothalamus, or pituitary. The difference in the receptor binding capacity is clearly related to the number of receptor sites, and not to the affinity of the receptor for [^{3}H]radioligand, RU 28362. Moreover, the difference occurs in glucocorticoid receptors, but not the mineralocorticoid receptor sites (measured using either radiolabeled aldosterone or B, plus a 50-fold excess of cold RU 28362). Finally, using *in situ* hybridization with probes selective for either the glucocorticoid or mineralocorticoid receptor mRNA, we[68] found that glucocorticoid receptor mRNA expression (grains/cell) was higher throughout the hippocampus of H compared with NH animals. There were no differences in mineralocorticoid receptor mRNA expression.

The difference in hippocampal glucocorticoid receptor density appears to be related to the more efficient suppression of poststress HPA activity in the H animals. Chronic administration of B results in a 30–45% down-regulation of hippocampal glucocorticoid receptor binding sites.[69,70] The effect is highly specific to the hippocampus, such that receptor binding capacity in the hypothalamus and pituitary is unaffected. In one experiment H animals were treated for five days with B and were allowed two days for steroid clearance.[58] Hippocampal glucocorticoid receptor density was down-regulated in the H + B animals to levels that were indistinguishable from those of NH animals, and significantly less than those of the H + vehicle animals. There were no differences in glucocorticoid receptor density in the hypothalamus or pituitary. When the animals in these groups were exposed to a 20-minute period of restraint, we found that the H + B animals, like the NH animals, hypersecreted B 60 and 120 minutes poststress in comparison to the H + vehicle, control animals. These data suggest that the difference in negative-feedback efficiency between H and NH is related to the differences in hippocampal glucocorticoid receptor density. Thus, the chronic B treatment reversed both the handling-induced increase in hippocampal glucocorticoid receptor binding capacity and the difference in poststress HPA activity.

It appears that the increase in glucocorticoid receptor sites in the hippocampus is a critical feature for the handling effect on HPA function. The increase in receptor density appears to increase the sensitivity of the hippocampus to circulating glucocorticoids, enhancing the efficacy of negative-feedback inhibition over HPA activity, and serving to reduce poststress secretion of ACTH and B in H animals.

The effect of postnatal handling on HPA negative-feedback likely involves glucocorticoid receptor differences in at least one other region. Handling also increases glucocorticoid receptor density in the frontal cortex.[66] We recently provided evidence for the role of the frontal cortex in the regulation of stress-induced HPA activity.[71] Medial prefrontal cortex lesions produced increased levels of ACTH and B both during and after the termination of stress. B implants placed directly into this region produce a 40–50% decrease in stress-induced ACTH and B levels. Interestingly, these effects are apparent only with more moderate stimuli, in this case restraint. Neither the medial prefrontal cortex lesions nor B implants into this region had any effect on ACTH or B levels observed using ether stress; a more severe stressor associated with 2–3 times higher levels of ACTH. Moreover, these effects were observed only during or following stress; neither treatment altered basal ACTH or B levels at any point over the diurnal cycle. These findings suggest that the handling effect on HPA function may involve altered glucocorticoid receptor density in the frontal cortex.

THE NATURE OF THE GLUCOCORTICOID NEGATIVE-FEEDBACK SIGNAL

In recent studies we have provided a more detailed description of plasma ACTH responses to ether and restraint stress in H and NH animals.[62] The results of these studies have shown that very shortly after the onset of stress, plasma ACTH levels are higher in the NH rats. Although ACTH levels rise in both groups, the increase is greater in the NH animals. Thus, the integrated (hormone levels × time) plasma ACTH response in the NH rats is generally about twofold greater than in the H animals. At this point it is important to note that H and NH animals do not differ in glucocorticoid fast feedback sensitivity, the inhibitory signal associated with the rapidly increasing levels of plasma B.[62]

These data raise an interesting set of problems. First, assuming that differences in fast feedback are not relevant here, the other important negative-feedback signal in determining the magnitude of the plasma ACTH response to stress is that associated with basal glucocorticoid levels. Moreover, although we previously showed that basal B levels do not differ in H versus NH rats, there are differences in glucocorticoid receptor levels in brain regions known to regulate HPA activity. Inasmuch as the increased receptor density confers a greater sensitivity to B, it remains possible that the basal glucocorticoid feedback signal might be stronger in the H rats.

The second problem concerns the differences in poststress levels of HPA activity. H and NH rats differ in poststress plasma levels of B; NH animals show elevated B levels for a considerably longer period of time. Thus, the termination of the adrenocortical response to stress in the H animals occurs more efficiently than in NH animals. We assumed that this difference is associated with the differences in negative-feedback sensitivity between H and NH rats and that the relevant signal was the elevated B levels achieved during stress. We believed that the high levels of B served to provide a strong negative-feedback signal which, in turn, inhibited HPA activity once the drive associated with the stressor was terminated. However, the adrenal is known to respond to the integrated ACTH signal. The integrated ACTH level determines not only the peak in B secretion, but also the duration of the response; higher levels of ACTH not only result in greater levels of B, but also in a longer period of elevated B. Therefore, the poststress differences in plasma B that are observed in the NH animals could occur in response to the amount of ACTH secreted during stress.

One very interesting question that emerges here concerns the nature of the relevant glucocorticoid feedback signal. There are at least two obvious signals: basal B levels before stress and the elevated B levels occurring during stress. Stress-induced elevations in B could serve as the signal for the termination of the stress response once the activational effect of the stress has been removed. Alternatively, the increase in plasma ACTH could be associated with differences in the tonic negative-feedback signal associated with basal B levels.

In order to examine this question we[62] compared ACTH responses to restraint in H and NH (1) ADX animals, which lack any glucocorticoid negative-feedback signal; (2) ADX animals, which provide the equivalent of a basal B signal (ADX + B), but lack the negative-feedback signal associated with stress-induced increases in B; and (3) intact, sham-operated animals (SHAM), which possess both basal and stress-induced glucocorticoid signals. These animals were studied five days after ADX. At this time the HPA axis has generally stabilized in ADX + B animals (see refs. 12 and 72). The B pellets provided circulating hormone levels of about 5 μg/dL, equivalent to the integrated basal level of B over the diurnal cycle. Basal plasma ACTH and anterior pituitary POMC mRNA levels were substantially increased by ADX in both H and NH rats, and these effects were effectively reversed with B pellet implants in both groups of animals. Thus, the B pellet was equally effective in reversing the effects of ADX on basal HPA activity in H and NH rats.

No differences existed in the plasma ACTH responses to restraint in ADX/NH versus ADX/H animals. This was an important finding because it suggests that in the absence of a glucocorticoid negative-feedback signal, ACTH responses to stress are comparable in H and NH rats, thereby confirming that the differences in HPA responses to stress observed in intact H and NH animals are associated with differences in glucocorticoid negative-feedback sensitivity. As expected, plasma ACTH levels during and after restraint in the intact NH animals were significantly greater than in the H animals. Surprisingly, differences in plasma ACTH between H and NH animals were also observed in the ADX animals provided with basal B replacement (FIG. 1). In the ADX + B/NH rats, the plasma ACTH response to restraint was comparable to that in the ADX/NH animals. In contrast, in the ADX + B/H rats the plasma ACTH response to restraint was significantly reduced compared to ADX/H rats, and significantly lower than in ADX + B/NH animals. Thus, basal B replacement was sufficient to reinstate the differences between H and NH rats.

It is also important to note the specificity of this effect. The B replacement regimen used in this study was sufficient to greatly attenuate the adrenalectomy-induced increase in pituitary POMC mRNA, basal ACTH, and plasma CBG in both H and NH animals, but altered stress-induced ACTH secretion only in the H animals. A number of previous studies have shown that in laboratory rats B-pellet replacement of this order of magnitude is sufficient to correct basal ACTH secretion[72-74] and CBG production,[75] but not stress-induced increases in plasma ACTH; these findings are comparable to our data with ADX + B/NH rats. By contrast, basal B replacement did attenuate the ACTH hypersecretion with stress in ADX + B/H rats. The reduced ACTH secretion in response to stress in the ADX + B/H animals is consistent with previous data showing increased glucocorticoid negative-feedback sensitivity in H animals. Taken together, these data indicate that differences in HPA response to stress between H and NH animals are dependent upon the presence of glucocorticoids, but are not dependent upon stress-induced elevations in glucocorticoid levels.

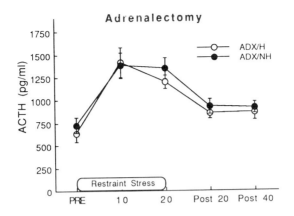

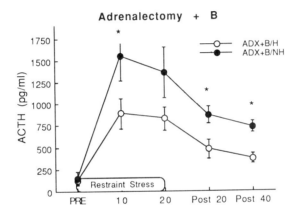

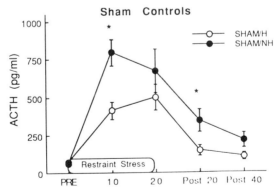

FIGURE 1. Plasma ACTH levels before, during, and at various times after a 20-minute restraint in adrenalectomized (ADX), ADX corticosterone-replaced (ADX + B), and intact, sham-operated (SHAM) handled (H) and nonhandled (NH) animals. Asterisk indicates values that differ at $p < 0.05$. Integrated values for plasma ACTH (pg/mL/min): SHAM/H = 326 ± 68; SHAM/NH = 448 ± 83; ADX/H = 1031 ± 61; ADX/NH = 1070 ± 111; ADX + B/H = 609 ± 142; ADX + B/NH = 1091 ± 111.

These findings also suggest that negative-feedback differences between H and NH animals can occur in response to basal B levels. These differences appear to be reflected in differences in median eminence content of various ACTH secretagogues. We found that under resting state conditions median eminence levels of CRF and AVP (but not oxytocin) are significantly higher in NH compared with H rats.[62] We also recently found that hypothalamic CRF mRNA levels are about 2.5-fold higher in NH compared with H animals.[76] Thus, under resting conditions, hypothalamic CRF and AVP synthesis appears to be elevated in NH rats, a difference that occurs in the presence of basal glucocorticoid levels.

The differences in median eminence levels of CRF and AVP offer an important insight into understanding the nature of the differences in glucocorticoid negative-feedback between H and NH animals. Because H and NH animals do not differ in basal levels of ACTH or B,[58,60] it seems likely that the differences in CRF and AVP represent differences in readily releasable storage pools of these peptides in axon terminals of PVN neurons located in the median eminence. The excitatory signal at the level of the paraventricular nucleus of the hypothalamus associated with stress likely results in greater CRF and AVP release in the NH animals. This, in turn, would result in a greater plasma ACTH signal. This idea is consistent with the finding that H and NH animals differ in plasma ACTH responses to a wide variety of stimuli. Indeed, the differences in the terminal pools of CRF and AVP suggest that H and NH animals would differ in stressors mediated by either secretagogue. Note, however, that pituitary ACTH responses to both restraint and ether stress appear to be mediated by dynamic variations in both CRF and AVP.[5,6] This hypothesis has been at least partially confirmed in one recent study. Plotsky and Meaney[76] found that CRF release from the median eminence in response to restraint was significantly greater in NH compared with H rats.

It is also important to note that ADX + B animals do not differ in corticotrope sensitivity to CRF[77] and that differences in ACTH release in response to stress most likely reflect differences in neural regulatory components of ACTH secretion (also see ref. 73). This idea is also consistent with available information on the role of the hippocampus in mediating glucocorticoid inhibition of HPA activity. Hippocampal lesions result in a prolonged elevation of B after stress.[31] Herman et al.[33] found that hippocampal lesions resulted in increased CRF and AVP mRNA levels in the hypothalamus under basal B conditions. Moreover, Sapolsky et al.[34] found that portal concentrations CRF and AVP were negatively correlated with hippocampal glucocorticoid receptor occupancy. Interestingly, hippocampal glucocorticoid receptor occupancy was significantly correlated with resting (prestress) portal concentrations of both CRF and AVP. These findings suggest that an increased glucocorticoid receptor signal at the level of the hippocampus is associated with decreased levels of hypophyseal CRF and AVP.

On the basis of these data, it seems reasonable to propose that (1) H and NH animals differ in delayed negative-feedback[58] and that this difference is reflected in differential rates of CRF and AVP synthesis in the PVN of the hypothalamus, (2) differences in negative-feedback regulation are apparent even in response to basal B signals and occur as a result of the increased glucocorticoid receptor density in the hippocampus (and perhaps the medial prefrontal cortex), (3) in response to stress there is a greater release of CRF and/or AVP in the NH animals (see ref. 76), giving rise to a greater increase in plasma ACTH levels and a greater increase in plasma B levels which persists for a longer period of time (i.e., higher poststress plasma B levels in the NH animals). Thus, differences between H and NH animals in HPA activity both during and after stress can occur independently of the stress-induced increase in plasma B. In our view, the central feature of the handling effect on HPA responsivity to stress involves the changes in hippocampal glucocorticoid receptor gene expression (FIG. 2).

EFFECTS OF POSTNATAL HANDLING ON HPA RESPONSES TO CHRONIC STRESS

Thus far, studies on the effects of early environmental regulation of neuroendocrine responses to stress have focused largely on responses to acute stress. The need

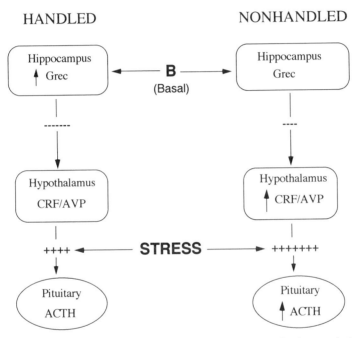

FIGURE 2. A summary of our current understanding of the mechanisms underlying the differences in HPA responses to acute stress in handled and nonhandled animals. The increased glucocorticoid receptor levels confer greater sensitivity to corticosterone (B) in hippocampal tissue from handled animals. Therefore, even under basal corticosterone levels (which do not differ in young, adult handled and nonhandled rats), there is a greater tonic inhibitory signal (−) on hypothalamic corticotropin-releasing factor (CRF) and vasopressin (AVP) synthesis in handled rats. In response to the neural signals associated with stress and impinging upon the hypothalamus, a greater release of CRF/AVP into portal circulation (+) occurs in the nonhandled rats, resulting in greater ACTH release.

for studies using chronic stress paradigms is based on the considerations (1) that the more demanding conditions associated with chronic stress are likely to emphasize the differences associated with early environment, revealing underlying vulnerability that may not be apparent with the less challenging conditions of acute stress, and (2) that the chronic stress condition is likely to be more relevant to conditions associated with the development of pathology.

There are two prominent effects of chronic stress on the HPA axis. First, some adaptation to the stressor occurs with repeated exposure. Second, there is a potentiation, or facilitation,[78] to a novel stressor. The latter effect is reflected in higher plasma ACTH responses in animals that have been exposed to chronic stress than in animals with no recent stressful experience.

In a recent series of studies we[79] examined the HPA response to chronic stress in H and NH animals. In these studies we used daily exposure to a cold (4–6 °C) chamber for 4 hours for 21 consecutive days as the chronic stress. Note that this paradigm involves repeated, intermittent chronic stress and not continuous chronic stress (such as 24 h/day of cold). Animals exposed to the 4 hours per day of cold are able to defend their normal body temperature. The advantage of this form of stress is that it is the only stressor we have found to date that does not distinguish between H and NH animals (i.e., the plasma ACTH and B response to acute exposure to 4 h of cold is comparable in H and NH animals). This allowed us to examine the effects of chronic exposure to stress in H and NH animals without the complication of differences on day 1 of testing. Thus, plasma ACTH responses to 4 hours of cold did not differ on day 1 between H and NH animals. However, after 21 consecutive days of exposure to cold, plasma ACTH responses in H animals had diminished significantly, and to a greater extent than in NH animals. These data suggest that adaptation to repeated, intermittent cold stress was greater in the H animals.

On day 22 of testing, chronically stressed H and NH animals, along with their nonstressed controls, were exposed to a novel stressor (20-min restraint). Exposure to chronic stress facilitated HPA responses to restraint in the NH, but not in the H animals. NH previously exposed to cold stress on days 1–21 secreted significantly higher levels of both ACTH and B compared with NH controls. No reliable differences were present in plasma ACTH and B responses to restraint between the chronically stressed and control H animals. Thus, chronic stress did not serve to facilitate subsequent HPA responses to acute stress in the H animals.

These data reflect the differences in HPA responses to stress between H and NH animals at the level of chronic stress. We should bear in mind that these differences emerged in response to a specific form of chronic stress, and it may well be that the pattern adaptation/facilitation that occurs is specific to the type of stress. Indeed, in a provocative review on the topic of chronic stress, Dallman and colleagues[79] concluded that the critical neural sites for facilitation are distal to the PVN. If this is indeed true, then we might well expect that different forms of chronic stress might vary in their ability to facilitate HPA responses to novel stressors. Nevertheless, our findings reveal that the differences between H and NH animals are observable within a chronic stress paradigm.

EFFECTS OF PROLONGED PERIODS OF MATERNAL SEPARATION ON HPA RESPONSES TO STRESS

These studies show that the HPA response to stress is modified by early handling. However, handling represents an interesting manipulation. The procedure involves separating the pup from the dam for a period of 3–15 minutes (depending upon the lab) and exposing the pup to a novel array of sensory stimuli. It is noteworthy that in the course of normal mother-pup interactions the dam is regularly away from the nest and the pups, for periods of 20–30 minutes. Thus, the handling manipulation does not seem to represent any abnormal period of separation or loss of maternal care. What about much longer periods of separation where there is a loss of maternal care (including the nutritional and thermal needs met by the mother)?

Indeed, there seems to be good reason to believe that the effects of short periods of perturbation, such as handling, are *qualitatively* different from more severe forms of maternal separation. Kuhn and colleagues[80] found that prolonged periods of maternal separation (>2 h) result in a suppression of plasma growth hormone. In contrast, brief periods of separation (15 min) or handling result in an *increase* in plasma growth hormone levels. This finding is of considerable importance because it suggests that different forms of environmental stimulation can have very different effects on neuroendocrine systems.

What about differences in the long-term consequences of these manipulations? We[76] began our studies on this topic by examining the effects of repeated maternal separation of varying durations. From day 2 until day 14 of life, pups were separated from their mothers once per day for 0, 15, 60, 180 or 360 minutes. The animals were otherwise reared under identical conditions. At 120 days of age the animals were exposed to restraint. In a manner comparable to the experiments of Kuhn *et al.,* the data show that the long-term effects of HPA responses to stress were qualitatively different depending upon the duration of maternal separation. Compared to 0-minute controls (animals reared in the same manner as NH animals), the 15-minute period of separation (or handling) resulted in animals that showed reduced plasma B levels during and following stress. In contrast, animals separated for 180 or 360 minutes per day showed *increased* plasma B levels both during and following stress. Thus, neonatal handling was associated with a 40% reduction in B secretion as compared to the NH rats, whereas maternal separation was associated with a 40% increase in the B response as compared to the NH group. These findings underscore the very different sequela associated with handling versus maternal separation. Adult male rats that had been maternally separated (MS) for 180 minutes per day also exhibited hypersecretion of ACTH and B to a novel environment as compared to the NH and H groups.

We then compared these animals using a dexamethasone suppression test as an indication of negative-feedback sensitivity. Administration of dexamethasone (10 μg/100 g body weight) at 0900 hours completely suppressed B secretion (<1 μg/dL) in the H ($n = 6$) and NH ($n = 6$) groups at 3, 6, and 9 hours after administration. B levels of rats in the MS group were also suppressed at 3 hours and 6 hours after dexamethasone; however, by 9 hours circulating B levels had "escaped" to 4.5 ± 0.3 μg/dL ($n = 6$), suggesting that the efficiency of glucocorticoid negative-feedback was reduced by repeated periods of maternal separation during early life.

Could the effects of maternal separation involve alteration in the development of CRF systems? To date, we have demonstrated changes in hypothalamic CRF mRNA and in CRF content in adult rats exposed to handling or maternal separation as neonates. Pups that had experienced maternal separation for 180 minutes/day exhibited a marked increase in hypothalamic CRF mRNA as compared to either H or NH pups. Furthermore, stalk median eminence CRF peptide content paralleled the changes in hypothalamic mRNA. These preliminary studies are consistent with the idea that the hypothalamic CRF neurons are a target for regulation by neonatal experience and that this regulation results in permanent alteration of the HPA axis. The changes observed provide a central molecular basis for the differences in HPA function observed in adult rats differing in early life experience.

EFFECTS OF NEONATAL ENDOTOXIN EXPOSURE ON HPA RESPONSES TO STRESS

In an effort to examine the effects of rather general and common early life events on the development of the HPA response to stress, we[81] examined the effects of early illness. In order to address this question we exposed rat pups on days 3 and 5 of life with a low dose of an endotoxin. The dose was chosen in order to induce illness, but at a level that was not life-threatening, that is, none of the 100–110 pups treated died within the next two weeks. The endotoxin treatment elevated plasma glucose levels, severely dampened behavioral activity, and increased body temperature.

When the animals were examined as adults, the results were surprising. The endotoxin-treated animals showed significantly increased plasma ACTH and B responses to restraint in comparison to both saline-treated and untreated controls. In accordance with our previous findings, these animals also differed in glucocorticoid negative-feedback sensitivity. An injection of 10 μg/100 g bw of dexamethasone 3 hours prior to restraint completely abolished plasma ACTH responses in the controls (100% suppression). In the endotoxin-treated animals, the plasma ACTH response to restraint was only partially suppressed (∼ 40% suppression). Likewise, resting state levels of median eminence CRF were significantly higher in the endotoxin-treated animals compared with controls. Thus, the endotoxin treatment in early life produced an effect that was functionally the opposite to that of handling. Again, we find evidence of differences in adult hypothalamic CRF activity as a function of early life events.

EFFECTS OF PRENATAL STRESS ON HPA FUNCTION

In a series of recent studies we[82] began to examine the effects of exposure to prenatal stress on the development of HPA responses to stress. In these studies we used a form of prenatal stress that focuses on the third trimester of pregnancy. In these studies pregnant females were exposed to restraint for 1 hour per day for days 15–20 of gestation. The offspring were examined as fully mature adults, beginning at 120 days of life.

The effects of prenatal stress were very clearly sexually dimorphic; the effects were far more pronounced on females than on males.[82] Among the adult females, prenatal stress resulted in increased plasma ACTH and B responses to restraint. Virtually no effect of prenatal stress was evident on HPA responses in males. Likewise, in females, but not males, resting state levels of median eminence CRF were greater in the offspring of dams exposed to restraint. Interestingly, these effects are consistent with the effects of prenatal alcohol exposure on HPA development (see Weinberg, this volume). In these studies, prenatal alcohol resulted in increased HPA responses to stress in females, but not males.

Using the results of the handling studies, we then exhaustively studied mineralocorticoid and glucocorticoid receptor concentrations in brain and pituitary, but to no avail; the development of the corticosteroid receptor systems are unaffected by prenatal stress. Interestingly, Weinberg and colleagues found that prenatal alcohol exposure does not alter corticosteroid receptor development in the brain or pituitary. However, we did find that plasma CBG levels were clearly altered. In females, but not males, plasma CBG levels were elevated by about 50% in the prenatally stressed animals.

This finding suggests that although total (CBG-bound + free) B levels in the prenatally stressed female animals might be higher in response to stress, the increased CBG levels might serve to offset this difference. Indeed, when we calculated free B levels on the basis of the plasma CBG levels in these animals, there was little difference in the corticoid response to stress. It should be noted that it is the free form of the steroid that is biologically active and that determines the level of steroid receptor occupancy.

Such differences in plasma CBG are also likely to account for the increased plasma ACTH response to stress in the prenatally stressed animals. The difference in plasma CBG levels occurs under resting state conditions. At the same time there are no apparent differences in basal B between prenatal stress and control animals. Thus, the basal free B levels in the controls are higher than in the prenatal stress animals, and this should provide a stronger, resting-state negative-feedback signal in the controls. This difference appears to us as the most likely explanation for the increased hypothalamic CRF synthesis in the prenatal stress animals and the increased plasma ACTH response to stress.

CONCLUSIONS

Handling during the early postnatal period leads to increased glucocorticoid receptor binding in the hippocampus and is associated with enhanced negative-feedback control over HPA function. Ultimately, the CRF and CRF/AVP neurons in the PVN of the hypothalamus are the target for these differences in glucocorticoid negative feedback. In turn, the altered hypothalamic CRF/AVP activity serves as the mechanism by which differences in negative feedback are transduced into differences in HPA responses to stress. Likewise, each of the early environmental manipulations studied to date has served to alter resting-state hypothalamic CRF activity, although the changes at the level of the CRF neuron can occur as result of different processes (i.e., altered hippocampal glucocorticoid receptor density in the case of handling; increased plasma CBG levels in the prenatally stressed females). It is likely that this plasticity reflects a basic process whereby the early environment is able to "fine-tune" the sensitivity and efficiency of certain neuroendocrine systems that mediate the animal's response to stimuli that threaten homeostasis. It is also evident that this fine-tuning can occur at different levels of the HPA axis depending upon the nature of the environmental stimulation, as well as the gender and the developmental phase of the animal.

REFERENCES

1. SEYLE, H. 1950. The Physiology and Pathology of Exposure to Stress. Acta. Montreal.
2. ANTONI, F. A. 1986. Endocr. Rev. **7**: 351–370.
3. GIBBS, D. M. 1986. Psychoneuroendocrinology **11**: 131–140.
4. PLOTSKY, P. M. 1987. Ann. N.Y. Acad. Sci. **512**: 205–217.
5. LINTON, E. A., F. J. H. TILDERS, S. HODGKINSON, F. BERKENBOSCH, I. VERMES & P. J. LOWRY. 1985. Endocrinology **116**: 966–970.
6. NAKANE, T., T. AUGHYA, N. KANIE & C. S. HOLLANDER. 1985. Proc. Natl. Acad. Sci. USA **82**: 1247–1251.
7. RIVIER, C. & W. W. VALE. 1983. Regul. Pept. **7**: 253–258.
8. RIVIER, C. & P. M. PLOTSKY. 1986. Annu. Rev. Physiol. **48**: 475–489.
9. RIVIER, C., M. BROWNSTEIN, J. SPIESS, J. RIVIER & W. W. VALE. 1982. Endocrinology **110**: 272–278.
10. BRINDLEY, D. & Y. ROLLAND. 1989. Clin. Sci. **77**: 453–461.
11. MUNCK, A., P. M. GUYRE & N. J. HOLBROOK. 1984. Endocr. Rev. **5**: 25–44.
12. DALLMAN, M. F., S. AKANA, C. S. CASCIO, D. N. DARLINGTON, L. JACOBSON & N. LEVIN. 1987. Recent Prog. Horm. Res. **43**: 113–173.
13. JONES, M. T., B. GILLHAM, B. D. GREENSTEIN, U. BECKFORD & M. C. HOLMES. 1982. *In* Current Topics in Neuroendocrinology. D. Ganten & D. Pfaff, Eds. Vol. **2**: 45–68. Springer. New York, NY.

14. KELLER-WOOD, M. & M. F. DALLMAN. 1984. Endocr. Rev. **5:** 1–24.
15. PLOTSKY, P. M. & W. W. VALE. 1984. Endocrinology **114:** 164–169.
16. PLOTSKY, P. M., S. OTTO & R. M. SAPOLSKY. 1986. Endocrinology **119:** 1126–1130.
17. VAN LOON, G. R. & E. B. DE SOUZA. 1987. Ann. N.Y. Acad. Sci. **512:** 300–307.
18. LIGHTMAN, S. L. & W. S. YOUNG. 1987. J. Physiol. **394:** 23–39.
19. BEYER, H. S., S. G. MATTA & B. M. SHARP. 1988. Endocrinology **123:** 2117–2123.
20. SWANSON, L. W. & D. M. SIMMONS. 1989. J. Comp. Neurol. **285:** 413–435.
21. WOLFSON, B., R. W. MANNING, L. G. DAVIS, R. ARENTZEN & F. BALDRINO. 1985. Nature **315:** 59–61.
22. YOUNG, W. S., E. MEZEY & R. E. SEIGEL. 1986. Mol. Brain Res. **1:** 231–241.
23. MERCHENTHALER, I., S. VIGH, P. PETRUSZ & A. V. SCHALLY. 1983. Regul. Pept. **5:** 295–305.
24. SWANSON, L. W., P. E. SAWCHENKO, C. RIVIER & W. W. VALE. 1983. Neuroendocrinology **36:** 165–186.
25. KISS, J. Z., E. MEZEY & L. SKIRBOLL. Proc. Natl. Acad. Sci. USA **81:** 1854–1858.
26. PLOTSKY, P. M. & P. E. SAWCHENKO. 1987. Endocrinology **120:** 1361–1369.
27. JACOBSON, L. & R. M. SAPOLSKY. 1991. Endocr. Rev. **12:** 118–134.
28. FELDMAN, S. & N. CONFORTI. 1976. Horm. Res. **7:** 56–60.
29. FELDMAN, S. & N. CONFORTI. 1980. Neuroendocrinology **30:** 52–55.
30. FISCHETTE, C. T., B. R. KOMISURAK, H. M. EDINER, H. H. FEDER & A. SIEGAL. 1980. Brain Res. **195:** 373–380.
31. SAPOLSKY, R. M., L. C. KREY & B. S. MCEWEN. 1984. Proc. Natl. Acad. Sci. USA **81:** 6174–6177.
32. WILSON, M., M. GREER & L. ROBERTS. 1980. Brain Res. **197:** 344–351.
33. HERMAN, J. P., M. K.-H. SCHAFER, E. A. YOUNG, R. THOMPSON, J. DOUGLASS, H. AKIL & S. J. WATSON. 1989. J. Neurosci. **9:** 3072–3082.
34. SAPOLSKY, R. M., M. P. ARMANINI, D. R. PACKAN, S. W. SUTTON & P. M. PLOTSKY. 1990. Neuroendocrinology **51:** 328–336.
35. MCEWEN, B. S., E. R. DE KLOET & W. H. ROSTENE. 1986. Physiol. Rev. **66:** 1121–1150.
36. MEANEY, M. J., S. R. BODNOFF, D. O'DONNELL, A. SARRIEAU, N. P. V. NAIR, D. M. DIAMOND, G. M. ROSE, J. POIRIER & J. R. SECKL. *In* Restorative Neurology, Vol. 6. C. Cuello, Ed. Elsevier. New York, NY. In press.
37. SAPOLSKY, R. M. & M. J. MEANEY. 1986. Brain Res. Rev. **11:** 65–76.
38. GOLDMAN, L., C. WINGET, G. HOLLINSHEAD & S. LEVINE. 1978. Neuroendocrinology **12:** 199–211.
39. BEAUMONT, K. & D. D. FANESTIL. 1983. Endocrinology **113:** 2043–2051.
40. EMADIAN, S. M., W. G. LUTTGE & C. L. DENSMORE. 1986. J. Steroid Biochem. **24:** 953–961.
41. FUNDER, J. W. & K. SHEPPARD. 1987. Annu. Rev. Physiol. **49:** 397–412.
42. REUL, J. M. & E. R. DE KLOET. 1985. Endocrinology **117:** 2505–2511.
43. REUL, J. M. & E. R. DE KLOET. 1986. J. Steroid Biochem. **24:** 269–272.
44. REUL, J. M., F. R. VAN DEN BOSCH & E. R. DE KLOET. 1987. J. Endocrinol. **115:** 459–467.
45. REUL, J. M., F. R. VAN DEN BOSCH & E. R. DE KLOET. 1987. Neuroendocrinology **45:** 407–412.
46. SARRIEAU, A., M. DUSSAILLANT, M. MOGUILEWSKY, D. COUTABLE, D. PHILIBERT & W. H. ROSTENE. 1988. Neurosci. Lett. **92:** 14–20.
47. CASCIO, C. S., L. JACOBSON, S. F. AKANA, R. M. SAPOLSKY & M. F. DALLMAN. 1989. Endocr. Soc. Abstr. **71:** 459.
48. MEANEY, M. J., V. VIAU, S. BHATNAGAR & D. H. AITKEN. 1988. Brain Res. **445:** 198–203.
49. BRADBURY, M. & M. F. DALLMAN. 1989. Soc. Neurosci. Abstr. **19:** 716.
50. RATKA, A., W. SUTANTO, M. BLOEMERS & E. R. DE KLOET. 1989. Neuroendocrinology **50:** 117–123.
51. AKANA, S. F., C. S. CASCIO, J. Z. DU, N. LEVIN & M. F. DALLMAN. 1986. Endocrinology **119:** 2325–2332.
52. ADER, R. & L. J. GROTA. 1969. Physiol. Behav. **4:** 303–305.
53. HESS, J. L., V. H. DENENBERG, M. X. ZARROW & W. D. PFEIFER. 1969. Physiol. Behav. **4:** 109–112.
54. LEVINE, S. 1957. Science **126:** 405–406.
55. LEVINE, S. 1962. Science **135:** 795–796.

56. LEVINE, S., G. C. HALTMEYER, G. G. KARAS & V. H. DENENBERG. 1967. Physiol. Behav. **2:** 55–63.
57. MEANEY, M. J., D. H. AITKEN, S. BHATNAGAR, C. VAN BERKEL & R. M. SAPOLSKY. 1988. Science **238:** 766–768.
58. MEANEY, M. J., D. H. AITKEN, S. SHARMA, V. VIAU & A. SARRIEAU. 1989. Neuroendocrinology **50:** 597–604.
59. GROTA, L. J. 1975. Dev. Psychobiol. **9:** 211–215.
60. MEANEY, M. J., D. H. AITKEN, S. SHARMA & V. VIAU. 1992. Neuroendocrinology **55:** 205–213.
61. PARTRIDGE, W. M., R. SAKIYAMA & H. L. JUDD. 1983. J. Clin. Endocrinol. Metab. **57:** 160–166.
62. VIAU, V., S. SHARMA, P. M. PLOTSKY & M. J. MEANEY. 1993. J. Neurosci. **13:** 1097–1105.
63. ZARROW, M. X., P. S. CAMPBEL & V. H. DENENBERG. 1972. Proc. Soc. Exp. Biol. Med. **356:** 141–143.
64. SARRIEAU, A., S. SHARMA & M. J. MEANEY. 1988. Dev. Brain Res. **43:** 158–162.
65. MEANEY, M. J. & D. H. AITKEN. 1985. Dev. Brain Res. **22:** 301–304.
66. MEANEY, M. J., D. H. AITKEN, S. R. BODNOFF, L. J. INY, J. E. TATAREWICZ & R. SAPOLSKY. 1985. Behav. Neurosci. **99:** 760–765.
67. MEANEY, M. J., D. H. AITKEN & R. M. SAPOLSKY. 1987. Neuroendocrinology **45:** 278–283.
68. LAROCQUE, S., D. O'DONNELL, C. GIANOULAKIS, J. R. SECKL & M. J. MEANEY. 1992. Soc. Neurosci. Abstr. **18:** 479.
69. SAPOLSKY, R. M., L. C. KREY & B. S. McEWEN. 1984. Stress down-regulated corticosterone receptors in a site-specific manner. Endocrinology **114:** 287–292.
70. TORNELLO, S., E. ORTI, A. F. DeNICOLA, T. C. RAINBOW & B. S. McEWEN. 1982. Neuroendocrinology **35:** 411–417.
71. DIORIO, D., V. VIAU & M. J. MEANEY. J. Neurosci. In press.
72. BRADBURY, M. J., C. S. CASCIO, K. A. SCRIBNER & M. F. DALLMAN. 1991. Endocrinology **129:** 99–108.
73. AKANA, S. F., L. JACOBSON, C. S. CASCIO, J. SHINSAKO & M. F. DALLMAN. 1988. Endocrinology **122:** 1337–1342.
74. JACOBSON, L., S. F. AKANA, C. S. CASCIO, J. SHINSAKO & M. F. DALLMAN. 1988. Endocrinology **122:** 1342–1348.
75. LEVIN, N., S. F. AKANA, L. JACOBSON, R. W. KUHN, P. K. SIITERI & M. F. DALLMAN. 1987. Endocrinology **121:** 1104–1110.
76. PLOTSKY, P. M. & M. J. MEANEY. 1993. Mol. Brain Res. **18:** 195–200.
77. AKANA, S. F., C. S. CASCIO, J.-Z. DU, N. LEVIN & M. F. DALLMAN. 1986. Endocrinology **119:** 2325–2332.
78. BHATNAGAR, S., N. SHANKS & M. J. MEANEY. 1992. Soc. Neurosci. Abstr. **18.**
79. DALLMAN, M. F., S. F. AKANA, K. A. SCRIBNER, M. J. BRADBURY, C.-D. WALKER, A. M. STRACK & C. S. CASCIO. J. Neuroendocrinol. In press.
80. KUHN, C. M., J. PAUK & S. M. SCHANBERG. 1990. Dev. Psychobiol. **23:** 395–410.
81. SHANKS, N. & M. J. MEANEY. 1992. Soc. Neurosci. Abstr. **18:** 1011.
82. McCORMICK, C. M., J. SMYTHE & M. J. MEANEY. 1992. Soc. Neurosci. Abstr. **18:** 1008.

Neuroendocrine Effects of Prenatal Alcohol Exposure[a]

JOANNE WEINBERG

Department of Anatomy, Faculty of Medicine
The University of British Columbia
2177 Wesbrook Mall
Vancouver, British Columbia, Canada V6T 1Z3

Children born to women with chronic alcoholism may exhibit multiple birth defects that together are termed the fetal alcohol syndrome (FAS).[1] The characteristic features of FAS include intrauterine and postnatal growth retardation, specific craniofacial abnormalities, and central nervous system dysfunction. Although some of these features may occur in normal infants or in infants exposed to other prenatal insults, it is the cluster of these characteristics that is diagnostically important for FAS. Furthermore, as our knowledge of the teratogenic effects of alcohol on the developing organism has progressed over the past 20 years, it has become apparent that alcohol may have adverse effects on almost every system of the body. In this review, data on the effects of fetal alcohol exposure on endocrine development of offspring will be discussed, with a specific focus on research on the hypothalamic-pituitary-adrenal (HPA) axis and the β-endorphin (β-EP) system. The role of alcohol-induced disturbances in endocrine balance as a possible mediator of the teratogenic effects of alcohol on the developing organism will also be discussed. In addition, evidence indicating an association between fetal alcohol exposure and immune system dysfunction will be examined, focusing specifically on the concept of alcohol as an immunoteratogenic agent.

EFFECTS OF FETAL ALCOHOL EXPOSURE ON THE HYPOTHALAMIC-PITUITARY-ADRENAL AXIS AND THE β-ENDORPHIN SYSTEM

It has been known for many years that alcohol can alter endocrine function in the adult organism. Acting directly on the endocrine glands themselves, and/or at the level of the pituitary or brain, alcohol has been shown to alter secretory activity and responsiveness of the adrenal cortex and medulla, the ovaries and testes, and the thyroid, and to affect plasma levels of a number of pituitary hormones including prolactin, luteinizing hormone, follicle stimulating hormone, adrenocorticotropic hormone, vasopressin, and growth hormone.

It is noteworthy that much of the work on alcohol and endocrine function has been done in males. Only a few investigators have examined the effects of alcohol on endocrine function of the female.[2–4] Furthermore and particularly relevant to this review, studies have only recently begun to examine the effects of alcohol on

[a]The work reported in this review was supported by previous grants from the British Columbia Health Research Foundation and the Medical Research Council of Canada, and since 1988, by a grant from the National Institute on Alcohol Abuse and Alcoholism. This review is based, in part, on previously published work.

endocrine function during pregnancy.[5-7] Alcohol-induced changes in maternal endocrine function could affect the female's ability to maintain a successful pregnancy. In addition, altered maternal endocrine function will disrupt the hormonal interactions between maternal and fetal systems and thus alter the normal maternal-fetal hormone balance.[8] The development of fetal endocrine function as well as fetal metabolic or physiological functions could thus be affected *in utero*. Moreover, because alcohol can readily cross the placenta, maternal alcohol consumption could result in direct stimulation or suppression of fetal endocrine activity.

Although clinical studies have established that alcohol consumption markedly alters hypothalamic-pituitary-adrenal function in chronic alcoholics,[9] few clinical studies have investigated the effects of drinking during pregnancy on the HPA axis of the developing child. A case study of four children with FAS (ages 9–14 yr) indicated that plasma cortisol levels are within normal limits.[10] However, there is no doubt that alcohol can have a stimulatory effect on the HPA axis of the newborn. A case study by Binkiewicz *et al.*,[11] for example, reported pseudo-Cushing's syndrome in an infant exposed to alcohol via breast milk. Similarly, animal studies strongly support the suggestion that alcohol (i.e., ethanol) consumption during pregnancy can have major effects on the HPA axis of the maternal female, as well as on the development and function of the HPA axis and β-EP system of the offspring exposed *in utero*.

In the pregnant female, ethanol consumption increases maternal adrenal weights, basal corticosterone levels, the adrenocortical response to stress, and the corticoid stress increment[6,12] compared to that in control females. Ethanol-induced activation of the maternal HPA axis occurs as early as day 11 of pregnancy, persists throughout gestation, may increase as gestation progresses, and occurs even with low concentrations of ethanol in the diet. Moreover, this activation appears to be specific to ethanol because maternal nutritional status has no major impact on these effects.[6] In an early study on pituitary-adrenal activity in females consuming moderate doses of ethanol throughout pregnancy, we suggested that ethanol may act on the pregnant female to raise the set point of the homeostatic feedback mechanisms that regulate pituitary-adrenal function.[12] Our more recent data[6] indicate that regular consumption of high doses of ethanol not only raises the set point of pituitary-adrenal function by increasing both basal and stress corticosterone levels during pregnancy, but may also make the HPA axis hyperresponsive to certain stressors. The additional finding[6] that binding capacity of plasma corticosterone binding globulin (CBG) in ethanol-consuming females is similar to or less than that in control group females supports the conclusion that ethanol consumption results in both hypersecretion and hyperresponsiveness of the HPA axis during pregnancy. Furthermore, we have shown that the stimulatory effects of ethanol on the maternal female may continue through parturition.[13] Consistent with the data on pregnant females, we found that relative adrenal weights as well as basal corticosterone levels and the adrenocortical response to stress are also increased in ethanol-consuming dams at parturition. Furthermore, CBG binding capacity does not differ among groups at this time, supporting our suggestion that this increased HPA activation represents a functionally important increase in hormone levels.

The mechanisms of the effects of ethanol on the maternal female remain to be determined. Data suggest that the primary site of action of ethanol is at the level of the hypothalamus; release of endogenous corticotropin-releasing factor (CRF) is an essential mediator of the acute effects of ethanol on pituitary-adrenal activity.[14] However, it has been shown that ethanol may also directly stimulate adrenocorticotropin (ACTH) release from rat anterior pituitary cells *in vitro*.[15,16] *In vitro* studies have further shown that ethanol or acetaldehyde can directly stimulate corticosterone production and secretion from perfused rat adrenal glands.[17] Together, these data suggest that the effects of maternal ethanol consumption on HPA activity during pregnancy probably result from a combination of central and direct actions.

Because the pregnant female and the fetus constitute an interrelated functional unit, the data on ethanol-induced changes in maternal hormonal activity during pregnancy clearly have implications for fetal hormonal development. Ethanol can cross the placenta and directly activate the fetal HPA axis, which is functional before birth.[18] Alternatively, ethanol can act indirectly through effects on maternal HPA activity. Because corticoids can cross the placenta in both directions,[18] an alcohol-induced increase in maternal corticoids could suppress the fetal HPA axis and possibly have permanent organizational effects on neural structures that regulate pituitary-adrenal activity throughout life.[19] The complex interaction of these two prenatal influences is apparent in offspring in the perinatal period. Ethanol-exposed fetuses (E) were found to have greater relative adrenal weights but lower plasma corticosterone levels than pair-fed (PF) and control (C) fetuses on day 21 of gestation.[13] Immediately after parturition, neonates exposed to ethanol *in utero* have elevated plasma and brain concentrations of corticosterone as well as elevated plasma levels and reduced pituitary content of β-EP compared to controls.[13,20–22] Furthermore, during the preweaning period (approximately the first three weeks of life), E offspring exhibit suppressed adrenocortical and β-EP responses to a wide range of stressors including ether, novelty, saline injection, and cold stress, as well as to drugs such as ethanol and morphine.[13,20,23] The meaning of this reduced hormonal responsiveness in E pups remains to be determined. Evidence from our work indicates that in addition to the reduced adrenocortical response to stressors, plasma CBG binding capacity is also reduced in E compared to PF and C pups during the first week of life.[13] It is known that a large proportion of circulating corticosterone is bound to CBG, and it is generally accepted that biological activity is limited to only the unbound form of this hormone[24] (although under certain conditions the bound form of the hormone may be active[25]). Therefore, it is possible that although the adrenocortical stress response is reduced in pups that were exposed to ethanol, the ratio of bound to free steroids may not be altered. That is, a reduction in CBG binding capacity may represent a compensatory response to maintain normal neuroendocrine function in E offspring.

Interestingly, the reduced HPA and β-EP responsiveness observed in E pups during the preweaning period is a transient phenomenon. Our data[13] and that of others[20,23] indicate that stress responsiveness is normalized by the second to third week of life. Moreover, from weaning age on, E animals are typically hyperresponsive to stressors. Enhanced pituitary-adrenal activation to footshock, ether, neurogenic stressors, and drugs such as ethanol and morphine, and a significant increase in CRF biosynthesis and expression, as well as significantly increased β-EP responses to cold and ether stress have been reported in E animals compared to controls.[12,20,26–29] Furthermore, E animals may exhibit more prolonged corticosterone elevations after stress, suggesting deficits in adrenocortical response inhibition or recovery to basal levels.[29,30]

An interesting finding in many of the studies cited above is that females appear to be more vulnerable than males to the effects of *in utero* ethanol exposure on stress responsiveness. Data from Taylor and coworkers demonstrating HPA hyperresponsiveness in E animals were derived primarily from females.[28,31,32] Studies in our laboratory found deficits in adrenocortical response inhibition or recovery following restraint stress only in E females; E males were similar to their respective controls.[29] Similarly, a recent study by Kelly *et al.*[33] reported that early postnatal ethanol exposure results in adrenocortical hyperresponsiveness in a forced swimming task in female but not male offspring. However, our more recent data[30] suggest that under appropriate conditions, pituitary-adrenal hyperresponsiveness and/or deficits in recovery after stress may be demonstrated in E males as well. In previous studies, acute rather than chronic stressors and/or stressors of relatively short duration were typically used. We found that in response to a prolonged stressor (4-h restraint stress), although E males are not different from controls in their initial response to restraint, they show a greater and more prolonged corticosterone elevation over the 4-hour stress period. Interestingly, under these conditions, E females do not differ significantly from their controls.

Further studies suggest that prenatal exposure to ethanol may differentially affect male and female offspring at different levels of the HPA axis and β-EP system. In a series of experiments,[34,35] we examined the effects of fetal ethanol exposure on the response to repeated exposures to a stressor (60 min daily restraint stress for 5 or 10 days). Data indicated that males from E, PF, and C conditions do not differ significantly from each other in plasma corticosterone or adrenocorticotropin (ACTH) levels following either single or multiple exposures to restraint. However, E males exhibit a significantly greater β-EP response than controls after repeated restraint. In contrast, E females show significantly greater corticosterone and ACTH levels than controls after repeated restraint stress, but do not differ from controls in their β-EP response. Thus it appears that the parameters of the test situation, the nature and intensity of the stressor, the time course that is measured, and the level of the stress axis that is examined all play a role in determining whether E offspring differ from controls in stress responsiveness and whether differential effects of fetal ethanol exposure are observed in males and females.

In addition to alterations in pituitary-adrenal activation and recovery following stress, E offspring also appear to exhibit deficits in ability to use or respond to environmental cues. For example, we found that when allowed access to water in a novel environment, E females show a significantly smaller decrease in plasma corticosterone levels than PF and C females.[29] Previous data indicate that it is the psychological rather than the physiological aspects of consummatory behavior that modulate the pituitary-adrenal stress response to a novel environment. For example, exposure to cues associated with eating or drinking, or opportunity to chew a nonnutritive inert substance, is as effective as eating or drinking in reducing adrenocortical activity in food or water-deprived animals.[36–38] The finding that E females show deficits in pituitary-adrenal response inhibition in a consummatory task suggests that E females may have a deficit in their ability to use the cues associated with drinking to reduce their adrenocortical response to the novel environment. Further evidence for a deficit in ability to use environmental cues comes from another study demonstrating that the plasma corticosterone response of E females to predictable (PRED) and unpredictable (UNPRED) restraint stress differs from that of C females.[39] We found that C females have higher basal corticosterone levels if previously subjected to PRED restraint than if previously subjected to UNPRED restraint, whereas they have higher stress levels of corticosterone in response to UNPRED restraint than in response to PRED restraint. E females do not show this differential responsiveness. In this task, E males do not differ significantly from their controls. Together, the data from these two studies suggest that prenatal ethanol exposure may alter adrenocortical responsiveness to psychological stressors, and may result in deficits in the development of expectancies or in the ability to use or respond to behavioral or environmental cues. Furthermore, it appears that these deficits in responsiveness to behavioral cues occur selectively in E females.

These data may have important clinical implications. Children prenatally exposed to alcohol are known to be hyperactive, uninhibited, impulsive in behavior, and to have attentional deficits that may reflect an inability to inhibit responses.[40,41] These behavioral deficits are particularly noticeable in challenging or stressful situations.[41] The data presented above suggest that hyperresponsiveness of the HPA axis and/or deficits in HPA response inhibition or recovery after stress could accompany or perhaps even exacerbate these behavioral deficits, because CRF, ACTH, and the glucocorticoids are known to have modulatory effects on behavioral responses to stressful situations.[42]

The mechanisms underlying hyperresponsiveness of the HPA axis and β-EP system of E offspring are unknown at present. One possibility is that prenatal ethanol exposure results in a deficit in feedback control of pituitary-adrenal activity. The hippocampus is the principal site for glucocorticoid feedback in the brain and plays a critical role in terminating the pituitary-adrenal response to stress.[42,43] We hypothesized that an ethanol-induced decrease in hippocampal glucocorticoid receptor concentration might, at least in part, mediate the increased stress responsiveness, as well as the deficits in recovery from stress that occur in E offspring. To test this hypothesis, the concentration of hippocampal cytosolic glucocorticoid receptors in adult offspring from E and control conditions was measured.[44] Data indicated that no significant differences exist in specific binding or binding affinity of glucocorticoid receptors among animals from E, PF, and C groups tested under basal (i.e., nonstressed) conditions. However, these data do not preclude the possibility that receptor binding capacity may be differentially affected in E animals compared to controls during stress. This possibility is currently being investigated. It is also possible that feedback control of the HPA axis is intact at the level of the hippocampus but is deficient at the level of the hypothalamus or pituitary. Two studies by Taylor and coworkers[31,32] provide support for this possibility. In one study,[32] it was found that E animals show more prolonged elevations of plasma ACTH than PF and C animals after footshock stress. In a subsequent study,[31] ACTH levels after two episodes of footshock stress, separated by a 5-minute interval, were measured. The peak ACTH response occurred at 5 minutes after the second shock in all groups; however, ACTH levels in E rats were significantly higher than levels in PF and C rats at this time. By 10 minutes after the second shock, ACTH levels in all groups had declined and no longer differed from each other. These data indicate that the ACTH response of E rats to multiple stress presented in the time domain of fast feedback is enhanced. Together, these studies support the hypothesis that feedback inhibition is either impaired or delayed in E rats compared to animals in the control groups.

Fetal ethanol exposure may also alter responsiveness of the HPA axis through its effects on central neurotransmitter systems that regulate HPA function. Hypothalamic CRF is the major central mediator of ACTH secretion, although it is known to act in concert with other hypophysiotropic factors such as vasopressin and epinephrine. Data indicate that CRF release is stimulated by acetylcholine and epinephrine in a dose-dependent manner and by low doses of norepinephrine, and is inhibited by γ-aminobutyric acid (GABA), β-EP, and dynorphin.[45,46] Acetylcholine, norepinephrine, and epinephrine also appear to be stimulatory to ACTH secretion at the level of the pituitary.[46] Data from a recent study[47] indicate that cortical and hypothalamic norepinephrine content is reduced in E animals compared to controls. If this decrease in catecholamine content is indicative of depletion of norepinephrine resulting from an increase in neuronal activity (turnover), then it is possible that an alteration in catecholaminergic regulation of CRF secretion induced by fetal ethanol exposure may play a role in mediating the increased HPA activity observed in E offspring. Some support for this hypothesis is provided by data from Lee et al.,[26] indicating that the increased stress-induced ACTH response of E compared to control offspring is accompanied by significantly elevated CRF mRNA levels in the hypothalamus.

EFFECTS OF FETAL ALCOHOL EXPOSURE ON IMMUNOCOMPETENCE

The issue of immune dysfunction in association with FAS has only recently begun to receive attention. In clinical studies, an increased incidence of serious illnesses such as pneumonia and meningitis, and of minor infections such as otitis media, gastroenteritis, urinary tract infections, and recurrent upper respiratory tract infections have been observed in children with FAS.[48,49] In addition, immune system abnormalities such as reduced numbers of total circulating lymphocytes, diminished responsiveness of lymphocytes to mitogens, and hypogammaglobulinemia have been reported.[48]

Studies of immune status in animals exposed to ethanol *in utero* have substantiated the clinical evidence of impaired immunity associated with FAS. Using flow cytometry, several investigators have shown that in mice, prenatal or early postnatal ethanol exposure may alter the development of T lymphocyte populations, resulting in a general decrease in thymus cell number in the fetus, as well as reduced numbers of T-helper and T-cytotoxic/suppressor lymphocytes both in the fetus and in mice of weaning age.[50–52] Adverse effects of ethanol on cell-mediated immune functions such as contact hypersensitivity and graft-versus-host response have also been observed in adult mice after prenatal exposure.[53] Offspring of female rats exposed to high doses of ethanol throughout gestation were shown to have reduced numbers of thymocytes, a reduced proliferative response of splenic and thymic T lymphocytes to mitogens, and reduced responsiveness of splenic and thymic T lymphoblasts to interleukin-2 (IL-2), a cytokine necessary for lymphocyte proliferation.[54–56] Impaired responsiveness to cytokines would be expected to have a profound effect on the immunocompetence of the host because cytokines play key roles in stimulating and promoting a variety of immune responses. Importantly, our data[56] are the first to report a long-term sex difference in the effects of ethanol on the immune system of offspring exposed *in utero*. We found that fetal ethanol-exposed females are relatively normal in immunocompetence compared to their respective controls, whereas fetal ethanol-exposed males show long-term immunological impairments, primarily in T-cell responses. In addition, we have recently shown (unpublished data) that prenatal ethanol exposure may alter receptor expression of specific lymphocyte populations. In adulthood, E animals show increased pan T lymphocyte receptor expression in peripheral blood, stress-induced increases in CD8 receptor expression in the lymph node, and decreased CD4 receptor expression in the thymus, compared to controls. Prenatal ethanol exposure has also been shown to disrupt the development of synaptic elements of the sympathetic nervous system, and to do so selectively in lymphoid organs. Reduced norepinephrine levels and β-adrenoceptor density in lymphoid organs[57] as well as altered noradrenergic synaptic transmission in the spleen and thymus[53] are observed, all of which may affect immune responsiveness.

The immunosuppression noted in adult animals in response to ethanol consumption has been shown to be mediated partially by adrenocorticosteroids.[58,59] The role of adrenocorticosteroids in mediating the immunosuppressive effects of prenatal ethanol exposure remains to be elucidated. As discussed, maternal ethanol consumption markedly alters development and responsiveness of the HPA axis in the offspring. Hyperresponsiveness of the HPA axis and/or deficits in recovery after stress could have adverse consequences for metabolic and immune system functions and could thus play some role in mediating the immunological impairments noted in fetal ethanol-exposed animals. Alternatively, in view of the finding that fetal ethanol exposure appears to have greater effects on immune function of male than of female offspring, it is possible that the sex hormones may be involved in mediating the immunosuppressive effects of ethanol. The complex influence of sex hormones on the immune system is beginning to be appreciated. It has been suggested that a hypothalamic-pituitary-gonadal (HPG)-thymic axis exists that results in regulation of the immune system through alterations in thymic hormone production.[60,61] Prenatal exposure to ethanol is known to have adverse effects on the HPG axis of both males and females.[62] Thus it is possible that ethanol exposure *in utero* may act on the developing HPG-thymic axis to disturb the hormone balance in this system, resulting in deficits in immunocompetence. Finally, it is possible that altered neurotransmitter levels, β-adrenergic receptors, and/or noradrenergic synaptic transmission within the lymphoid organs, as described by Gottesfeld and coworkers,[53,57] mediate, at least in part, the immunological deficits observed in E animals.

EARLY EXPERIENCE MAY ALTER EFFECTS OF FETAL ALCOHOL EXPOSURE

Experiences that occur during sensitive periods in the development of an organism can markedly alter developmental processes, as well as subsequent behavioral and physiological reactivity, and even susceptibility to disease and ultimate survival. One of the simplest and most frequently studied forms of early experience is infantile stimulation or early handling.[63] In the typical early handling procedure, the maternal female is removed from the home cage and pups are then removed into separate holding compartments for a short time (periods of 3–15 min have been used). The dam and pups are then returned to the home cage. This procedure is usually repeated daily during the preweaning period, although the critical period for effects of early handling appears to be approximately the first 10–14 days of life. Animals handled in infancy typically mature more rapidly and show an earlier onset of the adrenocortical circadian rhythm.[63] When tested in adulthood, handled (H) animals explore more than nonhandled (NH) animals in open-field and hole-board tasks,[64,65] perform better in some avoidance learning paradigms, and are less reactive in reaction-to-handling tests.[66] Moreover, the corticosterone response of H animals is generally lower than that of NH animals in response to mild stressors (e.g., novelty), whereas after severe stressors (e.g., shock), H animals respond more quickly, with a greater initial corticoid elevation, and show a faster recovery toward basal levels.[67] These data suggest that H animals are less emotional and show more adaptive responses to stressors than NH animals.

Data from our laboratory indicate that early handling may attenuate both behavioral and physiological deficits shown by fetal ethanol-exposed animals. For example, we have studied the effects of early handling on performance of E, PF, and C animals in a passive avoidance task in which animals had to learn to stay up on a small platform in order to avoid shock.[68] We found that all animals learn the task equally well. However, on the extinction test day, NH E offspring have more step-down attempts than NH PF and C offspring. Early handling attenuates this deficit, that is, no significant differences in performance exist among H animals from the three prenatal treatment groups.

Early handling also appears to attenuate the degree of ethanol-induced hypothermia exhibited by E animals.[69] After a challenge dose (2 g/kg, i.p.) of ethanol, all animals show a significant hypothermic response. For NH males, however, hypothermia is greater in E and PF than in C animals. Early handling eliminates the differences among groups. In contrast, E, PF, and C females in both the H and NH conditions are not significantly different from each other in their hypothermic response to ethanol. These data suggest that fetal ethanol exposure may affect males more than females in terms of vulnerability to the hypothermic effects of ethanol challenge in adulthood. Furthermore, the finding that PF males show a response similar to that of E males indicates that ethanol-induced nutritional effects play a role in mediating these adverse effects of fetal ethanol exposure.

Finally, we have shown that early handling may alter adrenocortical responsiveness of E animals to restraint stress.[70] In this study, E females were exposed to a 3-hour restraint stress, and a plasma corticosterone time course was determined. NH E females showed a significantly greater corticoid response to restraint at 30 minutes and higher corticoid levels at 180 minutes compared to NH PF and C females. Early handling attenuated the hyperresponsiveness of E females at 30 minutes, but not the higher corticoid levels found at 180 minutes. Thus it appears that early handling can modulate some but not all aspects of the adrenocortical response to stressors in females prenatally exposed to ethanol.

CONCLUDING REMARKS

The data presented in this review clearly demonstrate the impact of maternal ethanol consumption on endocrine and immune function of the offspring. Proper maternal-fetal hormone balance is essential to insure a successful pregnancy outcome; the female's ability to maintain a normal pregnancy and the balanced hormonal interactions between maternal and fetal systems may be compromised by ethanol-induced disruption of maternal endocrine activity.[8] In addition, ethanol readily crosses the placenta and thus may have direct effects on fetal metabolic and physiological functions. Clearly, altered endocrine balance induced directly or indirectly by maternal ethanol consumption may be one of the factors mediating abnormal physiological and behavioral development in offspring prenatally exposed to ethanol. In addition, the data presented in this review indicate that ethanol may be teratogenic to the developing immune system. The mechanisms responsible have not yet been identified; however, a combination of variables is likely involved, including direct effects of ethanol on the ontogeny of immune system components and the disruption of the bidirectional communication that occurs between the immune and neuroendocrine systems.[71] The evidence clearly suggests that the immunoteratogenic effects of ethanol result in long-lasting immunological impairments.

The studies described in this review further demonstrate that male and female offspring may be differentially affected by prenatal exposure to ethanol depending upon the developmental period during which exposure occurs, the parameters of the test situation, and the end-points measured. If only male or only female offspring are utilized in studies of fetal ethanol exposure, the true impact of the teratogenic effects of alcohol may be underestimated or misinterpreted.

Finally, the data presented here indicate that deficits that occur in fetal ethanol-exposed offspring may be subtle or may become apparent only when the offspring are challenged, either physically or psychologically. When tested under basal or non-stressed conditions, E offspring are often similar to controls in behavioral and physiological responsiveness. However, when challenged with stressors, hormones or pharmacological agents, or when placed in behaviorally challenging situations, deficits or alterations in responsiveness are revealed. Moreover, data indicate that early (preweaning) experience can modulate the impact of fetal ethanol exposure on both behavioral and physiological development. Further research will enable us to begin to unravel the mechanisms underlying the effects of *in utero* ethanol exposure on offspring development. Clearly, the study of ethanol-induced endocrine disturbances in maternal and offspring systems can provide important insight into factors that may mediate some of the long-term effects of ethanol on behavioral and physiological development of offspring.

REFERENCES

1. JONES, K., D. SMITH, C. ULLELAND & A. STREISSGUTH. 1973. Pattern of malformation in offspring of chronic alcoholic mothers. Lancet 1: 1267–1271.
2. MELLO, N. K., J. H. MENDELSON & S. K. TEOH. 1989. Neuroendocrine consequences of alcohol abuse in women. Ann. N.Y. Acad. Sci. 562: 211–240.
3. VAN THIEL, D. H. & J. S. GAVALER. 1982. The adverse effects of ethanol upon hypothalamic-pituitary-gonadal function in males and females compared and contrasted. Alcohol. Clin. Exp. Res. 6: 179–185.
4. KRUGER, W. A., W. J. BO & P. K. RUDEEN. 1983. Estrous cyclicity in rats fed an ethanol diet for four months. Pharmacol. Biochem. Behav. 19: 583–585.
5. LEE, M. & K. WAKABAYASHI. 1986. Pituitary and thyroid hormones in pregnant alcohol-fed rats and their fetuses. Alcohol. Clin. Exp. Res. 10: 428–431.
6. WEINBERG, J. & S. BEZIO. 1987. Alcohol-induced changes in pituitary-adrenal activity during pregnancy. Alcohol. Clin. Exp. Res. 11: 274–280.
7. YLIKORKALA, O., U-H. STENMAN & E. HALMESMAKI. 1988. Testosterone androstenedione, dehydroepiandrosterone sulfate and sex hormone binding globulin in pregnant alcohol abusers. Obstet. Gynecol. 71: 731–735.
8. ANDERSON, R. A. 1981. Endocrine balance as a factor in the etiology of the fetal alcohol syndrome. Neurobehav. Toxicol. Teratol. 3: 89–104.
9. MERRY, J. & B. MARKS. 1973. Hypothalamic-pituitary-adrenal function in chronic alcoholics. In Alcohol Intoxication and Withdrawal: Experimental Studies. Advances in Experimental Medicine and Biology. M. M. Gross, Ed. Vol. 35: 167– 179. Plenum Press. New York, NY.
10. ROOT, A. W., E. O. REITER, M. ANDRIOLA & G. DUCKETT. 1975. Hypothalamic-pituitary function in the fetal alcohol syndrome. J. Pediatr. 87: 585–588.
11. BINKIEWICZ, A., M. J. ROBINSON & B. SENIOR. 1978. Pseudo-Cushing syndrome caused by alcohol in breast milk. J. Pediatr. 6: 965–967.
12. WEINBERG, J. & P. V. GALLO. 1982. Prenatal ethanol exposure: Pituitary-adrenal activity in pregnant dams and offspring. Neurobehav. Toxicol. Teratol. 4: 515–520.
13. WEINBERG, J. 1989. Prenatal ethanol exposure alters adrenocortical development of offspring. Alcohol. Clin. Exp. Res. 13: 73–83.
14. RIVIER, C., T. BRUHN & W. VALE. 1986. Effect of ethanol on the hypothalamic-pituitary-adrenal axis in the rat: Role of corticotropin releasing factor (CRF). J. Pharmacol. Exp. Ther. 237: 59–64.
15. REDEI, E., B. J. BRANCH & A. N. TAYLOR. 1986. Direct effect of ethanol on adrenocorticotropin (ACTH) release in vitro. J. Pharmacol. Exp. Ther. 237: 59–64.
16. KEITH, L. D., J. C. CRABBE, L. M. ROBERTSON & J. W. KENDALL. 1986. Ethanol-stimulated endorphin and corticotropin secretion in vitro. Brain Res. 367: 222–229.
17. COBB, C. F., D. H. VAN THIEL, S. GAVALER & R. LESTER. 1981. Effects of ethanol and acetaldehyde on the rat adrenal. Metabolism 30: 537–543.
18. EGUCHI, Y. 1969. Interrelationships between the foetal and maternal hypophyseal-adrenal axes in rats and mice. In Physiology and Pathology of Adaptation Mechanisms. E. Bajusz, Ed.: 3–27. Pergamon Press. New York, NY.
19. LEVINE, S. & R. F. MULLINS. 1966. Hormonal influences on brain organization in infant rats. Science 152: 1585–1592.
20. ANGELOGIANNI, P. & C. GIANOULAKIS. 1989. Prenatal exposure to ethanol alters the ontogeny of the β-endorphin response to stress. Alcohol. Clin. Exp. Res. 13: 564–571.
21. TAYLOR, A. N., B. J. BRANCH, N. KOKKA & R. E. POLAND. 1983. Neonatal and long-term neuroendocrine effects of fetal alcohol exposure. Monogr. Neural Sci. 9: 140–152.
22. KAKIHANA, R., J. C. BUTTE & J. A. MOORE. 1980. Endocrine effects of maternal alcoholization: Plasma and brain testosterone, dihydrotestosterone, estradiol, and corticosterone. Alcohol. Clin. Exp. Res. 1: 57–61.
23. TAYLOR, A. N., B. J. BRANCH, L. R. NELSON, L. A. LANE & R. E. POLAND. 1986. Prenatal ethanol and ontogeny of pituitary-adrenal responses to ethanol and morphine. Alcohol 3: 255–259.
24. BALLARD, P. L. 1979. Delivery and transport of glucocorticoids to target cells. In

Monographs on Endocrinology. Glucocorticoid Hormone Action. J. D. Barter & G. G. Rousseau, Eds. Vol. **12:** 25–45. Springer-Verlag. Berlin.

25. ROSNER, W. & R. HOCHBERG. 1972. Corticosteroid-binding globulin in the rat. Isolation and studies of its influence on cortisol action in vivo. Endocrinology **91:** 626–632.

26. LEE, S., T. IMAKI, W. VALE & C. RIVIER. 1990. Effect of prenatal exposure to ethanol on the activity of the hypothalamic-pituitary-adrenal axis of the offspring: Importance of the time of exposure to ethanol and possible modulating mechanisms. Mol. Cell. Neurosci. **1:** 168–177.

27. NELSON, L. R., A. N. TAYLOR, J. W. LEWIS, R. E. POLAND, E. REDEI & B. J. BRANCH. 1986. Pituitary-adrenal responses to morphine and footshock stress are enhanced following prenatal alcohol exposure. Alcohol. Clin. Exp. Res. **10:** 397–402.

28. TAYLOR, A. N., B. J. BRANCH, S. H. LIU & N. KOKKA. 1982. Long-term effects of fetal ethanol exposure on pituitary-adrenal responses to stress. Pharmacol. Biochem. Behav. **16:** 585–589.

29. WEINBERG, J. 1988. Hyperresponsiveness to stress: Differential effects of prenatal ethanol on males and females. Alcohol. Clin. Exp. Res. **12:** 647–652.

30. WEINBERG, J. 1992. Prenatal ethanol effects: Sex differences in offspring stress responsiveness. Alcohol **9:** 219–223.

31. TAYLOR, A. N., B. J. BRANCH, J. E. VAN ZUYLEN & E. REDEI. 1988. Maternal alcohol consumption and stress responsiveness in offspring. *In* Mechanisms of Physical and Emotional Stress. Advances in Experimental Medicine and Biology. G. P. Chrousos, D. L. Loriaux & P. W. Gold, Eds. Vol. **245:** 311–317. Plenum Press. New York, NY.

32. TAYLOR, A. N., B. J. BRANCH, J. E. VAN ZUYLEN & E. REDEI. 1986. Prenatal ethanol exposure alters ACTH stress response in adult rats. Alcohol. Clin. Exp. Res. **10:** 120.

33. KELLY, S. J., J. C. MAHONEY, A. RANDICH & J. R. WEST. 1991. Indices of stress in rats: Effects of sex, perinatal alcohol and artificial rearing. Physiol. Behav. **49:** 751–756.

34. WEINBERG, J. & C. GIANOULAKIS. 1991. Fetal ethanol exposure alters glucocorticoid and β-endorphin responses to stress. Soc. Neurosci. Abstr. **17:** 1596.

35. WEINBERG, J., A. N. TAYLOR & C. GIANOULAKIS. Prenatal ethanol exposure alters pituitary-adrenal and β-endorphin responses to stress. In preparation.

36. COOVER, G. D., B. R. SUTTON & J. P. HEYBACH. 1977. Conditioning decreases in plasma corticosterone level in rats by pairing stimuli with daily feedings. J. Comp. Physiol. Psychol. **91:** 716–726.

37. HENNESSY, M. B. & T. FOY. 1987. Nonedible material elicits chewing and reduces the plasma corticosterone response during novelty exposure in mice. Behav. Neurosci. **101:** 237–245.

38. WEINBERG, J. & R. WONG. 1983. Consummatory behavior and adrenocortical responsiveness in the hamster. Physiol. Behav. **31:** 7–12.

39. WEINBERG, J. 1992. Prenatal ethanol exposure alters adrenocortical response to predictable and unpredictable stressors. Alcohol **9:** 427–432.

40. STREISSGUTH, A. N., H. M. BARR, P. D. SAMPSON, J. C. PARRISH-JOHNSON, G. L. KIRCHNER & D. C. MARTIN. 1986. Attention, distraction and reaction time at age 7 years and prenatal alcohol exposure. Neurobehav. Toxicol. Teratol. **8:** 717–725.

41. STREISSGUTH, A. N., S. K. CLARREN & K. L. JONES. 1985. Natural history of the fetal alcohol syndrome: A 10-year follow-up of eleven patients. Lancet **1:** 85–92.

42. MCEWEN, B. S., E. R. DEKLOET & W. ROSTENE. 1986. Adrenal steroid receptors and actions in the nervous system. Physiol. Rev. **66:** 1121–1188.

43. SAPOLSKY, R. M., L. C. KREY & B. MCEWEN. 1984. Glucocorticoid-sensitive hippocampal neurons are involved in terminating the adrenocortical stress response. Proc. Natl. Acad. Sci. USA **81:** 6174–6177.

44. WEINBERG, J. & T. D. PETERSEN. 1991. Effects of prenatal ethanol exposure on glucocorticoid receptors in rat hippocampus. Alcohol. Clin. Exp. Res. **15:** 711–716.

45. ASSENMACHER, I., A. SZAFARCZYK, G. ALONSO, G. IXART & G. BARBANEL. 1987. Physiology of neural pathways affecting CRH secretion. Ann. N.Y. Acad. Sci. **512:** 149–161.

46. PLOTSKY, P. M. 1987. Regulation of hypophysiotropic factors mediating ACTH secretion. Ann. N.Y. Acad. Sci. **512:** 205–217.

47. RUDEEN, P. K. & J. WEINBERG. Prenatal ethanol exposure: changes in regional brain catecholamine content following stress. J. Neurochem. In press.
48. JOHNSON, S., R. KNIGHT, D. J. MARMER & R. W. STEELE. 1981. Immune deficiency in fetal alcohol syndrome. Pediatr. Res. **15:** 908–911.
49. STEINHAUSEN, H.-C., V. NESTLER & H.-L. SPHOR. 1982. Development and psychopathology of children with the fetal alcohol syndrome. J. Dev. Behav. Ped. **3:** 49–54.
50. EWALD, S. J. 1989. Lymphocyte populations in fetal alcohol syndrome. Alcohol. Clin. Exp. Res. **13:** 485–489.
51. EWALD, S. J. & W. W. FROST. 1987. Effect of prenatal exposure to ethanol on development of the thymus. Thymus **9:** 211–215.
52. GIBERSON, P. K. & B. R. BLAKELY. Effect of postnatal ethanol exposure on expression of differentiation antigens on murine splenic lymphocytes. Alcohol. Clin. Exp. Res. In press.
53. GOTTESFELD, Z., R. CHRISTIE, D. L. FELTEN & S. J. LEGRUE. 1990. Prenatal ethanol exposure alters immune capacity and noradrenergic synaptic transmission in lymphoid organs of the adult mouse. Neuroscience **35:** 185–194.
54. NORMAN, D. C., M. P. CHANG, S. C. CASTLE, J. E. VAN ZUYLEN & A. N. TAYLOR. 1989. Diminished proliferative response of Con A-blast cells to interleukin 2 in adult rats exposed to ethanol in utero. Alcohol. Clin. Exp. Res. **13:** 69–72.
55. REDEI, E., W. R. CLARK & R. F. MCGIVERN. 1989. Alcohol exposure in utero results in diminished T cell function and alterations in brain corticotropin-releasing factor and ACTH content. Alcohol. Clin. Exp. Res. **13:** 439–443.
56. WEINBERG, J. & T. R. JERRELLS. 1991. Suppression of immune responsiveness: Sex differences in prenatal ethanol effects. Alcohol. Clin. Exp. Res. **15:** 525–531.
57. GOTTESFELD, Z., B. MORGAN & J. R. PEREZ-POLO. 1990. Prenatal alcohol exposure alters the development of sympathetic synaptic components and of nerve growth factor receptor expression selectivity in lymphoid organs. J. Neurosci. Res. **26:** 308–316.
58. JERRELLS, T. R., C. A. MARIETTA, F. F. WEIGHT & M. J. ECKARDT. 1990. Effect of adrenalectomy on ethanol-associated immunosuppression. Int. J. Immunopharmacol. **12:** 435–442.
59. MUNCK, A., P. M. GUYRE & N. J. HOLBROOK. 1984. Physiological functions of glucocorticoids in stress and their relation to pharmacological actions. Endocr. Rev. **5:** 25–44.
60. GROSSMAN, C. J. 1985. Interactions between the gonadal steroids and the immune system. Science **227:** 257–261.
61. GROSSMAN, C. J. 1990. Are there underlying immune-neuroendocrine interactions responsible for immunological sexual dimorphism? Prog. NeuroEndocrinImmunol. **3:** 75–82.
62. WEINBERG, J. 1993. Prenatal alcohol exposure: Endocrine function of offspring. In Alcohol and the Endocrine System. S. Zakhari, Ed. NIAAA Research Monograph **23:** 363–382. U.S. Department of Health and Human Services, NIH, NIΛΛΛ. Bethesda, MD.
63. LEVINE, S. 1960. Stimulation in infancy. Sci. Am. **202:** 80–86.
64. LEVINE, S., G. C. HALTMEYER, G. KARAS & V. DENENBERG. 1967. Physiological and behavioral effects of infantile stimulation. Physiol. Behav. **2:** 55–59.
65. WEINBERG, J., E. A. KRAHN & S. LEVINE. 1978. Differential effects of handling on exploration in male and female rats. Dev. Psychobiol. **11:** 251–259.
66. ADER, R. 1965. Effects of early experience and differential housing on behavior and susceptibility to gastric erosions in the rat. J. Comp. Physiol. Psychol. **60:** 233–238.
67. LEVINE, S. 1962. Plasma-free corticosteroid response to electric shock in rats stimulated in infancy. Science **135:** 795–796.
68. GALLO, P. V. & J. WEINBERG. 1982. Neuromotor development and response inhibition following prenatal ethanol exposure. Neurobehav. Toxicol. Teratol. **4:** 505–513.
69. WEINBERG, J. 1990. Early handling modifies hypothermic responses of rats exposed to ethanol in utero. Soc. Neurosci. Abstr. **16:** 755.
70. WEINBERG, J. 1989. Early handling effects on adrenocortical responsiveness following prenatal ethanol exposure. Alcohol. Clin. Exp. Res. **13:** 321.
71. GIBERSON, P. K. & J. WEINBERG. 1992. Fetal alcohol syndrome and functioning of the immune system. Alcohol Health and Research World **16:** 29–38.

Effect of Peripheral and Central Cytokines on the Hypothalamic-Pituitary-Adrenal Axis of the Rat[a]

CATHERINE RIVIER

The Clayton Foundation Laboratories for Peptide Biology
The Salk Institute
La Jolla, California 92037

An essential requisite for the survival of mammalian organisms is the maintenance of homeostasis. Among the homeostatic systems, the immune and the endocrine axes have special relevance for restoring the physiological balance when challenged by antigens. Although long considered virtually independent of each other, these axes are now known to communicate via common ligands and receptors.[1–3] Thus it is believed that the occurrence of immune activation must be conveyed to the brain in order to allow the coordination of the appropriate metabolic, behavioral, and endocrine changes necessary for the restoration of homeostasis. In this concept, the hypothalamus, a brain area containing many of the peptides that modulate neuroendocrine functions,[4] is considered central to the bilateral functional communication pathways between the immune and the neuroendocrine axes.

Increased production of interleukins or cytokines, proteins released by activated macrophages upon presentation of an antigen,[5,6] represents an essential feature of the early events of immune activation called the "acute-phase response."[7] Although a primary function of these proteins is directed towards expansion of the immunologic mass and activity by stimulating the production of growth factors, cytokines also reach the general circulation, and thus can act on distant endocrine organs. Specifically, increased release of hormones such as ACTH and corticosteroids in response to immune challenges is considered important in eliciting the negative-feedback mechanism that prevents overproduction of interleukins.[8–12]

The first demonstration of a possible link between the immune system and the hypothalamic-pituitary-adrenal (HPA) axis came from the report that rats injected with sheep red blood cells showed increases in plasma corticosterone levels that paralleled their immune response.[13] This led to the proposal that activated immune cells released "signals" (now known to be interleukins, ILs), which stimulate the activity of the HPA axis. We reasoned that if this hypothesis were correct, we should be able to demonstrate that increased levels of endogenous ILs such as those caused by the administration of endotoxins,[14] or the injection of exogenous ILs, should release ACTH and corticosterone. Indeed, we[15–17] and others[18–20] reported that both endotoxins (lipopolysaccharides, LPS) and IL-1α or IL-1β caused dose-related increases in plasma ACTH and corticosterone levels. The inability of IL-1 to acutely stimulate ACTH secretion by pituitary cells cultured in the absence of endotoxin suggested that ILs acted within the central nervous system (CNS), and, indeed, we observed significant increases in corticotropin-releasing factor (CRF) concentrations

[a] This work was supported by NIH grant DK26741.

97

in the portal circulation of rats injected with IL-1α.[21] In agreement with the importance of endogenous CRF in mediating the stimulatory action of IL on the HPA axis, we subsequently found that immunoneutralization of CRF,[21] or lesions of the paraventricular nucleus (PVN) of the hypothalamus[22] (the primary source of CRF released to the pituitary[23]), significantly blunted IL-1-induced ACTH secretion.

POSSIBLE MECHANISMS—CATECHOLAMINES AND PROSTAGLANDINS

Several questions then arose: Do ILs act directly on CRF perikarya, or is their stimulatory action mediated through secretagogues? Furthermore, can ILs reach the PVN, or do they primarily release CRF from nerve terminals in the median eminence?

Evidence exists that ILs stimulate CRF release by isolated hypothalamic fragments[24,25] or upon direct infusion into the hypothalamus,[26] thus supporting a direct effect of these cytokines on CRF-secreting cells. However, this does not necessarily mean that activation of other pathways is not also relevant. In particular, we investigated the potential mediating role of circulating catecholamines (which are released by ILs[17] and stimulate the HPA axis both at the level of the pituitary[27,28] and the CNS[29]); and that of prostaglandins (PGs), which are also elevated in the presence of increased IL secretion.[5,30,31]

We observed that blockade of adrenergic receptors, a treatment that totally abolished epinephrine-induced ACTH secretion, did not measurably alter the stimulatory effect of IL-1α.[17] Thus an increase in circulating catecholamines does not appear as a major mechanism of IL-1-induced activation of the HPA axis. The effect of IL on CRF released by isolated hypothalamic fragments is blocked by indomethacin,[32,33] suggesting the importance of eicosanoid pathways in this process. Indeed, several investigators have reported that in the rat, acute treatment with indomethacin totally abolished the effect of IL on the HPA axis.[34-36] Subsequent studies from our laboratory, however, have suggested that the role of PGs is only partial and may depend on the corticosteroid milieu.[37] Furthermore, a recent report showed that at least in mice, the route of IL administration is important in determining whether activation of PG-dependent pathways is involved.[38] We therefore conducted a series of studies aimed at investigating whether this was also true in rats. We carried out several experiments using three routes of injection in each: intravenous (i.v.), intraperitoneal (i.p.), and intracerebroventricular (i.c.v.). All three routes caused significant increases in circulating ACTH levels, although neither the vehicle (FIG. 1) nor indomethacin alone (not shown) measurably stimulated ACTH release. After i.v. or i.c.v. injection of IL-1β, we consistently observed that injection of 10 mg/kg indomethacin 15 minutes prior to administration of the cytokine virtually blocked ACTH secretion at all times studied (FIG. 1). In contrast, results from i.p. injections were inconsistent. As illustrated in FIG. 2, the ability of indomethacin to interfere with the effect of IL-1β was variable over the different experiments. Although at present the reasons for these discordant results are not clear, there is no doubt that prior injuries (such as those resulting from inserting the cannulas we use for blood sampling[17]) can release endogenous cytokines and alter the response of the HPA axis to subsequent immune challenges.[39] Whether this phenomenon, or others such as the undocumented presence of infectious or inflammatory processes, might explain our results remains to be determined. These observations nevertheless emphasize the existence of multiple potential pathways in mediating the stimulatory action of ILs on the HPA axis, and suggest that the dependence of the effect of ILs on specific secretagogues might at least in part be related to the nature of the immune challenge.

SITES OF ACTION OF INTERLEUKINS

Another question raised by our results concerns the sites of action of ILs and the potential entry of these large proteins beyond the blood-brain barrier. We showed that lesions of the PVN abolished the stimulatory action of i.c.v. injected IL-1β on the HPA axis.[22] These results, coupled with our observation that the i.c.v. injection of IL-1β caused a significant increase in c-*fos* immunoreactivity in CRF-positive cells of the PVN,[40] strongly support the hypothesis that central administration of IL-1β primarily relies on direct activation of the PVN in order to increase ACTH secretion.

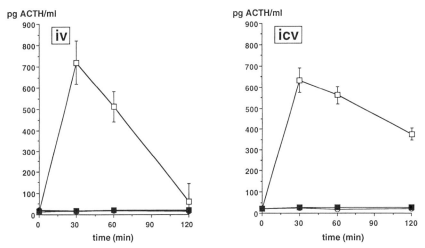

FIGURE 1. Effect of prior (−15 min) injection of indomethacin (10 mg/kg, i.v.) on the stimulatory effect of IL-1β, injected intravenously (300 ng/kg; *left panel*) or intracerebroventricularly (300 ng/kg; *right panel*), on ACTH secretion. Each point represents the means ± SEM of 5–7 rats. *Open squares,* IL-1β; *solid squares,* IL-1β + indomethacin.

In contrast, the i.v. administration of IL-1β, which significantly elevates ACTH levels, does not cause an immediate increase in c-*fos* protein.[40] This led us to propose that peripherally administered IL-1β acts at the level of the median eminence to induce the release of CRF from nerve terminals, a hypothesis supported by the ability of direct infusion of IL-1 into this structure to release ACTH.[41] There is little doubt that during prolonged exposure to cytokines, such as that which occurs during true immune stimulation, both the median eminence and the PVN represent sites at which ILs can stimulate the production of CRF. Increasing evidence also exists that pituitary cells (both corticotropes and folliculo-stellate cells[42,43]) respond to long-term exposure to cytokines[44–46] and could participate in the activation of the HPA axis.[47] Finally, peptides other than CRF, in particular vasopressin, oxytocin, and possibly VIP,[48–52] represent potential and still unexplored modulators of the short- and long-term effect of ILs on the HPA axis.

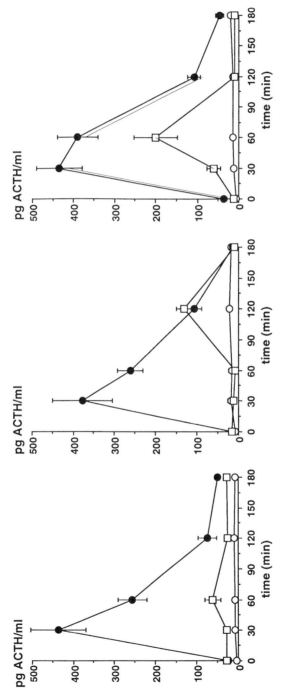

FIGURE 2. Effect of prior (−15 min) injection of indomethacin (10 mg/kg, i.v.) on the stimulatory effect of IL-1β, injected intraperitoneally. Each point represents the means ± SEM of 5–6 rats. *Open circles,* vehicle; *solid circles,* 300 ng IL-1β/kg; *open squares,* IL-1β + indomethacin.

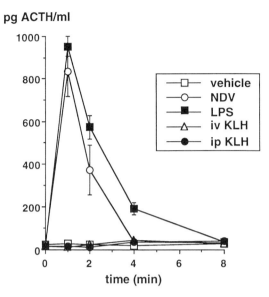

FIGURE 3. Effect of the injection of endotoxin (LPS, 80 μg/kg, i.v.), NDV (7000 HU/kg, i.v.) or KLH (250 μg/kg, i.v. or i.p.) on ACTH secretion. Each point represents the means ± SEM of 5–6 rats.

IMMUNE ACTIVATION AND STIMULATION OF THE HPA AXIS—IS THERE AN OBLIGATORY FUNCTIONAL RELATIONSHIP?

As discussed in the introduction, true immune activation has been linked to activation of the HPA axis.[11,53,54] However, we have been consistently unable to measure any changes in plasma ACTH or corticosterone levels in rats injected with sheep red blood cells obtained from commercial sources (unpublished). We therefore used two other antigens to probe the possible relationship between administration of an antigen and the response of the HPA axis: Newcastle disease virus (NDV)

FIGURE 4. Effect of immunoneutralization of endogenous CRF on NDV-induced ACTH secretion. Blood samples were obtained 1 hour after treatment. Each bar represents the means ± SEM of 5 rats. *Open rectangles,* NSS; *solid rectangles,* anti-CRF serum. $**p < 0.01$.

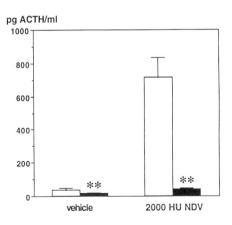

and keyhole limpet hemacyanin coupled to phosphocholine (KLH). As previously reported in mice,[55,56] the i.v. injection of NDV caused a rapid increase in ACTH secretion with a time course of action similar to that of endotoxin (FIG. 3). In support of the observation that the rapid stimulatory effect of NDV on the HPA axis is modulated by endogenous IL-1,[56] we found that immunoneutralization of endogenous CRF completely abolished NDV-induced ACTH release (FIG. 4). The i.v. or i.p. administration of KLH, on the other hand, did not acutely activate the HPA axis (FIG. 3). Monitoring the appearance of specific gamma globulins indicated a peak of IgM values seven days after injection of both 250 and 1000 μg/kg KLH, followed by increasing levels of IgG.[57] However, only injection of the higher dose of KLH was accompanied by a very modest increase in plasma corticosterone (but not ACTH) levels on day 5. These results do not support the hypothesis of an obligatory activation of the HPA axis during the immune response. Our findings, however, must not be interpreted as invalidating the concept of an immune-endocrine loop. As can be intuitively conceived, it may not be beneficial for the organism to undergo significant increases in corticosteroids after each and every moderate stimulation of the immune system. In contrast, when sufficient cell growth factors have already been produced for the clonal expansion of the antigen-committed cells, massive antigen challenges may require activation of the HPA axis to suppress excessive recruitment of noncommitted immune cells, and overproduction of cytokines which might in itself threaten homeostasis.

CONCLUSION

The concept of the intercellular communication between the immune and the neuroendocrine axes via peptide and protein signals has provided the conceptual framework for the investigation of the bilateral communication pathways between these axes. In particular, studies have shown the existence of functional connections between activated macrophages and the HPA axis, in which immune cells serve a sensory function for stimuli such as viruses and bacteria, and provide information relayed by interleukins to the brain. The descending arm of this functional loop provides, when necessary, a negative feedback on the number and function of immune cells; this influence is exerted through the increased release of corticosteroids and other immunologically relevant hormones. Thus, the immune system (through cytokines produced by activated macrophages) and the HPA axis (through CRF released by the hypothalamus and the subsequent increase in ACTH and corticosteroid secretion) appear functionally linked in providing a coordinated response to immune challenges.

ACKNOWLEDGMENTS

We thank Dr. S. Gillis for the gift of IL-1β and Dr. A. Dunn for the gift of NDV.

REFERENCES

1. WEIGENT, D. A. & J. E. BLALOCK. 1987. Interactions between the neuroendocrine and immune systems: Common hormones and receptors. Immunol. Rev. 100: 79–108.
2. BLALOCK, J. E. 1989. A molecular basis for bidirectional communication between the immune and neuroendocrine systems. Physiol. Rev. 69: 1–32.

3. BLALOCK, J. E., D. HARBOUR-MCMENAMIN & E. M. SMITH. 1985. Peptide hormones shared by the neuroendocrine and immunologic systems. J. Immunol. **135:** 858s–861s.
4. SWANSON, L. W. 1987. The hypothalamus. *In* Handbook of Chemical Neuroanatomy. A. Bjorklund, P. Hokfelt & L. W. Swanson, Eds. Vol. **5:** 1–124. Elsevier. Amsterdam.
5. DINARELLO, C. A. 1988. Biology of interleukin 1. FASEB **2:** 108–115.
6. DINARELLO, C. A. 1992. Role of interleukin-1 in infectious diseases. Immunol. Rev. **127:** 119–146.
7. KUSHNER, I. 1982. The phenomenon of the acute phase response. Ann. N.Y. Acad. Sci. **389:** 39–48.
8. BESEDOVSKY, H., A. DEL REY, E. SORKIN & C. A. DINARELLO. 1986. Immunoregulatory feedback between interleukin-1 and glucocorticoid hormones. Science **233:** 652–654.
9. KROEMER, G., H. P. BREZINSCHEK, R. FAESSLER, K. SCHAUENSTEIN & G. WICK. 1988. Physiology and pathology of an immunoendocrine feedback loop. Immunol. Today **9:** 163–165.
10. BATEMAN, A., A. SINGH, T. KRAL & S. SOLOMON. 1989. The immune-hypothalamic-pituitary-adrenal axis. Endocr. Rev. **10:** 92–112.
11. SHEK, P. N. & B. H. SABISTON. 1983. Neuroendocrine regulation of immune processes: Change in circulating corticosterone levels induced by the primary antibody response in mice. Int. J. Immunopharmacol. **5:** 23–33.
12. BESEDOVSKY, H. O. & A. DEL REY. 1992. Immuno-neuroendocrine circuits: Integrative role of cytokines. Front. Neuroendocrinol. **13:** 61–94.
13. BESEDOVSKY, H. & E. SORKIN. 1975. Changes in blood hormone levels during the immune response. Proc. Soc. Exp. Biol. Med. **150:** 466–470.
14. SHALABY, M. R., A. WAAGE, L. AARDEN & T. ESPEVIK. 1989. Endotoxin, tumor necrosis factor-α and interleukin 1 induce interleukin 6 production *in vivo*. Clin. Immunol. Immunopathol. **53:** 488–498.
15. RIVIER, C. 1989. Role of endotoxin and interleukin-1 in modulating ACTH, LH and sex steroid secretion. *In* Proceedings of Circulating Regulatory Factors and Neuroendocrine Function. J. C. Porter & D. Jezova, Eds.: 295–301. Plenum Press. New York, NY.
16. RIVIER, C. & S. RIVEST. 1993. Mechanisms mediating the effects of cytokines of neuroendocrine functions in the rat. *In* Proceedings of Ciba Foundation Symposium No. 172. K. Ackrill, Ed.: 204–225.
17. RIVIER, C., W. VALE & M. BROWN. 1989. In the rat, interleukin-1α and -β stimulate adenocorticotropin and catecholamine release. Endocrinology **125:** 3096–3102.
18. YASUDA, N. & M. A. GREER. 1978. Evidence that the hypothalamus mediates endotoxin stimulation of adrenocorticotropic hormone secretion. Endocrinology **102:** 947–953.
19. MAKARA, G. B., E. STARK & T. MESZAROS. 1971. Corticotrophin release induced by *E. coli* endotoxin after removal of the medial hypothalamus. Endocrinology **88:** 412–414.
20. MOBERG, G. P. 1974. Site of action of endotoxins on hypothalamic-pituitary-adrenal axis. Am. J. Physiol. **220:** 397–400.
21. SAPOLSKY, R., C. RIVIER, G. YAMAMOTO, P. PLOTSKY & W. VALE. 1987. Interleukin-1 stimulates the secretion of hypothalamic corticotropin-releasing factor. Science **238:** 522–524.
22. RIVEST, S. & C. RIVIER. 1991. Influence of the paraventricular nucleus of the hypothalamus in the alteration of neuroendocrine functions induced by physical stress or interleukin. Endocrinology **129:** 2049–2057.
23. SWANSON, L. W., P. E. SAWCHENKO, J. RIVIER & W. W. VALE. 1983. Organization of ovine corticotropin releasing factor (CRF)-immunoactive cells and fibers in the rat brain: An immunohistochemical study. Neuroendocrinology **36:** 165–186.
24. TSAGARAKIS, S., G. GILLIES, L. H. REES, M. BESSER & A. GROSSMAN. 1989. Interleukin-1 directly stimulates the release of corticotrophin releasing factor from rat hypothalamus. Neuroendocrinology **49:** 98–101.
25. CAMBRONERO, J. C., F. J. RIVAS, J. BORRELL & C. GUAZA. 1992. Release of corticotropin-releasing factor from superfused rat hypothalami induced by interleukin-1 is not dependent on adrenergic mechanism. Eur. J. Pharmacol. **219:** 75–80.
26. BARBANEL, G., G. IXART, A. SZAFARCZYK, F. MALAVAL & I. ASSENMACHER. 1990. Intrahypothalamic infusion of interleukin-1β increases the release of corticotropin-

releasing hormone (CRH 41) and adrenocorticotropic hormone (ACTH) in free-moving rats bearing a push-pull cannula in the median eminence. Brain Res. **516:** 31–36.

27. VALE, W., G. GRANT, M. AMOSS, R. BLACKWELL & R. GUILLEMIN. 1972. Culture of enzymatically dispersed anterior pituitary cells. Functional validation of a method. Endocrinology **91:** 562–572.

28. VALE, W., J. VAUGHAN, M. SMITH, G. YAMAMOTO, J. RIVIER & C. RIVIER. 1983. Effects of synthetic ovine CRF, glucocorticoids, catecholamines, neurohypophysial peptides and other substances on cultured corticotropic cells. Endocrinology **113:** 1121–1131.

29. PLOTSKY, P., E. T. J. CUNNINGHAM & E. P. WIDMAIER. 1989. Catecholaminergic modulation of corticotropin-releasing factor and adrenocorticotropin secretion. Endocr. Rev. **10:** 437–458.

30. DINARELLO, C. A. 1984. Interleukin-1 and the pathogenesis of the acute-phase response. N. Engl. J. Med. **311:** 1413–1418.

31. DINARELLO, C. A. 1985. An update on human interleukin-1: From molecular biology to clinical relevance. J. Clin. Immunol. **5:** 287–297.

32. NAVARRA, P., S. TSAGARAKIS, M. S. FARIA, L. H. REES, G. M. BESSER & A. B. GROSSMAN. 1991. Interleukins-1 and -6 stimulate the release of corticotropin-releasing hormone-41 from rat hypothalamus *in vitro* via the eicosanoid cyclooxygenase pathway. Endocrinology **128:** 37–45.

33. LYSON, K. & S. M. MCCANN. 1992. Involvement of arachidonic acid cascade pathways in interleukin-6-stimulated corticotropin-releasing factor release *in vitro*. Neuroendocrinology **55:** 708–713.

34. MORIMOTO, A., N. MURAKAMI, T. NAKAMORI, Y. SAKATA & T. WATANABE. 1989. Possible involvement of prostaglandin E in development of ACTH response in rats induced by human recombinant interleukin-1. J. Physiol. **411:** 245–256.

35. WATANABE, T., A. MORIMOTO, Y. SAKATA & N. MURAKAMI. 1990. ACTH response induced by interleukin-1 is mediated by CRF secretion stimulated by hypothalamic PGE. Experientia **46:** 481–484.

36. KATSUURA, G., P. E. GOTTSCHALL, R. R. DAHL & A. ARIMURA. 1988. Adrenocorticotropin release induced by intracerebroventricular injection of recombinant human interleukin-1 in rats: Possible involvement of prostaglandin. Endocrinology **122:** 1773–1779.

37. RIVIER, C. & W. VALE. 1991. Stimulatory effect of interleukin-1 on ACTH secretion in the rat: Is it modulated by prostaglandins? Endocrinology **129:** 384–388.

38. DUNN, A. J. & H. E. CHULUYAN. 1992. The role of cyclo-oxygenase and lipoxygenase in the interleukin-1-induced activation of the HPA axis: Dependence on the route of injection. Life Sci. **51:** 219–225.

39. DERIJK, R. H., N. VAN ROOIJEN & F. BERKENBOSCH. 1992. The role of macrophages in the hypothalamic-pituitary-adrenal activation in response to endotoxin (LPS). Res. Immunol. **143:** 224–229.

40. RIVEST, S., G. TORRES & C. RIVIER. 1991. Differential effects of central and peripheral injection of interleukin-1β on brain c-fos expression and hypothalamo-pituitary-adrenal axis activity. Annual Meeting of the Society for Neurosciences. New Orleans, LA. Nov. 10–15. **17:** 475.61197.

41. MATTA, S. G., J. SINGH, R. NEWTON & B. M. SHARP. 1990. The adrenocorticotropin response to interleukin-1β instilled into the rat median eminence depends on the local release of catecholamines. Endocrinology **127:** 2175–2182.

42. TATSUNO, I., A. SOMOGYVARI-VIGH, K. MIZUNO, P. E. GOTTSCHALL, H. HIDAKA & A. ARIMURA. 1991. Neuropeptide regulation of interleukin-6 production from the pituitary: Stimulation by pituitary adenylate cyclase activating polypeptide and calcitonin gene-related peptide. Endocrinology **129:** 1797–1804.

43. VANKELECOM, H., P. CARMELIET, J. VAN DAMME, A. BILLIAU & C. DENEF. 1989. Production of interleukin-6 by folliculo-stellate cells of the anterior pituitary gland in a histiotypic cell aggregate culture system. Neuroendocrinology **49:** 102–106.

44. KOENIG, J. I., K. SNOW, B. D. CLARK, R. TONI, J. G. CANNON, A. R. SHAW, C. A. DINARELLO, S. REICHLIN, S. L. LEE & R. M. LECHAN. 1990. Intrinsic pituitary

interleukin-1β is induced by bacterial lipopolysaccharide. Endocrinology **126:** 3053–3058.

45. SPANGELO, B. L., W. D. JARVIS, A. M. JUDD & R. M. MACLEOD. 1991. Induction of interleukin-6 release by interleukin-1 in rat anterior pituitary cells *in vitro*: Evidence for an eicosanoid-dependent mechanism. Endocrinology **129:** 2886–2894.
46. SPANGELO, B. L., A. M. JUDD, P. C. ISAKSON & R. M. MACLEOD. 1991. Interleukin-1 stimulates interleukin-6 release from rat anterior pituitary cells *in vitro*. Endocrinology **128:** 2685–2692.
47. KEHRER, P., D. TURNILL, J.-M. DAYER, A. F. MULLER & R. C. GAILLARD. 1988. Human recombinant interleukin-1-beta and -alpha, but not recombinant tumor necrosis factor alpha stimulate ACTH release from rat anterior pituitary cells *in vitro* in a prostaglandin E_2 and cAMP independent manner. Neuroendocrinology **48:** 160–166.
48. KASTING, N. W., M. F. MAZUREK & J. B. MARTIN. 1985. Endotoxin increases vasopressin release independently of known physiological stimuli. Am. J. Physiol. **248:** E420–E424.
49. CHRISTENSEN, J. D., E. W. HANSEN & B. FJALLAND. 1989. Interleukin-1β stimulates the release of vasopressin from rat neurohypophysis. Eur. J. Pharmacol. **171:** 233–235.
50. NAITO, Y., J. FUKATA, K. SHINDO, O. EBISUI, N. MURAKAMI, T. TOMINAGA, Y. NAKAI, K. MORI, N. W. KASTINGH & H. IMURA. 1991. Effects of interleukins on plasma arginine vasopressin and oxytocin levels in conscious, freely moving rats. Biochem. Biophys. Res. Commun. **174:** 1189–1195.
51. HANSEN, E. W. & J. D. CHRISTENSEN. 1992. Endotoxin and interleukin-1 β induces fever and increased plasma oxytocin in rabbits. Pharmacol. & Toxicol. **70:** 389–391.
52. BRANDTZAEG, P., O. OKTEDALEN, P. KIERULF & P. K. OPSTAD. 1989. Elevated VIP and endotoxin plasma levels in human gram-negative septic shock. Regul. Pept. **24:** 37–44.
53. BESEDOVSKY, H., E. SORKIN, D. FELIX & H. HAAS. 1977. Hypothalamic changes during the immune response. Eur. J. Immunol. **7:** 323–325.
54. BESEDOVSKY, H., A. DEL REY, E. SORKIN, M. DA PRADA, R. BURRI & C. HONEGGER. 1983. The immune response evokes changes in brain noradrenergic neurons. Science **221:** 564–566.
55. DUNN, A. J., M. L. POWELL, W. V. MORESHEAD, J. M. GASKIKN & N. R. HALL. 1987. Effects of Newcastle disease virus administration to mice on the metabolism of cerebral biogenic amine, plasma corticosterone, and lymphocyte proliferation. Brain, Behav. & Immunol. **1:** 216–230.
56. BESEDOVSKY, H. O. & A. D. REY. 1989. Mechanism of virus-induced stimulation of the hypothalamus-pituitary-adrenal axis. J. Steroid Biochem. **34:** 235–239.
57. STENZEL-POORE, M., W. W. VALE & C. RIVIER. 1993. Relationship between antigen-induced immune stimulation and activation of the hypothalamic-pituitary-adrenal axis in the rat. Endocrinology **132:** 1313–1318.

Neuropeptides, the Stress Response, and the Hypothalamo-Pituitary-Gonadal Axis in the Female Rhesus Monkey[a]

MICHEL FERIN

Center for Reproductive Sciences, and
Departments of Physiology and Obstetrics and Gynecology
College of Physicians and Surgeons
Columbia University
New York, New York 10032

In most animal species, conditions of stress are known to reduce reproductive proficiency.[1-4] With the original observation by Selye[5] that activation of the hypothalamo-pituitary-adrenal (HPA) axis characteristically underlies the response of the organism to stress comes the hypothesis that hormones of the HPA axis may themselves alter the secretory activity of the hypothalamo-pituitary-gonadal axis. However, the mechanisms by which one endocrine axis may influence the activity of another one have not been well studied until recently. This review will focus on work from our research laboratory performed in a nonhuman primate, the female rhesus monkey. This animal provides a good model because its menstrual cycle is similar in most aspects to that of the human. After a brief discussion of the hypothalamo-pituitary-gonadal axis in the monkey, we will report our initial attempts at studying the neuroendocrine signals by which activation of the hypothalamo-pituitary-adrenal axis is translated into abnormal function of the hypothalamo-pituitary-gonadal axis.

THE HYPOTHALAMO-PITUITARY-GONADAL AXIS—THE GnRH PULSE GENERATOR

The dynamic relationships between the different levels of the reproductive axis in the female are such that the reproductive process occurs in a cyclic fashion in an orderly sequence of events. This sequence involves a remarkable coordination between hormonal secretion and morphological changes in various organs, including the hypothalamus, the pituitary, and the ovaries.[6] In the primate, this cycle (the menstrual cycle) lasts approximately one month and comprises two phases. The *follicular* phase is the period during which growth of an estradiol-secreting follicle occurs and which culminates in ovulation when a mature oocyte is released into the reproductive tract for fertilization. During the *luteal* phase, a newly formed corpus luteum secretes progesterone in preparation for implantation of the fertilized egg. Morphological and secretory changes in the ovary are controlled by the pituitary gonadotropins, which are themselves driven by an hypothalamic hormone, gonadotropin-releasing hormone (GnRH). GnRH release into the hypothalamo-pituitary portal circulation is essential for proper gonadotropin secretion. For example, abnormal migration of GnRH-producing neurons from the olfactory placodes (where

[a]The research presented in this review was supported by NIH grants DK39144 and HD05077.

they originate)[7] to their proper hypothalamic locations in contact with the portal circulation, such as occurs in Kallmann's syndrome, results in hypogonadotropic hypogonadism.[8] Not only must GnRH reach the gonadotrope, but it must also be released in a pulsatile manner for normal gonadotropin release to proceed. Thus, the concept of the GnRH pulse generator[9]: each GnRH pulse entrains a pulse of luteinizing hormone (LH) and follicle-stimulating hormone (FSH).

In the human, three conditions have been identified which frequently induce abnormalities of the menstrual cycle, ranging from inadequate luteal phase to anovulation, and which may produce the hypothalamic amenorrhea syndrome.[10,11] These include abnormal nutrition, intense exercise, and psychological or physical stress. What unites these three conditions is that they impinge upon the normal activity of the GnRH pulse generator and reduce GnRH pulse frequency[11-14] with resultant cyclic dysfunction. Interference with GnRH pulsatile activity can be profound and usually parallels the intensity of the causal agent. However, normal pulsatile activity and cyclicity are readily restored after removal of the condition, such as eliminating the stress, improving the diet or reducing the intensity of exercise. That reduced GnRH pulse frequency may lead to abnormal menstrual cycles is not surprising in view of recent experimental evidence demonstrating that optimal follicular growth requires a proper GnRH pulse frequency. Indeed, in monkeys lacking endogenous GnRH and receiving pulsatile GnRH infusions,[15] it was shown that a pulse frequency lower than circhoral results in stunted follicular growth, the severity of which increases with a decreasing GnRH pulse frequency. At first, submaximal follicular growth with ensuing inadequate luteal phase may occur, whereas a greater decrease in pulse frequency may lead to a complete arrest of follicular growth and of estradiol secretion. In both cases, fertility will be compromised.

A ROLE FOR CORTICOTROPIN-RELEASING FACTOR

A major advancement in our understanding of how a stress condition may influence gonadotropin secretion comes from the recent demonstration that corticotropin-releasing factor (CRF), the major neurohormonal stimulus to the pituitary-adrenal axis, influences the GnRH pulse generator. Indeed, intraventricular or intravenous administration of CRF to ovariectomized rhesus monkeys results in a rapid inhibition of pulsatile LH and FSH secretion.[16] An immediate decrease in LH secretion, similar to that which follows administration of CRF, also characterizes the response to a stressful condition, such as a sudden, unexpected noise, in the ovariectomized rhesus monkey (unpublished observation).

CRF administration, of course, also activates the pituitary-adrenal axis and produces an increase in cortisol release. However, although it has been shown in the human that glucocorticoid excess may be associated with the development of hypogonadotropic hypogonadism[17] and in the male monkey that gonadotropin secretion is decreased after a cortisol infusion,[18] cortisol does not mediate the acute inhibitory effect of CRF on LH. Indeed, a study comparing the effects of CRF on gonadotropin secretion in the ovariectomized monkey before and after adrenalectomy clearly indicates that the adrenal glands are not required for the acute CRF effect; similar decrements in gonadotropins are observed in the adrenalectomized monkey.[19] Indirect evidence in support of this conclusion is also provided by the observation that ACTH infusions do not interfere with normal pulsatile gonadotropin secretion.[20] Inasmuch as these infusions also result in large increases in cortisol, one may conclude that overall stimulation of the pituitary-adrenal axis in itself does not acutely interfere with pituitary-gonadal function. The above-reported observations of inhibitory effects of glucocorticoids on gonadotropin secretion in the human and monkey most probably reflect the chronic administration of the compound. For instance, in the orchidectomized monkey treated with hydrocortisol acetate, LH and FSH levels begin to decline only 35 days after initiation of the treatment.[18]

THE IMMUNE SYSTEM AND THE ADRENAL AXIS

The fundamental response to infection or injury includes the production and release of several immunoregulatory cytokines. A key inducer of the acute phase appears to be interleukin-1 (IL-1). In addition to its immunological properties, IL-1 may also be an important messenger between the immune system and several endocrine pathways. In the rodent, IL-1 has been reported to activate the adrenal axis.[21,22] In view of our previous observations of CRF effects on LH in the ovariectomized monkey, we began investigations of the use of IL-1α as a tool to activate the HPA axis. We have clearly demonstrated that intraventricular administration of IL-1α results in an increase in cortisol secretion,[23] which is inhibited by the concomitant administration of a CRF antagonist [(D-PHE,[12] NLE,[21,38] CαMe LEU[37]) CRF$_{12-41}$]. IL-1α also inhibits LH and FSH secretion in the ovariectomized monkey. Significantly, the inhibition of gonadotropins by IL-1α is causally related to the activation of CRF release, because in the presence of the CRF antagonist pulsatile LH release undistinguishable from that observed in the control animal continues unabated.[23] What physiological relevance these effects of IL-1α may have in the primate remains to be determined, but it is known that states in which the immunological system is activated and in which IL-1 is released may be accompanied by reproductive deficiency. Unknown, of course, are the potential cellular sources of IL-1 in the primate brain, such as whether the cytokine is released from stimulated macrophages entering the brain or from specialized cells intrinsic to the brain.[24-26]

A ROLE FOR VASOPRESSIN

Although the main function of arginine vasopressin (AVP) is related to its antidiuretic action on the kidney, AVP has also been shown to participate with CRF in the neuroendocrine control of the adrenal axis.[27-30] In contrast to its antidiuretic action, which involves the classical AVP magnocellular pathways, this synergistic action on ACTH most likely implicates parvicellular pathways that have been described in the primate[31] and rodent.[32] Various challenges in the rodent, including IL-1α administration or insulin-induced hypoglycemia, increase AVP release.[33,34] However, the action of AVP on the gonadal axis has not been substantially investigated, except for a report in the orchidectomized rat of an inhibition of LH release by this neuropeptide, albeit to a lesser degree than that seen after CRF.[35] Our results in the ovariectomized monkey demonstrate for the first time that endogenously released AVP is involved in the process through which IL-1α inhibits gonadotropin secretion. Indeed, although IL-1α acutely reduces LH concentrations and LH pulse frequency, the concomitant infusion of the AVP antagonist [(deamino-Pen,[1] O-Me-Tyr,[2] Arg[8]) vasopressin] prevents this inhibitory effect and restores LH pulsatile secretion.[36]

Our results in the monkey clearly suggest a role for the two main neuropeptides of the adrenal axis in the processes that modulate the effects of challenges to the reproductive axis. This may not be surprising in view of the neuroanatomical evidence of copackaging of CRF and AVP in the same neurosecretory granules of some CRF axons.[37-39] However, not all CRF axons contain AVP, and the particular subtype of parvicellular neuron active in these responses remains unknown.

In contrast to our results with the CRF antagonist, coadministration of the AVP antagonist does not affect the IL-1α–induced cortisol increase.[36] This observation suggests that, in the primate, adrenocortical activation in response to IL-1 does not require AVP. This result diverges from that in the rodent, in which CRF and AVP appear to synergize to produce the adrenal response, and from the sheep in which AVP appears to be the predominant neuropeptide in regard to ACTH secretion.[29,30]

Because both AVP and CRF are probably released by IL-1α, the observation may imply that AVP and CRF must act synergistically to inhibit GnRH secretion. Yet, this conclusion is difficult to reconcile with observations that the exogenous administration of *either* neuropeptide (ref. 16 and unpublished observation) results in a gonadotropin decrease. It is possible, however, that these results simply reflect the presence of a sufficient basal activity of the other neuropeptide. Alternatively, recent *in vitro* observations[40] suggest that a stepwise mechanism whereby the two neuropeptides may act in sequence may be relevant. These mechanisms are presently under study.

ADRENAL AXIS NEUROPEPTIDE-GnRH PATHWAYS

It is unlikely that the inhibitory actions of CRF and AVP on gonadotropin secretion are exerted at the level of the gonadotrope. Rather, a central hypothalamic site is indicated because administration of CRF results in a decrease of multiple unit electrical activity in the arcuate nucleus, which is thought to represent the activity of the GnRH pulse generator.[41] Observations in the rodent that IL-1 is ineffective *in vitro* in altering GnRH release from the median eminence but can modulate GnRH release from hypothalamic fragments[42] suggest that this effect is exerted at the neuronal cell body.

Recently, in an important development, evidence was provided for a possible direct pathway between adrenal axis neuropeptides and the GnRH neuron in the monkey: AVP immunoreactive boutons were reported to make symmetrical synapses onto GnRH cell bodies.[43] Of significance is that the AVP synapse appears to be the only other afferent, other than opioid or GnRH, that has been identified in the primate. Direct connections between CRF and GnRH neurons in the preoptic area have been observed in the rodent.[44] The relevance of the latter observation to the monkey, if confirmed in this species, is not clear because preoptic GnRH neurons do not appear to play a dominant role in the control of pulsatile gonadotropin secretion (see below).

A ROLE FOR THE ENDOGENOUS OPIOID PEPTIDES

A large body of evidence exists which demonstrates an intermediary role for the hypothalamic opioid peptides in the neuroendocrine control of the gonadal axis. Opioid peptides themselves are known to decrease LH and FSH secretion,[45] and β-endorphin appears to exert a robust monosynaptic influence on the GnRH neuron.[46]

Are the opioid peptides involved in decreasing LH during stress? It would appear so because CRF has been shown to release β-endorphin from the hypothalamus,[47] and pretreatment with naloxone prevents the inhibitory effect of CRF on LH and FSH release.[48] β-endorphin may be the principal opioid peptide involved in this process inasmuch as antiserum to β-endorphin prevents the induced LH inhibition in the ovariectomized monkey (unpublished observation) and rodent.[49] Whether CRF acts directly on the arcuate proopiomelanocortin (POMC) neurons (CRF receptors on these cells have not been identified) or via other hypothalamic neurotransmitter systems remains to be ascertained. It is also not known whether the endogenous opioid peptides also modulate the action of vasopressin. That an elevated endogenous opioid tone may underlie the hypothalamic amenorrhea syndrome is suggested by clinical observations of restored ovulatory menstrual cycles in some (but not all) patients with hypothalamic amenorrhea after infusions with naltrexone.[50]

A modulatory role by the endogenous opioid peptides on gonadotropin release may also explain why, in the primate, glucocorticoids, which are known to interfere with the corticotropic response to a CRF stimulus,[51] also prevent the inhibitory effect of CRF on gonadotropin secretion.[52] For example, it may be postulated that the absence of gonadotropin response to CRF that we observed in monkeys pretreated with large doses of glucocorticoids is the consequence of the interference by the steroid of the process of POMC cleavage, synthesis or release. An effect of glucocorticoids on POMC mRNA has been demonstrated at the hypothalamic level.[53] Of interest is the observation that the inhibitory action of morphine on LH persists in these animals,[52] suggesting that glucocorticoids do not prevent opiate-receptor interactions. These results involving large doses of glucocorticoids must be placed in proper perspective, however. Indeed, a similar action of physiologically elevated glucocorticoid levels in response to stress-induced CRF release would in fact effectively eliminate the ability of the organism to respond to stressful stimuli by inhibiting the reproductive process, which in itself constitutes an important aspect of the adaptational response to such stimuli. This is clearly not the case, because, as seen in our previous examples, the inhibitory action of CRF upon gonadotropin secretion can be sustained in the presence of acutely elevated but physiological levels of cortisol.

It should be noted that, in addition to their role in the physiopathology of gonadotropin secretion, endogenous opioid peptides play a crucial *physiological* role in the phenomenon of cyclicity in the rhesus monkey.[54,55] This is because the hypothalamic opioid center in the arcuate nucleus mediates the effect of progesterone on LH pulse frequency during the luteal phase and thereby prepares the gonadal axis for the next cycle. In brief, progesterone, secreted by the corpus luteum under the stimulation of LH, increases β-endorphin release from the endogenous hypothalamic opiate center during the luteal phase.[55] This enhanced hypothalamic β-endorphin activity is then directly responsible for the decreased LH pulse frequency which is characteristic of the luteal phase;[56] naloxone administration during this phase of the cycle results in an increase in LH pulse frequency to one that is more comparable to that seen in the follicular phase.[57,58] Experimental evidence in the monkey suggests that the striking deceleration of pulse frequency in the luteal phase may be an important determinant of cycle quality. Indeed, significant disturbances in the menstrual cycle of the monkey follow imposed changes in the normal frequency pattern of the GnRH hypophysiotropic signal during the luteal phase.[59]

A ROLE FOR OTHER POMC-DERIVED PEPTIDES

In the hypothalamus, the C-terminal portion of POMC is processed primarily to β-endorphin, γ-lipotropin, ACTH, and α-melanocyte-stimulating hormone (α-

MSH). Although β-endorphin has been the major POMC product studied with respect to neuroendocrine effects, it has become evident that other POMC derivatives have a variety of effects that are opposite to those of β-endorphin. For instance, α-MSH has been shown to attenuate opioid-induced analgesia and to prevent the inhibitory effects of β-endorphin on several behavioral end points.[60–62] We have demonstrated that several of the endocrine effects of β-endorphin can also be blocked by α-MSH. For instance, the inhibition of LH and the release of prolactin provoked by β-endorphin can be prevented by the coadministration of α-MSH.[63] Additional results also show that central administration of α-MSH can block the inhibitory effects of CRF or IL-1α on gonadotropins, an action which most probably results from antagonism by α-MSH of the effect of endogenously released β-endorphin.[64] The data support the notion that the posttranslational processing of POMC represents an important step in the neuroendocrine processes that govern pituitary secretion. In regard to gonadotropin secretion, it is possible that the ratio of hypothalamic β-endorphin to α-MSH may be more important than the absolute β-endorphin concentration in determining the ultimate effect on LH and FSH secretion. This concept is presently under study.

MODULATION OF THE STRESS RESPONSE BY OVARIAN STEROIDS

At this point, the reader should be reminded that the preceding experimental data were all obtained in the ovariectomized monkey. This is important because ongoing experiments indicate that the characteristic gonadotropin response pattern to adrenal axis neuropeptides is profoundly modified by estradiol pretreatment (unpublished observations). In a first experiment, ovariectomized monkeys were treated for 4–5 days with estradiol in order to restore steroid concentrations in peripheral blood equal to those observed during the early follicular phase of the menstrual cycle. Surprisingly, the IL-1α inhibitory effect on LH was significantly blunted or lost, in contrast to the robust decrease observed in the monkey without steroid replacement. This observation suggests that the presence of estradiol during the menstrual cycle may provide "protection" against the detrimental effects of stress on the gonadal axis. This protective action occurs even though the adrenal axis continues to be activated by IL-1α, as evidenced by the increase in cortisol.

In a second experiment, a higher estradiol replacement dose was provided in order to increase estradiol concentrations to levels that are seen during the late follicular phase. In this situation, IL-1α administration resulted in a frank increase in LH secretion. This observation of a stimulatory effect on LH release in the estrogen-replaced ovariectomized monkey parallels data in the literature in which stress or neuropeptides were observed to facilitate LH release,[65] as well as observations of LH release after administration of vasopressin in the intact baboon.[66]

The nature of the neuroendocrine pathways activated by IL-1α in the steroid-replaced monkey, as well as the significance of these contrasting responses of the gonadal axis to adrenal axis activation under different ovarian endocrine conditions, remains to be thoroughly investigated. These divergent LH responses in the presence or absence of ovarian steroids are not unprecedented. N-methyl-D,L-aspartate[67] and neuropeptide-Y,[68] for instance, have also been shown to elicit varying responses under different endocrine conditions; usually expression of an excitatory LH response requires the presence of estradiol. Of interest is a recent report on the rodent demonstrating that administration of ACTH to estrogen-primed ovariectomized rats causes a significant elevation of LH, which is abolished by adrenalectomy.[69] This effect of ACTH appears to be mediated by progesterone released from the adrenal in response to the pituitary hormone. Although this phenomenon may play a role in the spontaneous ovulatory gonadotropin surge occurring at proestrus in the rat,[70] its role in the monkey remains to be determined.

THE PRIMATE VERSUS THE RODENT

The present review has dealt uniquely with our data obtained in a primate species. The subject of the relationships between stress and the function of the adrenal and gonadal axes and of the pathways that mediate these relationships in the rodent has been reviewed elsewhere[71] as well as in other parts of this volume. Many similarities are present between the two species. CRF exerts a stimulatory action on the adrenal axis and an inhibitory effect on the gonadal axis both in the rodent[72] and primate. IL-1 has similar actions on the adrenal and gonadal axes in both species.[73] Yet, there are significant differences in the action of these neuropeptides in the two species. (1) Although intravenous administration of CRF significantly decreases LH levels in the ovariectomized monkey, this route was ineffective in influencing LH secretion in the rat. This difference in response may reflect the more extended rostral-caudal migration of the GnRH neuron characteristic of the primate,[74] such that in this species the main relevant portion of GnRH neurons in regard to gonadotropin control resides within the medial basal hypothalamus within the arcuate nucleus.[75,76] This area may possibly be easier to access after intravenous injection than the preoptic area in the rodent. (2) Although CRF and IL-1 administration inhibits FSH as well as LH secretion in the monkey, it only affects LH secretion in the rodent. GnRH is well known to influence the secretion of both LH and FSH, and a parallel decrease in both gonadotropins in the monkey may suggest more direct inhibitory pathways to the arcuate GnRH pulse generator. The reasons for the discrepancy in LH and FSH responses in the rodent remain to be determined. (3) The inhibitory effects of IL-1 on LH secretion in the rodent do not appear to be mediated by CRF or vasopressin because neither antagonist prevents the decrease in this species. This observation is in sharp contrast with the monkey, and obviously suggests that different neuroendocrine pathways participate in these immune-neuroendocrine interactions in both species. The anatomical relationships between vasopressin and GnRH pathways recently described in the monkey[43] may begin to explain such differences, although the exact nature of the relationship or the origin of these vasopressin neurons remains to be investigated.

In fact, considerable research remains to be performed in order to delineate the pathways that mediate the effects of stress on gonadotropin secretion in both species. For example, CRF injection into the medial preoptic area significantly decreases plasma LH levels in the ovariectomized rat.[71] Yet, the location of the CRF perikarya from which derive the CRF-GnRH immunoreactive synapses formed in this area is unknown. Complete destruction of the paraventricular nucleus, an important source of CRF neurons, surprisingly fails to interfere with the inhibitory effect of stress on LH secretion in the rat.[77] The site of origin of the inhibitory stimulus thus remains unknown.

SUMMARY

In conclusion, we have demonstrated that in the primate increased activity of the immune system and the consequent IL-1 release result in the activation of neuropeptides of the adrenal axis, mainly CRF and AVP. These neuropeptides, through a direct effect on the GnRH pulse generator or indirectly through the hypothalamic endogenous opioid peptides, inhibit the GnRH pulse generator. Some of the POMC derivatives, such as α-MSH, may antagonize these effects. The consequential decrease in GnRH pulse frequency results in an acute decrease in LH and FSH secretion. This decrease in gonadotropin release may explain the deleterious effects of stress on the menstrual cycle. However, an acute decrease in gonadotropins following activation of the adrenal axis is not observed in the presence of estradiol. Thus, during the menstrual cycle, a relative protection against the deleterious effects of acute stress may exist. How potent this protective mechanism is against repetitive stress is not known.

REFERENCES

1. CHRISTIAN, J. J., J. A. LOYD & D. E. DAVIS. 1965. The role of endocrines in the self regulation of mammalian populations. Recent Prog. Horm. Res. **21:** 501–578.
2. HAGINO, N. 1968. Ovulation and mating behavior in female rats under various environmental stresses or androgen treatment. Jpn. J. Physiol. **18:** 350–355.
3. SAPOLSKY, R. M. & L. C. KREY. 1988. Stress-induced suppression of LH concentrations in wild baboons: Role of opiates. J. Clin. Endocrinol. & Metab. **66:** 722–726.
4. RIVIER, C., J. RIVIER & W. VALE. 1986. Stress induced inhibition of reproductive function: Role of endogenous CRF. Science **231:** 607–609.
5. SELYE, H. 1939. Effect of adaptation to various damaging agents on the female sex organs in the rat. Endocrinology **25:** 615–624.
6. FERIN, M., R. JEWELEWICZ & M. WARREN. 1993. The menstrual cycle. Oxford University Press. New York, NY.
7. SCHWANZEL-FUKUDA, M. & D. W. PFAFF. 1989. Origin of LHRH neurons. Nature **338:** 161–164.
8. SCHWANZEL-FUKUDA, M., D. BICK & D. W. PFAFF. 1989. Luteinizing hormone-releasing hormone (LHRH)-expressing cells do not migrate normally in an inherited hypogonadal (Kallmann) syndrome. Mol. Brain Res. **6:** 311–326.
9. KNOBIL, E. 1980. The neuroendocrine control of the menstrual cycle. Recent Prog. Horm. Res. **36:** 53–88.
10. LACHELIN, G. C. L. & S. S. C. YEN. 1978. Hypothalamic chronic anovulation. Am. J. Obstet. Gynecol. **130:** 825–831.
11. BERGA, S. L., J. F. MORTOLA, L. GIRTON, B. SU, G. LAUGHLIN, P. PHAM & S. S. C. YEN. 1989. Neuroendocrine aberrations in women with functional hypothalamic amenorrhea. J. Clin. Endocrinol. & Metab. **68:** 301–308.
12. LOUCKS, A. B., J. F. MORTOLA, L. GIRTON & S. S. C. YEN. 1989. Alterations in the hypothalamic-pituitary-ovarian and the hypothalamic-pituitary-adrenal axes in athletic women. J. Clin. Endocrinol. & Metab. **68:** 402–411.
13. REAME, N. E., S. E. SAUDER, G. D. CASE, R. P. KELCH & J. C. MARSHALL. 1985. Pulsatile gonadotropin secretion in women with hypothalamic amenorrhea: Evidence that reduced frequency of GnRH secretion is the mechanism of persistent anovulation. J. Clin. Endocrinol. & Metab. **61:** 851–858.
14. VELDHUIS, J. D., W. S. EVANS, L. M. DEMERS, M. O. THORNER, D. WAKAT & A. D. ROGOL. 1985. Altered neuroendocrine regulation of gonadotropin secretion in women distance runners. J. Clin. Endocrinol. & Metab. **61:** 557–563.
15. POHL, C. R., D. W. RICHARDSON, J. J. HUTCHISON, J. A. GERMAK & E. KNOBIL. 1983. Hypophysiotropic signal frequency and the functioning of the pituitary ovarian system in the rhesus monkey. Endocrinology **112:** 2076–2080.
16. OLSTER, D. H. & M. FERIN. 1987. Corticotropin-releasing hormone (CRH) inhibits gonadotropin secretion in the ovariectomized rhesus monkey. J. Clin. Endocrin. & Metab. **65:** 262–267.
17. MCADAMS, M. R., R. H. WHITE & B. E. CHIPPS. 1986. Reduction of serum testosterone levels during chronic glucocorticoid therapy. Ann. Intern. Med. **104:** 648–651.
18. DUBEY, A. K. & T. M. PLANT. 1985. A suppression of gonadotropin secretion by cortisol in castrated male rhesus monkeys (*Macaca mulatta*) mediated by the interruption of hypothalamic gonadotropin-releasing hormone release. Biol. Reprod. **33:** 423–431.

19. XIAO, E., J. LUCKHAUS, W. NIEMANN & M. FERIN. 1989. Acute inhibition of gonadotropin secretion by corticotropin-releasing hormone (CRH) in the primate: Are the adrenal glands involved? Endocrinology **124:** 1632–1637.
20. XIAO, E. & M. FERIN. 1988. The inhibitory action of corticotropin-releasing hormone on gonadotropin secretion in the ovariectomized rhesus monkey is not mediated by adrenocorticotropic hormone. Biol. Reprod. **38:** 763–767.
21. BATEMAN, A., A. SINGH, T. KRAL & S. SOLOMON. 1989. The immunohypothalamic-pituitary-adrenal axis. Endocr. Rev. **10:** 92–112.
22. RIVIER, C., W. VALE & M. BROWN. 1989. In the rat, interleukin-1α and -β stimulate adrenocorticotropin and catecholamine release. Endocrinology **125:** 3096–3102.
23. FENG, Y. J., E. SHALTS, L. XIA, J. RIVIER, C. RIVIER, W. VALE & M. FERIN. 1991. An inhibitory effect of interleukin-1α on basal gonadotropin release in the ovariectomized rhesus monkey: Reversal by a CRH antagonist. Endocrinology **128:** 2077–2082.
24. FONTANA, A., E. WEBER & J. M. DAYER. 1984. Synthesis of interleukin 1/endogenous pyrogen in the brain of endotoxin-treated mice: A step in fever induction? J. Immunol. **133:** 1696–1698.
25. GIULIAN, D., T. J. BAKER, L. N. SHIH & L. B. LACHMAN. 1986. Interleukin-1 of the central nervous system is produced by ameboid microglia. J. Exp. Med. **164:** 594–603.
26. BREDER, C. D., C. A. DINARELLO & C. B. SAPER. 1988. Interleukin-1 immunoreactive innervation of the human hypothalamus. Science **240:** 321–324.
27. RIVIER, C., J. RIVIER, P. MORMEDE & W. VALE. 1984. Studies of the nature of the interaction between vasopressin and corticotropin-releasing factor on adrenal corticotropin release in the rat. Endocrinology **115:** 882–886.
28. GAILLARD, R. C., A. M. RIONDEL, N. LING & A. F. MULLER. 1988. Corticotropin releasing factor activity of CRF 41 in normal man is potentiated by angiotensin-11 and vasopressin but not by desmopressin. Life Sci. **43:** 1935–1944.
29. SCACCIANOCE, S., L. A. A. MUSCOLO, G. CIGLIANA, D. NAVARRA, R. NICOLAI & L. ANGEUCCI. 1991. Evidence for a specific role of vasopressin in sustaining pituitary-adrenocortical stress response in the rat. Endocrinology **128:** 3138–3143.
30. LIU, J. P., P. J. ROBINSON, J. W. FUNDER & D. ENGLER. 1990. The biosynthesis and secretion of adrenocorticotropin by the ovine anterior pituitary is predominantly regulated by arginine vasopressin. Evidence that protein kinase C mediates the action of AVP. J. Biol. Chem. **265:** 14136–14142.
31. ZIMMERMAN, E. A., J. ANTUNES, P. W. CARMEL, R. DEFENDINI & M. FERIN. 1977. Magnocellular neurosecretory pathways in the monkey: Immunohistochemical studies of the normal and lesioned hypothalamus using antibodies to oxytocin, vasopressin and neurophysins. Trans. Am. Neurol. Assoc. **101:** 16–19.
32. PLOTSKY, P. M. 1991. Pathways to the secretion of adrenocorticotropin: A view from the portal. J. Neuroendocrinol. **3:** 1–9.
33. NAKATSURU, K., S. OHGO, Y. OKI & S. MATSUKURA. 1991. Interleukin-1 stimulates arginine vasopressin release from superfused rat hypothalamo-neurohypophyseal complexes independently of cholinergic mechanism. Brain Res. **554:** 38–45.
34. PLOTSKY, P. M., T. O. BRUHN & W. VALE. 1985. Hypophysiotropic regulation of adrenocorticotropin secretion in response to insulin-induced hypoglycemia. Endocrinology **117:** 323–329.
35. RIVIER, C. & W. VALE. 1985. Effects of corticotropin-releasing factor, neurohypophyseal peptides, and catecholamines on pituitary function. Fed. Proc. **44:** 189–195.
36. SHALTS, E., Y. J. FENG & M. FERIN. 1992. Vasopressin mediates the interleukin-1α-induced decrease in luteinizing hormone secretion in the ovariectomized rhesus monkey. Endocrinology **131:** 153–158.
37. WHITNALL, M. H. & H. GAINER. 1988. Major pro-vasopressin-expressing and pro-vasopressin-deficient subpopulations of corticotropin-releasing hormone neurons in normal rats. Neuroendocrinology **47:** 176–180.
38. WHITNALL, M. H. 1989. Stress selectively activates the vasopressin-containing subset of corticotropin-releasing hormone neurons. Neuroendocrinology **50:** 702–707.
39. DE GOEIJ, D. C. E., R. KVETNANSKY, M. H. WHITNALL, D. JEZOVA, F. BERKINBOSCH & F. J. H. TILDERS. 1991. Repeated stress-induced activation of corticotropin-releasing

factor neurons enhances vasopressin stores and colocalization with corticotropin-releasing factor in the median eminence of rats. Neuroendocrinology **53**: 150–159.

40. BURNS, G., O. F. X. ALMEIDA, F. PASSARELLI & A. HERZ. 1989. A two-step mechanism by which corticotropin-releasing hormone releases hypothalamic β-endorphin: The role of vasopressin and G-proteins. Endocrinology **125**: 1365–1372.

41. WILLIAMS, C. L., M. NISHIHARA, J. C. THALABARD, D. M. GROSSER, J. HOTCHKISS & E. KNOBIL. 1990. Corticotropin-releasing factor and gonadotropin-releasing hormone pulse generator activity in the rhesus monkey. Neuroendocrinology **52**: 133–137.

42. KALRA, P. S., A. SAHU & S. P. KALRA. 1990. Interleukin-1 inhibits the ovarian steroid-induced luteinizing hormone surge and release of hypothalamic luteinizing hormone-releasing hormone in rats. Endocrinology **126**: 2145–2152.

43. THIND, K. K., J. E. BOGGAN & P. C. GOLDSMITH. 1991. Interactions between vasopressin- and gonadotropin-releasing hormone-containing neuroendocrine neurons in the monkey supraoptic nucleus. Neuroendocrinology **53**: 287–297.

44. MACLUSKY, N. J., F. NAFTOLIN & C. LEVANTH. 1988. Immunocytochemical evidence for direct synaptic connections between corticotropin releasing hormone and GnRH-containing neurons in the preoptic area of the rat. Brain Res. **439**: 391–395.

45. FERIN, M., W. B. WEHRENBERG, N. Y. LAM, E. F. ALSTON & R. L. VANDE WIELE. 1982. Effects and site of action of morphine on gonadotropin secretion in the female rhesus monkey. Endocrinology **111**: 1652–1656.

46. THIND, K. K. & P. C. GOLDSMITH. 1988. Infundibular GnRH neurons are inhibited by direct opioid and autoregulatory synapses in juvenile monkeys. Neuroendocrinology **47**: 203–216.

47. NIKOLARAKIS, K. E., O. F. X. ALMEIDA & A. HERZ. 1986. Stimulation of hypothalamic β-endorphin release by corticotropin-releasing factor (in vitro). Brain Res. **399**: 152–157.

48. GINDOFF, P. R. & M. FERIN. 1987. Endogenous opioid peptides modulate the effect of corticotropin-releasing factor on gonadotropin release in the primate. Endocrinology **121**: 837–842.

49. PETRAGLIA, F., W. VALE & C. RIVIER. 1986. Opioids act centrally to modulate stress-induced decrease in luteinizing hormone in the rat. Endocrinology **119**: 2445–2450.

50. WILDT, L. & G. I. LEYENDECKER. 1987. Induction of ovulation by the chronic administration of naltrexone in hypothalamic amenorrhea. J. Clin. Endocrinol. & Metab. **64**: 1334–1335.

51. BRITTON, D. R., M. VARELA, A. GARCIA & M. ROSENTHAL. 1985. Dexamethasone suppresses pituitary-adrenal but not behavioral effects of centrally administered CRF. Life Sci. **38**: 211–216.

52. GINDOFF, P. R., E. XIAO, J. LUCKHAUS & M. FERIN. 1989. Dexamethasone treatment prevents the inhibitory effect of corticotropin-releasing hormone on gonadotropin release in the primate. Neuroendocrinology **49**: 202–206.

53. BEAULIEU, S., B. GAGNE & N. BARDEN. 1986. Glucocorticoid regulation of pro-opiomelanocortin (POMC) in RNA content of rat hypothalamus and amygdala (Abstract). First International Congress on Neuroendocrinology, San Francisco, CA.

54. FERIN, M., D. VAN VUGT & S. L. WARDLAW. 1984. The hypothalamic control of the menstrual cycle and the role of endogenous opioid peptides. Recent Prog. Horm. Res. **40**: 441–480.

55. WEHRENBERG, W. B., S. L. WARDLAW, A. G. FRANTZ & M. FERIN. 1982. β-endorphin in hypophyseal portal blood: Variations throughout the menstrual cycle. Endocrinology **111**: 879–881.

56. SOULES, M. R., R. A. STEINER, D. C. CLIFTON, N. L. COHEN, S. AKSEL & W. J. BREMNER. 1984. Progesterone modulation of pulsatile LH secretion in normal women. J. Clin. Endocrinol. & Metab. **58**: 378–383.

57. VAN VUGT, D. A., N. Y. LAM & M. FERIN. 1984. Reduced frequency of pulsatile luteinizing hormone secretion in the luteal phase of the rhesus monkey: Involvement of endogenous opiates. Endocrinology **115**: 1095–1101.

58. GINDOFF, P. R., R. JEWELEWICZ, W. HEMBREE, S. L. WARDLAW & M. FERIN. 1988.

Sustained effects of opioid antagonism during the normal human luteal phase. J. Clin. Endocrinol. & Metab. **66:** 1000–1004.

59. LAM, N. Y. & M. FERIN. 1987. Is the decrease in the hypophysiotropic signal frequency normally observed during the luteal phase important for menstrual cyclicity in the primate? Endocrinology **120:** 2044–2049.

60. CONTRERAS, P. C. & A. E. TAKEMORI. 1984. Antagonism of morphine-induced analgesia, tolerance and dependence by α-melanocyte-stimulating hormone. J. Pharmacol. Exp. Ther. **229:** 21–26.

61. SZEKELY, J. I., E. MIGLECZ, Z. DUNAI-KOVACS, I. TARNAWA, A. Z. RONAI, L. GRAF & S. BAJUSZ. 1979. Attenuation of morphine tolerance and dependence by α-melanocyte stimulating hormone. Life Sci. **24:** 1931–1938.

62. HUGHES, A. M., B. J. EVERITT & J. HERBERT. 1988. The effects of simultaneous or separate infusions of some pro-opiomelanocortin-derived peptides (β-endorphin, melanocyte-stimulating hormone, and corticotrophin-like intermediate polypeptide) and their acetylated derivatives upon sexual and ingestive behavior of male rats. Neuroscience **27:** 689–698.

63. WARDLAW, S. L. & M. FERIN. 1990. Interaction between β-endorphin and α-melanocyte-stimulating hormone in the control of prolactin and luteinizing hormone secretion in the primate. Endocrinology **126:** 2035–2040.

64. SHALTS, E., Y. J. FENG, M. FERIN & S. L. WARDLAW. 1992. α-Melanocyte-stimulating hormone antagonizes the neuroendocrine effects of corticotropin-releasing factor and interleukin-1α in the primate. Endocrinology **131:** 132–138.

65. LAWTON, I. 1972. Facilitatory feedback effects of adrenal and ovarian hormones on LH secretion. Endocrinology **90:** 575–579.

66. KOYAMA, T. & N. HAGINO. 1983. The effect of vasopressin on luteinizing hormone release in baboons. Horm. Metab. Res. **15:** 184–186.

67. REYES, A., L. XIA & M. FERIN. 1991. Modulation of the effects of N-methyl-D,L-aspartate on luteinizing hormone by the ovarian steroids in the adult rhesus monkey. Neuroendocrinology **54:** 405–411.

68. ADASHI, E. Y., C. E. RESNICK, M. E. SVOBODA & J. J. VAN WYK. 1986. Follicle-stimulating hormone enhances somatomedin-C binding to cultured rat granulosa cells: Evidence of cAMP-dependence. J. Biol. Chem. **261:** 3923–3928.

69. PUTNAM, C. D., D. W. BRANN & V. B. MAHESH. 1992. Acute activation of the adrenocorticotropin-adrenal axis: Effect on gonadotropin and prolactin secretion in the female rat. Endocrinology **128:** 2558–2566.

70. BUCKINGHAM, J., K. DOHLER & C. WILSON. 1978. Activity of the pituitary-adrenocortical system and thyroid gland during the oestrous cycle of the rat. J. Endocrinol. **78:** 359–366.

71. RIVIER, C. & S. RIVEST. 1991. Effect of stress on the activity of the hypothalamic-pituitary-gonadal axis: Peripheral and central mechanisms. Biol. Reprod. **45:** 523–532.

72. RIVIER, C. & W. VALE. 1984. Influence of corticotropin-releasing factor (CRF) on reproductive functions in the rat. Endocrinology **114:** 914–919.

73. RIVIER, C. & W. VALE. 1990. Cytokines act within the brain to inhibit luteinizing hormone secretion and ovulation in the rat. Endocrinology **127:** 849–856.

74. SILVERMAN, A. J., J. L. ANTUNES, G. ABRAMS, G. NILAVER, R. THAU, J. A. ROBINSON, M. FERIN & L. C. KREY. 1982. The luteinizing hormone-releasing pathways in the rhesus (*Macaca mulatta*) and pigtailed (*Macaca nemestrina*) monkeys: New observations using thick unembedded sections. J. Comp. Neurol. **211:** 309–317.

75. KREY, L. C., W. R. BUTLER & E. KNOBIL. 1975. Surgical disconnection of the medial basal hypothalamus and pituitary function in the rhesus monkey. I. Gonadotropin secretion. Endocrinology **96:** 1073–1087.

76. PLANT, T. M., L. C. KREY, J. MOOSSY, J. T. MCCORMACK, D. L. HESS & E. KNOBIL. 1978. The arcuate nucleus and the control of gonadotropin and prolactin secretion in the female rhesus monkey (*Macaca mulatta*). Endocrinology **102:** 52–62.

77. RIVEST, S. & C. RIVIER. 1991. Influence of the paraventricular nucleus of the hypothalamus in the alteration of neuroendocrine function induced by intermittent footshock or interleukin. Endocrinology **129:** 2049–2055.

Central Mechanisms and Sites of Action Involved in the Inhibitory Effects of CRF and Cytokines on LHRH Neuronal Activity[a]

SERGE RIVEST[b] AND CATHERINE RIVIER

The Clayton Foundation Laboratories for Peptide Biology
The Salk Institute
10010 North Torrey Pines Road
La Jolla, California 92037

A precise control of homeostasis is crucial for the survival of mammals. Thus, stimuli that threaten the organism, such as physical stress or pathogens, cause immune, endocrine, metabolic, and behavioral changes that are destined to restore and maintain the consistency of the *milieu intérieur*. However, the capacity of the neuroendocrine system to regulate and preserve homeostasis can be exceeded by the intensity of the stressful situation and, in turn, can induce pathological changes to the organism. The alteration of the reproductive system by stress can in fact generate pathological changes such as calcium bone resorption and can participate in the early induction of osteoporosis as well as many other conditions. The ability of severe and prolonged stress to interfere with human reproductive function has indeed long been recognized by clinicians and has been reviewed by us[1] and others[2,3] elsewhere. Although many investigators have studied the effects of various stressors, including infectious disease, psychiatric disorders, surgical trauma, and strenuous exercise on hypothalamic luteinizing hormone-releasing hormone (LHRH) release, plasma gonadotropin levels, sex steroid secretion, and the ovulatory process in various species of animals, the exact mechanisms through which stress alters reproductive function remain largely unknown. Nevertheless, several stress-related factors synthesized and released by different structures of the brain have been suggested as candidates that play a key role in inhibiting LHRH neuronal activity and in consequence interfere with reproduction. Among these stress-related factors, corticotropin-releasing factor (CRF), endogenous opioid peptides (EOP), and, more recently, cytokines are well recognized for their inhibitory action on the hypothalamic LHRH release. This paper will attempt to review the possible mechanisms by which these stress-related factors can interfere with the infundibular LHRH neuronal system in the rat.

[a]This research was supported by NIH grant HD-13527 and was conducted in part by the Foundation for Medical Research, Inc. S. R. is a postdoctoral fellow from the Medical Research Council of Canada (Centennial fellowship). C. R. is a Foundation for Medical Research Investigator.
[b]Corresponding author; present address: Laboratory of Molecular Endocrinology, CHUL Research Center, Centre Hospitalier de l'Université Laval, 2705, Boul. Laurier, Quebec GIV 4G2, Canada.

THE RAT LHRH NEURONAL SYSTEM

Reproduction in male and female mammals is critically dependent on the appropriate neurosecretion of LHRH. LHRH is released in pulses and triggers the production of gonadotropins that stimulate the growth and release of eggs by the ovary. This fact has been best illustrated by experiments in which the actions of the decapeptide have been blocked by immunoneutralization or receptor antagonist treatment which invariably leads to cessation or reduction of gonadotropin secretion, disruption of gonadal function, and infertility (see review, ref. 4). Sterility in mutant, non-LHRH-producing mice[5] and human infertility associated with LHRH insufficiency[6] have also provided a clear demonstration of the reproductive consequences of inappropriate or deficient LHRH neurosecretion. In the rat, administration of an LHRH antagonist during proestrus results in a rapid and complete inhibition of ovulation, which demonstrates the importance of this neuropeptide in reproductive function. Although it has been shown that 50–70% of LHRH neurons project to the infundibular system and, consequently, contribute to the control of LH secretion from the adenohypophysis,[7–9] the regulation of these neurons during normal and stressed conditions is still poorly understood. The fact that 30–40% of LHRH neurons spontaneously express immediate "early" genes such as c-*fos* and c-*jun* during a particular moment of proestrus is direct evidence that the stimulation of at least a proportion of LHRH neurons at that time takes place at the level of LHRH cell bodies.[10–13] We also observed by means of a retrograde tracing technique that a high percentage of LHRH neurons expressing c-*fos* protein during proestrus project to the infundibular system (Rivest *et al.*, in preparation). This endogenous process also provides a powerful tool for studying the activity of these neurons at the cellular level. However, the LHRH neuronal system remains one of the most difficult neuroendocrine systems to investigate. Rat LHRH perikarya are indeed distributed from the rostral division of the diagonal band of broca to the level of the retrochiasmatic area just above the supraoptic nucleus of the hypothalamus. Nevertheless, the medial preoptic area (MPOA) contains the highest density in LHRH cell bodies in a region extending about 2 mm on either side of the midsagittal plane.[14] Most of these cells are within a 1.5-mm block, which includes the optic chiasm and the area just dorsal and anterior to it.[14] The LHRH neurons located in this hypothalamic region also appear to be an important target for the inhibitory influence of CRF and IL-1 on the alteration of LHRH release and reproductive function (see below).[15,16] Because of the diverse distribution of the LHRH neuronal system, it is difficult to investigate precisely the activity of the neurons projecting to the median eminence (ME) and participating in the control of LH secretion from the adenohypophysis. In addition, the exact projections as well as the neurophysiological roles of the remainder of LHRH neurons, which do not send their axons to the ME, remain to be fully described.

Another major difficulty when studying the LHRH neuronal system is the number of factors (for example, classical neurotransmitters, neuropeptides, steroids, etc.) that have been reported to modulate directly or indirectly the LHRH neuronal system at the level of cell bodies or the ME (FIG. 1). It is quite conceivable that the interaction between several of these factors during stressful or normal circumstances modulates LHRH neuronal activity by complex cascade mechanisms which in turn inhibit the release of LHRH in the hypothalamic-pituitary portal vein. Our approach in investigating the mechanisms involved in the alteration of LHRH neuronal activity comprises five different levels (FIG. 2): (1) LHRH release is measured using a push-pull cannula implanted in the ME during proestrus in rats; (2) the site of action is analyzed by means of bilateral microinfusion cannulae located within various regions of the brain [paraventricular nucleus of the hypothalamus (PVN), arcuate nucleus (ARC), MPOA, . . .]; (3) the functional neuronal activity as well as the transduction and transcription mechanisms involved in LHRH gene expression are investigated *in vivo* by examining the expression of nuclear immediate early genes in neuronal cell bodies; (4) LHRH biosynthesis is estimated by means of *in situ* hybridization histochemistry; and (5) the cellular phenotype is demonstrated using single- and dual-immunocytochemistry. These contemporary *in vivo* techniques are

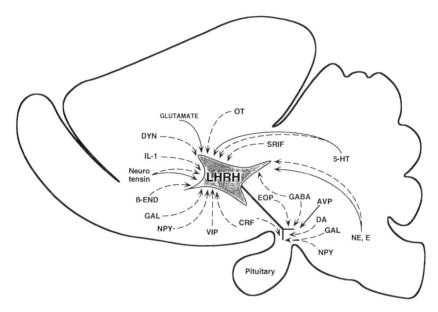

FIGURE 1. Summary of factors known for their ability to modulate LHRH neuronal activity from either LHRH cell bodies or nerve terminals. These factors, however, do not necessarily all have direct influence on LHRH neurons because of the absence of neuronal projections surrounding these cells. They can indirectly modulate the activity of the neurons responsible for the reproductive function via other neuronal pathways. Solid arrows indicate stimulatory effect; dashed arrows, inhibitory effect. *Abbreviations*: AVP, vasopressin; β-END, β-endorphin; CRF, corticotropin-releasing factor; DA, dopamine; DYN, dynorphin; E, epinephrine; EOP, endogenous opioid peptide; GABA, γ-aminobutyric acid; GAL, galanin; 5-HT, serotonin; IL-1, interleukin-1; NE, norepinephrine; NPY, neuropeptide Y; OT, oxytocin; SRIF, somatotropin release-inhibiting factor; VIP, vasoactive intestinal peptide.

employed as tools to clarify and yield a better understanding of the mechanisms participating in the inhibition of the infundibular LHRH neuronal system by various stress-related factors.

CORTICOTROPIN-RELEASING FACTOR AND LHRH NEURONAL ACTIVITY

As early as 1939, Selye[17] observed that stress is accompanied by both an increase in the activity of the hypothalamic-pituitary-adrenal (HPA) axis and a decrease in

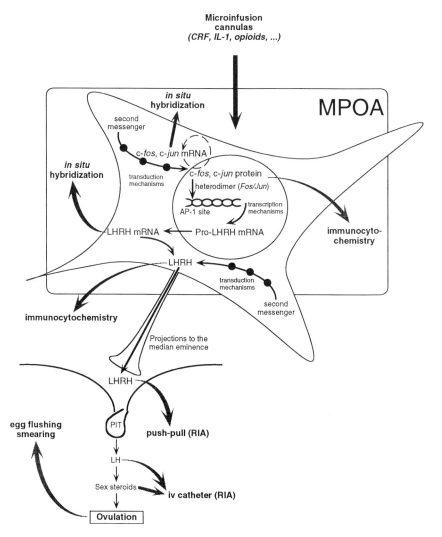

FIGURE 2. Representation of *in vivo* techniques used in our laboratory for the investigation of LHRH neuronal activity during normal and stress conditions. This schema also illustrates the possible involvement of the immediate "early" genes c-*fos* and c-*jun* in the regulation of LHRH gene expression as well as the LHRH release into the infundibular system during the proestrus surge of LH. *Abbreviations*: LHRH, luteinizing hormone-releasing hormone; LH, luteinizing hormone; MPOA, medial preoptic area of the hypothalamus; PIT, pituitary (adenohypophysis).

reproductive functions, a phenomenon he attributed to the necessity, in case of emergency, of preserving adrenal cortex function at the expense of gonadal activity. This observation suggested a possible inverse relationship between hormones of the HPA axis, which are markedly elevated during stress and immune challenge, and those of the hypothalamic-pituitary-gonadal (HPG) axis. It is now well known that intracerebroventricular (i.c.v.) injection of CRF suppresses the activity of the HPG axis.[18–21] Furthermore, the possibility that endogenous CRF might mediate stress-induced inhibition of LH release has also been suggested by a study showing that central injection of a CRF antagonist reverses these effects.[22] We also have reported that CRF attenuates LH secretion through a central mechanism involving the inhibition of LHRH neuronal activity within the MPOA of the hypothalamus.[15] In contrast, this stress-associated neuropeptide does not appear to have an inhibitory effect at the level of LHRH nerve terminals in the ME that secrete into the hypophyseal-portal system, because infusion of CRF directly into the ME did not significantly alter hypothalamic LHRH secretion during proestrus in rats.[15] In addition, as shown in FIGURE 3, bilateral infusion of CRF into two hypothalamic nuclei caudal to the MPOA, the hypothalamic PVN and the ARC, did not notably modify LHRH release measured via a push-pull cannula located in the ME.[15] Thus, the hypothalamic site of infusion appears to be critical for the inhibitory influence of CRF on the activity of the HPG axis in female rats.

Among hypothalamic structures, the MPOA of the rat contains the highest density of LHRH cell bodies making this the most likely site of action of CRF to influence the endogenous activity of LHRH neurons and the HPG axis. Moreover, it is well established that stimulation of the MPOA increases infundibular LHRH release and circulating LH levels, which can induce ovulation in female rats (see review, ref. 8). Additionally, direct anatomical connections exist between CRF axon

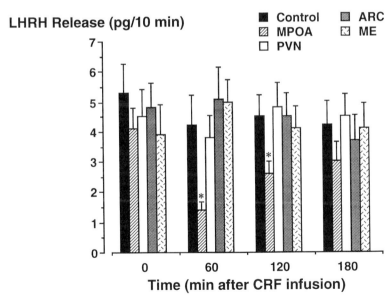

FIGURE 3. Infusion of rCRF into different hypothalamic regions on hypothalamic LHRH release during the afternoon of proestrus. rCRF was bilaterally infused in the hypothalamic medial preoptic area (MPOA), the paraventricular nucleus (PVN), the arcuate nucleus (ARC), and directly into the median eminence (ME) at a rate of 240 ng/10 nL/min over a period of 10 minutes. Animals without treatment were kept as a control group. *Significantly different ($p < 0.05$) from other treatments. Data obtained from ref. 15.

terminals and dendrites of LHRH-secreting neurons located in the MPOA,[23] suggesting a site for the inhibitory effect of stress-induced CRF release on reproductive function. Although CRF neurons appear to have projections to the MPOA and innervate LHRH perikarya, the origin of these fibers remains unclear. Cell bodies containing CRF-like immunoreactive material and messenger RNA (mRNA) are widely distributed in the central nervous system (CNS),[24,25] but little is known about the role played by CRF-containing neurons located in regions outside of the parvocellular PVN. In contrast, the importance of the PVN in controlling synthesis and release of ACTH/β-endorphin (β-END) from the pituitary is now established. That CRF released from parvocellular PVN neurons into the hypothalamic-pituitary portal blood is the primary stimulus to anterior pituitary ACTH secretion is accepted. Indeed, the parvocellular division of the hypothalamic PVN contains most of the CRF cell bodies projecting to the infundibular system.[24] Stressors as diverse as prolonged exercise, immobilization or exposure to mild footshocks markedly increases both c-*fos* expression in CRF-immunoreactive neurons and CRF mRNA in the PVN of rats.[25–27] However, this increase in CRF neuronal activity in the parvocellular division of the PVN does not seem to be related to the antireproductive effect of chronic physical stressors. Accordingly, we have recently observed that complete bilateral electrolytic lesion of the PVN failed to interfere with the inhibitory influence of prolonged stress on activity of the HPG axis in male rats.[28] The fact that the PVN does not notably contribute to innervation of the MPOA may explain the absence of effect of PVN lesions on stress-induced alteration of the HPG axis in rats. Although the PVN has efferents to different brain areas, such as the lateral hypothalamus, mesencephalic reticular formation, ventral tegmental area, and the locus coeruleus, this hypothalamic nucleus does not seem to project to the MPOA.[29] Mapping experiments have provided evidence for the existence of neural projections from the bed nucleus of the stria terminalis (BNST) and the central nucleus of the amygdala (CeA) to the MPOA,[30] but these neuronal connections are not well described. Interestingly, both the BNST and CeA contain a large number of CRF-like immunoreactive cells[31] and could theoretically participate in the innervation of some hypothalamic structures, such as the MPOA. Thus, an activation of putative CRF-containing projections from the BNST and the CeA to the MPOA might be involved in the alteration of LHRH neuronal activity during chronic stress. In addition, the MPOA itself encompasses numerous CRF-containing cell bodies.[31] The CRF-LHRH synapses could therefore in theory represent either local connections from CRF- and LHRH-containing cells located within the MPOA, or CRF neuronal projections coming from other hypothalamic structures and other areas of the brain, such as BNST and the CeA.

INTERACTION BETWEEN CRF AND ENDOGENOUS OPIOID PEPTIDES

It has previously been reported that inhibition of LHRH[18] and LH release[32] induced by i.c.v. injection of CRF was mediated, in part, by activation of the central EOP system. We also have shown that this action appears to take place at the level of the hypothalamic MPOA, because bilateral infusion of μ- or μ₁-opioid receptor antagonists into the MPOA partially inhibited the CRF-induced alteration of hypothalamic LHRH and pituitary LH release in ovariectomized and intact rats during the afternoon of proestrus.[15] In addition, the effect of EOP seems to be specifically via β-END, the major ligand for μ-receptors. The interaction between EOP and the LHRH-secreting system is well known and has been reviewed in detail.[1,33] EOP are able to decrease LHRH concentrations,[34] as well as decrease the release of LHRH into the hypophyseal portal system of the rat during proestrus,[35] and to alter the electrophysiological activity of the hypothalamic LHRH pulse generator in the rhesus monkey.[36] It has also been proposed that opioids act directly on LHRH neurons through specific μ-opioid receptors.[37,38] Almost 10% of synapses impinging on LHRH neurons present in the diagonal band/POA of the rat contain β-END.[39] Despite the approximately 3–4-fold more β-END input to the LHRH cells and processes in the female than in male rats, β-END exerts a robust synaptic influence on LHRH neurons in both sexes.[40] In addition, proopiomelanocortin (POMC) peptide-producing neurons capable of synthesizing β-END in the ventromedial ARC project to the MPOA of the hypothalamus, and some of these neurons establish direct contacts with LHRH-containing perikarya in the rat.[41] Although CRF is an important regulator of the synthesis of POMC-related peptides within the adenohypophysis[42–44] and the hypothalamus,[45] this stress-related neuropeptide does not seem to act within the ARC to increase the level of β-END in the MPOA. Indeed, no evidence exists that CRF can directly stimulate the activity of POMC neurons in the ARC, because there are no CRF binding sites in this hypothalamic region.[46] In addition, i.c.v. injection of CRF does not measurably activate the expression of the immediate early gene c-*fos* in the ARC (Rivest *et al.,* unpublished data), which is a good index for postsynaptic activation and signal transduction in the nervous system. Indeed, the proto-oncogene c-*fos* is expressed in numerous neuronal systems, and is now widely used as an anatomical marker of functional neuronal activity.[47] Rather, it is possible that CRF stimulates the release of β-END from POMC nerve terminals at the level of LHRH perikarya located in the MPOA. We also postulate that β-END is released from the POMC neurons originating from the ventromedial ARC of the hypothalamus. The release of β-END, in turn, would then activate mainly μ$_1$-opioid receptors and thus alter LHRH neuronal activity from the MPOA to the ME by a complex cascade mechanism.[15]

We have also shown that administration of μ- or μ$_1$-opioid receptor antagonists bilaterally into the MPOA failed to completely reverse the inhibitory influence of CRF on LHRH and LH release in female rats.[15] These results indicate that the effects of CRF on LHRH neurons located in the MPOA may also be due to a direct action and not to a prior activation of the β-END system. It is therefore possible that CRF alone and CRF-induced activation of POMC-derived peptide release, acting in a synergistic and additive way within the MPOA, may exert both a direct postsynaptic effect on LHRH neurons and influence LHRH synthesis and release during various stressors. In addition to the μ-opioidergic system, CRF may also modify the secretion of other peptidergic or aminergic systems present in the MPOA and, in turn, indirectly alter LHRH neuronal activity.

CYTOKINES AND ACTIVITY OF THE
HYPOTHALAMIC-PITUITARY-GONADAL AXIS

Besides CRF and POMC-derived peptides, cytokines appear to be involved in the alteration of reproductive functions induced by immune challenge and also other stressful situations. Among stress-related factors known for their inhibitory effects on LHRH neuronal activity, interleukin-1β (IL-1β) is certainly one of the most potent. Over the years, a large body of clinical evidence has indeed suggested possible connections between the immune and neuroendocrine systems.[48,49] However, the biochemical entities responsible for such communication pathways have long remained hypothetical. The characterization of proteins (called cytokines or interleukins) manufactured by macrophages during the early part of immune activation;[49,50] the demonstration that these proteins can stimulate neuropeptides (such as CRF[51-57]); and finally, the knowledge that subsequent activation of endocrine functions (such as adrenal steroid release) can in turn convey feedback signals to immune cells,[58] all have paved the way for a better understanding of the bilateral communication pathways that link the immune and the neuroendocrine systems. However, substantial evidence now exists to support the production of cytokines within the mammalian CNS (see reviews, refs. 59 and 60). These brain-derived cytokines may function to regulate specific challenges, such as immunological, trauma-induced, physical and emotional stress, to the CNS as well as to receive input from immune signals in the systemic circulation. In recent years, several landmark studies have provided evidence of the production and release of IL-1 (α and β), IL-2, IL-3, and IL-6 from neurons of various brain regions, including the hypothalamus.[59,60] The existence of IL-1 (α and β), IL-3, IL-6, TNFα, and IFNα within astrocytes after an immunological challenge has also been reported.[61,62] In the CNS, glial-derived IL-1 and IL-6 are thought to support trophic functions after brain injury from mechanical trauma, infection together with inflammation, induction of fever, regulation of slow wave-sleep patterns, in addition to possibly exerting paracrine and endocrine effects on production of other hypothalamic factors involved in the activity of the HPA and HPG axis.[59] Furthermore, the demonstration that microglia (resident macrophages) within the CNS are the counterparts of macrophages in systemic immunologic tissue suggests that the brain may contain its own phagocytic cell population. In 1988, Breder and colleagues[63] reported the presence of IL-1β in hypothalamic nerve fibers of postmortem human brain. Although identified in most hypothalamic nuclei, the IL-1β-immunopositive nerve fibers were concentrated within the PVN, the ARC, and the ME. More recent studies using colchicine treatment of rats followed by immunocytochemistry (ICC) with a specific antirat IL-1β antiserum identified dense IL-1β neuronal cell bodies in the magnocellular portion of the PVN, and fibers emanating from these cells were observed in the suprachiasmatic nucleus (SCh), ARC, ME, posterior pituitary, and parvocellular PVN.[64] In contrast to the widespread distribution of IL-1β in the rat brain, IL-1α appears to be confined to more discrete regions of the brain such as the diagonal band of Broca, the anterior hypothalamus (including the MPOA) and the hippocampus.[59,65] Interestingly, immobilization stress[66] and peripheral administration of immunogenic antigens, such as the endotoxin lipopolysaccharide (LPS), may induce brain IL-1 gene expression.[67] In contrast to the effects of systemic administration of IL-1 (α and β), these stressful situations alter the activity of the HPG axis,[68-71] which suggests that peripheral production of IL-1 is certainly not the primary mechanism involved in the alteration of LHRH neuronal activity during immune challenge and other prolonged stresses.

Recent studies have suggested that cytokines modulate neuroendocrine functions such as the activity of both the HPA and HPG axes (FIG. 4). Systemic administration of interleukin (IL)-1α and -β stimulates the activity of the HPA axis,[51-53,72] although this treatment does not modulate the release of plasma LH from the adenohypophysis of both castrated male and female rats.[51,73,74] In contrast, central infusion of IL-1 inhibits the spontaneous expression of nuclear c-fos protein that occurs in LHRH neurons during the afternoon of proestrus and interferes with the release of LHRH from the hypothalamus and LH from the adenohypophysis.[12,28,51,73,74] This treatment also activates nuclear c-fos expression within CRF-immunoreactive neurons of the PVN,[51,75] increases levels of CRF mRNA in this hypothalamic nucleus (Rivest et al., in preparation) and stimulates the release of

CRF from the ME[54] as well as into the hypophyseal-portal system.[52] However, this response of CRF does not appear to be related to the influence of IL-1 on the activity of the HPG axis. Indeed, we recently observed that central administration of two different types of CRF antagonists did not modify the ability of IL-1 to inhibit LHRH neuronal activity (FIG. 5, upper panel) or LH secretion (FIG. 5, lower panel),[12] a finding consistent with our previous demonstration that PVN lesions did not prevent IL-1-induced decrease in LH release in the male rat.[28]

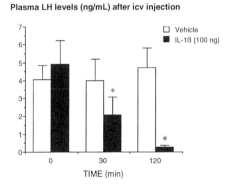

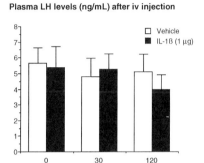

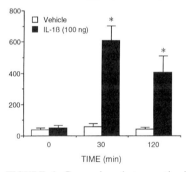

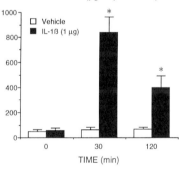

FIGURE 4. Comparison between the intracerebroventricular (i.c.v.) and intravenous (i.v.) route of administration of interleukin-1β (IL-1β) on plasma LH and ACTH secretion in castrated male rats. Results represent means ± SEM of 6 to 8 rats. *$p < 0.05$ from control rats. Data modified from ref. 51.

This confirms that the increase in CRF neuronal activity from the PVN is probably not directly related to the influence of IL-1β on the activity of LHRH neurons. It should be noted that in contrast to findings in rats exposed to physical stress,[25,27] no report shows that IL-1β can activate the CRF neuronal activity from brain regions other than the hypothalamic parvocellular subdivision of the PVN. This may explain the fact that CRF is involved in the antireproductive effects of physical stress,[22] but not those following IL-1 treatment.

SITE OF ACTION AND MEDIATORS OF IL-1 TO INTERFERE
WITH LHRH NEURONAL ACTIVITY

It is presently believed that IL-1β interferes with LHRH neuronal activity by acting at the level of LHRH perikarya rather than at the level of LHRH nerve terminals located in the ME. Furthermore, microinfusion of IL-1β bilaterally into the MPOA reduces LHRH release and the spontaneous expression of c-*fos* protein located within the nuclei of LHRH neurons in proestrus rats bearing a push-pull cannula within the ME.[16] These results indicate that the MPOA represents one of the target regions for central IL-1β in modulating the activity of LHRH neurons that project to the ME. Although it is possible that this cytokine acts directly on LHRH neurons, evidence exists that EOP,[76] prostaglandins,[69,77] and catecholamines[77] can mediate the effect of IL-1 on LHRH neuronal activity. Indeed, the administration of a nonselective opioid antagonist, naloxone, inhibits the influence of IL-1β on the LH secretion and ovulation,[73] whereas naloxone significantly reverses IL-1-induced suppression of LHRH release from incubated hypothalamic fragments.[76] Interestingly, endotoxins and IL-1 increase the levels of POMC-derived peptides in the blood and cerebrospinal fluid,[78,79] and stimulate POMC mRNA in the anterior pituitary.[55] Although the precise mechanisms by which opiates inhibit the activity of the HPG axis are still not well understood (see reviews, refs. 1 and 80), POMC-derived peptides are believed to participate in this effect.[33] As mentioned, the highest concentration of POMC-derived peptides is found in the ARC,[81] and it is known that these neurons innervate other rat hypothalamic regions such as the preoptic area.[39,41,82] In addition, we previously reported that central administration of IL-1β increases c-*fos* protein immunoreactivity in the ARC, which suggests that a number of cells are activated in this hypothalamic area.[51] We also observed that some of the POMC-immunoreactive cells in the ARC expressed Fos in their nuclei after i.c.v. injection of IL-1β, leading to the possibility that POMC neurons from the ARC to the MPOA may participate either directly or indirectly in the inhibition of LHRH neuronal activity during immune challenge or other types of stress activating the central IL-1 system. Nevertheless, the ARC does not appear to be the major target for IL-1 to interfere with the LHRH neuronal activity because bilateral microinfusion of the cytokine in this hypothalamic area did not markedly suppress the hypothalamic release of LHRH during the afternoon of proestrus in rat. Although the IL-1-induced activation of POMC neurons from their perikarya located in the ARC remains possible, a more likely mechanism seems to take place at the level of POMC nerve terminals located in the hypothalamic MPOA. Indeed, as we have already proposed for CRF,[15] it is possible that IL-1 activates the release of EOP, such as β-END, from POMC nerve terminals located in the MPOA and in turn interferes with LHRH neuronal activity. It is also possible that the hypothalamic ARC may be a transitory region for IL-1. In stimulating selective aminergic pathways from the brain stem or other brain structures, IL-1 could indirectly induce the activation of POMC

FIGURE 5. Influence of acute i.c.v. infusion of CRF antagonists and interleukin-1 (IL-1) on the activity of HPG axis in both female (*upper panel*) and male (*lower panel*) rats. The upper panel shows the hypothalamic LHRH release during the afternoon of proestrus in rats bearing a push-pull cannula into the median eminence (ME) whereas the lower panel illustrates the plasma LH levels of castrated male rats. The administration of two different types of CRF antagonists (α-helical CRF[9–41] and [D-PHE,[12] NLE[21,38] Cα Me LEU[37]] rCRF[12–41]) was performed 10 minutes before the i.c.v. infusion of IL-1. *Significantly different ($p < 0.05$) from vehicle-treated rats. Data obtained from ref. 12.

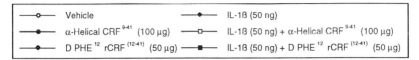

LHRH release (pg/10 min)

♀ **Proestrus**

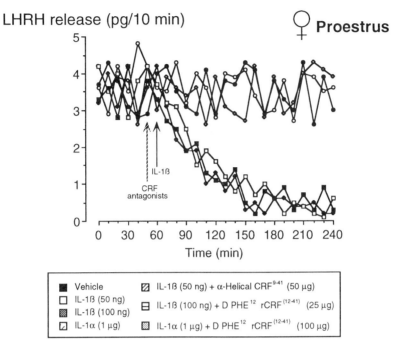

Plasma LH levels (ng/ml)

♂ **Castrated**

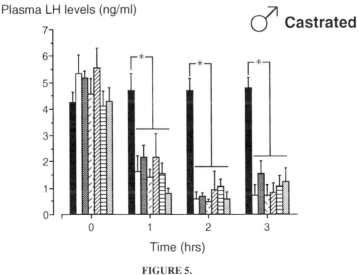

Time (hrs)

FIGURE 5.

neurons from the ARC and in turn increase the release of β-END at the level of the MPOA. The exact pathways by which IL-1 may communicate from one region to another remain, however, poorly understood. Nevertheless, it is important to point out that EOP may only partially mediate the inhibitory influence of IL-1 on the activity of the HPG axis in the rat. Consequently, other factors participate in the effects of these cytokines on the activity of LHRH neurons.

We recently observed that eicosanoid prostaglandins (PGs) play a crucial role in mediating the inhibitory effects of central IL-1β injection on the LHRH neuronal activity (FIG. 6). Indeed, administration of indomethacin, an inhibitor of the eicosanoid cyclooxygenase pathway, significantly reversed IL-1β-induced alteration of the HPG axis (FIG. 6).[69] In contrast, injection of a lipooxygenase inhibitor, nor-dihydroguaiaretic acid (NDGA), did not significantly modify the effect of IL-1β on plasma LH secretion.[69] Stimulation of various brain cells by cytokines primarily results in the release of PGE_2,[83] and this PG is reportedly elevated in the circulation during sepsis.[84] Upon observing that IL-1α blocked the release of PGE_2 evoked by exposure of mediobasal hypothalamic fragments to norepinephrine, Rettori et al.[77] proposed that the cytokine suppresses LH secretion through mechanisms that depend on the inhibition of PGE_2 production. This conclusion rests on the hypothesis that catecholamine-induced PG synthesis, which stimulates LHRH secretion,[85] represents a major step in mediating the ability of IL-1α to inhibit the activity of the HPA axis. Although evidence indeed exists that cytokines increase catecholaminergic tone within the CNS,[86] we have been so far unable to block the inhibitory effect of IL-1β by peripheral or central administration of prazosin and/or propanolol (unpublished results). In addition, the fact that indomethacin blocked the IL-1-induced inhibition of the HPG axis does not provide evidence that the possible decrease in the production of certain PGs is responsible for this effect but, in contrast, strongly suggests that the overall activation of PGs modulates the influence of IL-1 on LHRH neuronal activity. Inasmuch as PGs of the E type exert a marked stimulatory effect on the HPG axis whereas PGD_2 is inhibitory,[87] the consistent ability of cytokines to lower LHRH and LH secretion may imply complex interactions between the pattern of prostaglandins released by IL-1. In this context, our findings suggest that PGD_2 is the primary PG released after the central injection of IL-1β, or that in the net balance of the release of PGE_2, $PGF_{2\alpha}$, and PGD_2, this latter PG plays a dominant role. However, the exact mechanisms through which PGs may modulate the LHRH neuronal activity during immune challenge or other stressful situations have yet to be investigated.

Hence, the influence of IL-1α and β on the reproductive axis appears to involve complex cascade mechanisms that could originate from various structures of the brain or directly from the MPOA. Whether these mechanisms take place during physiological circumstances or during stress situations, such as meningitis, brain

---

FIGURE 6. Interaction between indomethacin (INDO) and interleukin-1β (IL-1β) on the activity of HPG axis in both female (*upper panel*) and male (*lower panel*) rats. The upper panel shows the hypothalamic LHRH release during the afternoon of proestrus in rats bearing a push-pull cannula into the median eminence (ME) whereas the lower panel illustrates the plasma LH levels of castrated male rats. IL-1β (50 ng) was infused i.c.v. 15 minutes after the i.v. injection of INDO (8 mg/kg). Control animals received the appropriate vehicle(s). Each point or bar represents the means ± SEM of 4–7 animals. *$p < 0.05$, significantly different from the other groups of animals. As shown by this FIGURE, INDO completely prevents the IL-1β-induced alteration of the HPG axis activity in both male and female rats. Data obtained from ref. 69.

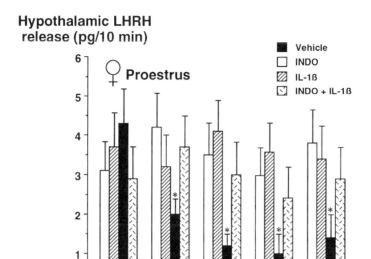

FIGURE 6.

damage, peripheral infection or physical stress, is not presently known. The number of IL-1α-immunoreactive neurons in the MPOA and the septum-diagonal band of Broca, two regions containing LHRH neurons,[8] significantly increases after systemic treatment with LPS[65] suggesting that the production of IL-1 in these regions may be stimulated during immune challenge. Similarly, Van Dam *et al.*[88] recently reported that peripheral administration of endotoxin resulted in the appearance of IL-1 in cells in the meninges, choroid plexus, brain blood vessels, and cells within the brain parenchyma. However, using monoclonal and polyclonal antibodies to macrophage and astrocyte antigens, the endotoxin-induced immunoreactive IL-1 (irIL-1) positive cells were identified as macrophages in the meninges and choroid plexus, perivascular cells, and ramified microglia cells but not in neuronal structures. Hardly any group of irIL-1 positive microglia was noted within the hypothalamus and other parts of the limbic system, except in areas located outside the blood-brain barrier at the circumventricular organs, such as the ME and the organum vasculosum of the lamina terminalis (OVLT), which contained large numbers of IL-1-positive microglial cells.[88] It is thus possible to postulate that the local secretion of IL-1 (α and/or β) in the OVLT or in regions surrounding it, such as the MPOA, by neuronal and/or glial structures during severe stressful situations could represent a mechanism involved in the alteration of reproductive function (FIG. 7).

The development of models of immune activation is actively sought as these would allow a better understanding of the mechanisms through which infectious diseases inhibit reproductive functions. Endotoxins are widely used to mimic some of the events that occur during sepsis,[59,89] and although not a true model of infection, they represent an accepted means of increasing the endogenous release of peripheral and central cytokines.[59,62,88–90] Interestingly, the peripheral administration of endotoxin, but not IL-1α or β, also significantly decreases circulating LH values,[69,91] a phenomenon partially reversed by antibodies against IL-1β.[68] This suggests that the increased production of IL-1 locally within the CNS, not from the periphery, participates in the alteration of LHRH neuronal activity after systemic endotoxin challenge. Though LPS decreases sex steroid secretion,[91] changes in gonadal hormones do not represent the primary mediator of the inhibitory action of LPS on gonadotropin release, because this effect is also observed in gonadectomized rats.[69] The use of antibodies specific for IL-1 receptors has suggested that these cytokines are at least in part responsible for several biological actions of peripherally injected LPS, and in particular their stimulatory effect on the HPA axis.[92] However, in contrast to the involvement of PGs in mediating the central IL-1-induced alteration of the HPG axis, indomethacin does not reverse the inhibitory effect of LPS injected i.v. on plasma LH levels, indicating that factors other than IL-1 are primarily responsible for the reduction of circulating LH levels in castrated rats after LPS treatment. In unpublished experiments, we also failed to observe any modulating effect of naloxone or anti-CRF serum on LPS-induced alteration of the activity of the HPG axis. Although the mechanisms responsible for the ability of endotoxins to decrease the activity of the HPG axis remain undetermined, it is possible to believe that central production of other cytokines could be involved in this process (FIG. 7).

IL-1 AND LHRH GENE EXPRESSION

As mentioned, LHRH neurons express the immediate "early" genes c-*fos*[10,12] and c-*jun*[11] during the proestrus surge of LH in rats (FIG. 8), a phenomenon totally inhibited by central infusion of IL-1β.[12] This provides direct evidence that stimulation of LHRH neurons during proestrus takes place at the level of LHRH cell bodies and that IL-1 is able to interfere strongly with this endogenous and spontaneous process (FIG. 9). Our results also indicate that the endogenous transsynaptic and intracellular transduction processes leading to Fos synthesis within the nucleus of LHRH neurons appear to be of very short duration, taking place probably between 1200 to 1430 h during the afternoon of proestrus.[12]

However, it is not known whether these spontaneous mechanisms will activate LHRH release and induce LH surge and ovulation. It can be postulated that the increase in amplitude of LHRH pulses during the proestrus afternoon[4] stimulates

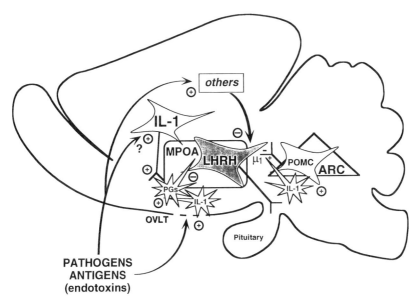

FIGURE 7. Schematic representation of the involvement of prostaglandins (PGs) and opioids (POMC) in modulating the influence of central interleukin-1 (IL-1) on LHRH neuronal activity. However, it is questionable whether the secretion of IL-1 from glial cells and/or neurons located in the MPOA or in structures surrounding it (such as the OVLT) is responsible for the inhibition of the HPG axis after systemic endotoxin administration (such as LPS). Although PGs play a major role in modulating the decrease of plasma LH after i.c.v. IL-1β administration, they do not appear to modulate the inhibitory influence of peripheral LPS treatment on the activity of HPG axis. Many other factors may participate in LPS-induced inhibition of the HPG axis activity in the rats. *Abbreviations*: ARC, arcuate nucleus of the hypothalamus; OVLT, organum vasculosum of the lamina terminalis; LPS, lipopolysaccharide (endotoxin).

expression of c-*fos* within LHRH cell bodies as a consequence of the decapeptide depletion in order to induce and increase LHRH gene transcription. It has been suggested that the regulation of LHRH synthesis is coupled to LHRH release and predicted that LHRH mRNA levels become elevated after a spontaneous surge of LHRH release from the ME.[93,94] Thus, it is possible that the transsynaptic signal stimulating the increase of LHRH pulse amplitude also activates indirectly LHRH gene transcription during the afternoon of proestrus. Inasmuch as IL-1β drastically suppresses LHRH release in the infundibular system, the lack of decapeptide

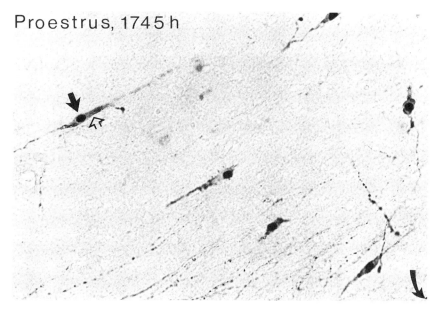

FIGURE 8. Representative example of LHRH neurons expressing c-*fos* protein in their nucleus during the afternoon of proestrus. Sprague-Dawley female rats were deeply anesthetized and rapidly perfused with 4% paraformaldehyde at 1745 h on the day of proestrus. The micrograph (250×) showing c-*fos* protein (*solid arrow*) and LHRH (*open arrow*) immunoreactivity detected by dual immunoperoxidase procedure. The black reaction (c-*fos*) was obtained by nickel sulfate intensification. Solid arrow, nuclear c-*fos* protein located within LHRH neuron; open arrow, LHRH-immunopositive neuron; curved arrow, direction of the organum vasculosum of the lamina terminalis. (Reduced to 70%.)

depletion could, in turn, prevent the activation of LHRH synthesis. This hypothesis remains purely speculative because the putative relationship between the alteration of c-*fos* protein within nuclei of the LHRH neuron and the inhibition of hypothalamic LHRH release has not yet been demonstrated. Indeed, it is likely that the release of LHRH is not necessarily always coupled to its synthesis, and it is possible that IL-1β inhibits the spontaneous expression of c-*fos*, which in turn could be related to the alteration in LHRH gene transcription by a distinct and independent mechanism controlling the release of LHRH. There is as yet no evidence that the IL-1β-induced alteration of endogenous c-*fos* expression in LHRH neurons is accompanied by a decrease in LHRH gene transcription, although central IL-1β injection also seems to reduce the LHRH mRNA levels in the rat hypothalamus. In fact, we observed by means of *in situ* hybridization histochemistry that the average number of silver grains (LHRH mRNA) in LHRH perikarya was significantly lower in IL-1-injected female rats than vehicle-treated animals, suggesting that the LHRH gene transcription is altered by IL-1 (Rivest *et al.*, unpublished data). The total LHRH mRNA levels measured by Northern blot analysis are also lower in chronically IL-1β-infused rats than in i.c.v. vehicle-administered female animals (Rivest *et al.*, unpublished data). Whether the IL-1-induced inhibition of the early gene c-*fos* is responsible for the alteration of LHRH gene expression is presently under investigation in our laboratory. Interestingly, the average number of silver grains (LHRH mRNA) within LHRH cell bodies appears to be higher in LHRH cells expressing c-*fos* protein than in non-Fos-immunoreactive neurons during the afternoon of proestrus in rat (Rivest *et al.,* unpublished data). It is, however, important to keep in mind that although the induction of nuclear Fos and Jun in LHRH neurons may direct the increase in LHRH gene transcription, it is possible that these early genes may increase gene expression of other proteins in LHRH neurons. In addition, a possible role for c-*fos* protein alone in regulating gene expression in LHRH neurons is implausible unless another immediate early gene product, such as Jun, can be identified in the same set of LHRH neurons. Indeed, homodimers of Fos bind with much lower affinity to the AP-1 site on DNA than do heterodimers of Fos with other immediate early genes containing leucine zipper motifs.[95–97] Among the leucine zipper-containing factors, c-*jun* and other members of the Jun protein family are consistently linked to c-*fos* function.[97] Fos/Jun heterodimers are implicated in gene expression in a number of systems including some neuropeptides.[98] However, as yet, no direct *in vivo* evidence exists that the expression of immediate early genes during proestrus is responsible for the activation of LHRH gene transcription. It is, however, possible that the Fos/Jun complex activates the transcription of LHRH gene during physiological situations such as the proestrus surge of LH, and by interfering with this endogenous process, IL-1 can attenuate the LHRH gene

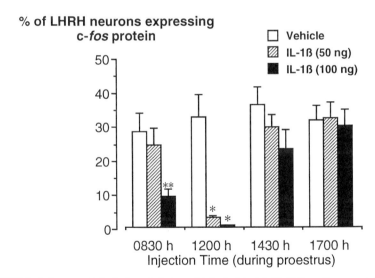

FIGURE 9. Influence of single i.c.v. infusion of interleukin-1β (IL-1β) on the expression of nuclear c-*fos* located within LHRH neurons between 1730 and 1800 h on the day of proestrus in Sprague-Dawley rats. Fifty or 100 ng IL-1β were infused in the lateral ventricle at either 0830, 1200, 1430, or 1700 h on the day of proestrus. The number of LHRH neurons expressing or not expressing c-*fos* in their nuclei was calculated from a 4-in-24 series sections. Then, the percentage (%) of LHRH neurons expressing c-*fos* protein in their nuclei was calculated as the number of LHRH cells containing c-*fos* per number of LHRH-like immunoreactive neurons. The bars represent mean ± SEM for 5–7 rats per group. Statistical analysis was performed using analysis of variance, which was followed by the Dunn-Sidak procedure for the post hoc comparisons. *Significantly different ($p < 0.05$) from vehicle-treated rats. **Significantly different ($p < 0.05$) from the vehicle and the 50-ng IL-1β-treated groups of rats. Data obtained from ref. 12.

expression and the decapeptide secretion. Whether the alteration of LHRH release is related to the inhibition of Fos expression as well as the LHRH synthesis or vice versa remains to be fully determined.

CONCLUSIONS

In women, a disorder called hypothalamic anovulation occurs when the hypothalamus does not produce LHRH, which in turn results in the absence of egg production and release by the ovaries. Similarly, if the LHRH secretion pattern is altered by prolonged stressful situations, a female will show symptoms of dysmenorrhea or amenorrhea whereas a male will reveal alteration of steroidogenesis as well as spermatogenesis. The incidence of secondary amenorrhea in elite female athletes participating in sports such as marathon running, gymnastics, ballet dancing, or others is an example of stress-induced alteration of reproductive function. However, whereas alterations in the secretion of LHRH in women are manifested dramatically and unequivocally as hypothalamic amenorrhea, the signs of hypogonadism in men may not be clinically apparent, although a deficiency in hypothalamic LHRH may exist.[99,100] Among the large amount of clinical evidence indicating that inhibition of reproductive function in women (that is, low levels of plasma estrogen) may cause or accelerate health problems, the increased risk of osteoporosis and subsequent fractures in older women after natural menopause is certainly the most well known.[101–103] The physical and emotional components of a prolonged stressful situation contribute to the stimulation of a series of cascade mechanisms, which in turn modulate the endogenous activity of LHRH neurons. Immune challenge is another powerful stressful circumstance able to perturb reproductive function and can involve similar or completely different mechanisms than those observed during other stresses. The action of the immune system–derived monokine, IL-1, to stimulate release of CRF from the hypothalamus and the consequent elaboration of ACTH release has provided an especially useful model to investigate the nature of the intercommunication of neuroendocrine and immunological pathways. In addition, when centrally injected, IL-1β is probably one of the most potent polypeptides in its ability to completely inhibit LHRH neuronal activity and the HPG axis. Finally, the physiological relevance as well as the exact involvement of the central IL-1 system on LHRH biosynthesis, LHRH release, gonadotropins, sex steroid production, and the ovulatory process during immune challenge and other types of stress are still open questions. Among the other stress-related factors produced and released by different structures of the brain, CRF and EOP most likely play an important role to perturb the reproductive function at the level of the CNS in altering the LHRH neuronal activity (FIG. 10). Although we are still far from understanding the exact neuromolecular mechanisms by which CRF and IL-1 interfere with the neurons responsible for reproduction, the data presented in this review have illustrated how these stress-related factors can independently modulate the reproductive function in the brain of female as well as of male rats. It remains, however, necessary to elucidate the neuroanatomical organization of these peptides and other stress-related factors and to determine whether these pathways can interfere with endogenous regulation of LHRH gene transcription, spontaneous early gene expression, and hypothalamic LHRH secretion, together with plasma gonadotropins, sex steroid concentrations, and the ovulatory process during stressful circumstances. Contemporary techniques of molecular neurobiology *in vivo* will certainly help us to elucidate mechanisms

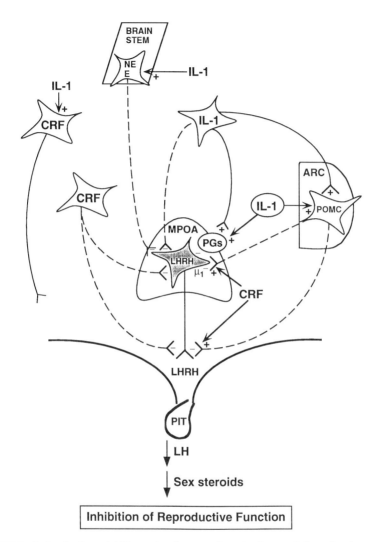

FIGURE 10. Synthesis model illustrating the central mechanisms and sites of action possibly involved in the inhibitory effects of CRF and IL-1 on the LHRH neuronal activity and in turn the reproductive function. Although CRF and IL-1 seem to interact in the brain (for example, IL-1-induced stimulation of CRF neurons from the hypothalamic PVN), these two peptides appear, however, to modulate independently the activity of LHRH neurons and the HPG axis. Arrows and solid axons indicate stimulatory effect; dashed axons, inhibitory effect. *Abbreviations:* ARC, arcuate nucleus of the hypothalamus; CRF, corticotropin-releasing factor; E, epinephrine; IL-1, interleukin-1; LH, luteinizing hormone; LHRH, luteinizing hormone-releasing hormone; MPOA, medial preoptic area of the hypothalamus; NE, norepinephrine; PGs, prostaglandins; PIT, pituitary; POMC, proopiomelanocortin.

participating in the control (activation and inhibition) of the neuroendocrine system responsible for regulation of reproductive function and will consequently improve our knowledge of infertility induced by various stressful situations, a phenomenon which has dramatically increased over the past decade. We have, however, a considerable challenge to study and understand the regulation of infundibular LHRH neurons because of the extreme complexity of this neuroendocrine system. It is also important to point out that the activation and the solicitation of different neural pathways and factors during stress are dependent on the intensity as well as the type of stress used during experimentation (for example, emotional, physical, immune, etc.), which makes generalizations about the mechanisms by which stress alters reproduction difficult.

ACKNOWLEDGMENTS

We thank Susan Johnson for her excellent technical assistance. We are very grateful to Dr. Robert Benoit from the Montreal General Hospital, McGill University (Quebec, Canada) for the gift of LHRH antibody (LR-1) and Dr. S. Gillis, Immunex (Seattle, WA) for the gift of IL-1β. We are also very grateful to Dr. David Parkes for his pertinent comments of this review.

REFERENCES

1. RIVIER, C. & S. RIVEST. 1991. Effect of stress on the activity of hypothalamic-pituitary-gonadal axis: Peripheral and central mechanisms. Biol. Reprod. **45:** 523–532.
2. COLLU, R., W. GIBB & J. R. DUCHARME. 1984. Effects of stress on the gonadal function. J. Endocrinol. Invest. **7:** 529–537.
3. RABIN, D., P. W. GOLD, A. N. MARGIORIS & G. P. CHROUSOS. 1988. Stress and reproduction: Physiologic and pathophysiologic interactions between the stress and reproductive axes. Adv. Exp. Med. Biol. **245:** 377–387.
4. LEVINE, J. E., A. C. BAUER-DANTOIN, L. M. BESECKE, L. A. CONAGHAN, S. J. LEGAN, J. M. MEREDITH, F. J. STROBL, J. H. URBAN, K. M. VOGELSON & A. M. WOLFE. 1991. Neuroendocrine regulation of the luteinizing hormone-releasing hormone pulse generator in the rat. Recent Prog. Horm. Res. **47:** 97–153.
5. SILVERMAN, A. J., E. A. ZIMMERMAN, M. J. GIBSON, M. J. PERLOW, H. M. CHARLTON, G. KOKORIS & D. T. KRIEGER. 1985. Implantation of normal fetal preoptic area into hypogonadal mutant mice: Temporal relationships of the growth of gonadotropin-releasing hormone neurons and the development of the pituitary/testicular axis. Neuroscience **16:** 69–84.
6. CROWLEY, W. F., M. FILICORI, D. I. SPRATT & N. F. SANTORO. 1985. The physiology of gonadotropin-releasing hormone (GnRH) secretion in men and women. Recent Prog. Horm. Res. **41:** 473–531.
7. SILVERMAN, A.-J., J. JHAMANDAS & L. P. RENAUD. 1987. Localization of luteinizing hormone-releasing hormone (LHRH) neurons that project to the median eminence. J. Neurosci. **7:** 2312–2319.
8. SILVERMAN, A. J. 1988. The gonadotropin-releasing hormone (GnRH) neuronal systems: Immunocytochemistry. *In* The physiology of reproduction. E. Knobil & J. Neil, Eds. Vol. **1:** 1283–1304. Raven Press. New York, NY.
9. MERCHENTHALER, S., G. SETALO, C. CSONTOS, P. PETRUSZ, B. FLERKO & A. NEGRO-VILAR. 1989. Combined retrograde tracing and immunocytochemical identification of luteinizing hormone- and somatostatin-containing neurons projecting to the median eminence of the rat. Endocrinology **125:** 2812–2821.
10. LEE, W. S., M. S. SMITH & G. E. HOFFMAN. 1990. Luteinizing hormone-releasing

hormone express Fos protein during the proestrus surge of luteinizing hormone. Proc. Natl. Acad. Sci. USA **87:** 5163–5167.

11. LEE, W. S., R. ABBUD, M. S. SMITH & G. E. HOFFMAN. 1992. LHRH neurons express c-*jun* protein during proestrus surge of luteinizing hormone. Endocrinology **130:** 3101–3103.

12. RIVEST, S. & C. RIVIER. 1993. Interleukin-1β inhibits the endogenous expression of the early gene c-*fos* located within the nucleus of LHRH neurons and interferes with hypothalamic LHRH release during proestrus in the rat. Brain Res. **613:** 132–142.

13. HOFFMAN, G. E., W. S. LEE, B. ATTARDI, V. YANN & M. D. FITZSIMMONS. 1990. Luteinizing hormone-releasing hormone neurons express c-*fos* antigen after steroid activation. Endocrinology **126:** 1736–1741.

14. WITKIN, J. W., C. M. PADEN & A. J. SILVERMAN. 1982. The luteinizing hormone-releasing hormone (LHRH) systems in the rat brain. Neuroendocrinology **35:** 429–438.

15. RIVEST, S., P. PLOTSKY & C. RIVIER. 1993. CRF alters the infundibular LHRH secretory system from the medial preoptic area of female rats: Possible involvement of opioid receptors. Neuroendocrinology. **57:** 236–246.

16. RIVEST, S. & C. RIVIER. 1992. Inhibitory influence of interleukin-1β on c-*fos* expression located in the LHRH neurons and hypothalamic LHRH release during proestrus in rats. *In* Proceeding of the 74th Annual Meeting of the Endocrine Society. **74:** 258. San Antonio, TX.

17. SELYE, H. 1939. Effect of adaptation to various damaging agents on the female sex organs in the rat. Endocrinology **25:** 615–624.

18. PETRAGLIA, F., S. SUTTON, W. VALE & P. PLOTSKY. 1987. Corticotropin-releasing factor decreases plasma LH levels in female rats by inhibiting gonadotropin-releasing hormone release into hypophysial-portal circulation. Endocrinology **120:** 1083–1088.

19. RIVIER, C. & W. VALE. 1984. Influence of corticotropin-releasing factor (CRF) on reproductive functions in the rat. Endocrinology **114:** 914–919.

20. ONO, N., M. D. LUMPKIN, W. K. SAMSON, J. K. McDONALD & S. M. McCANN. 1984. Intrahypothalamic action of corticotropin-releasing factor (CRF) to inhibit growth hormone and LH release in the rat. Life Sci. **35:** 1117–1123.

21. RIVEST, S., Y. DESHAIES & D. RICHARD. 1989. The effects of corticotropin-releasing factor on energy balance in rats are sex-dependent. Am. J. Physiol. **257:** R1417–R1422.

22. RIVIER, C., J. RIVIER & W. VALE. 1986. Stress-induced inhibition of reproductive functions: Role of endogenous corticotropin-releasing factor. Science **231:** 607–609.

23. MACLUSKY, N. J., F. NAFTOLIN & C. LERANTH. 1988. Immunocytochemical evidence for direct synaptic connections between corticotrophin-releasing factor (CRF) and gonadotrophin-releasing hormone (GnRH)-containing neurons in the preoptic area of the rat. Brain Res. **439:** 391–395.

24. SAWCHENKO, P. E. & L. W. SWANSON. 1990. Organization of CRF immunoreactive cells and fibers in the rat brain: Immunohistochemical studies. *In* Corticotropin-Releasing Factor: Basic and Clinical Studies of a Neuropeptide. E. B. DeSouza & C. B. Nemeroff, Eds.: 29–51. CRC Press, Inc. Boca Raton, FL.

25. IMAKI, T., J. L. NAHAN, C. RIVIER, P. E. SAWCHENKO & W. VALE. 1991. Differential regulation of corticotropin-releasing factor mRNA in rat brain regions by glucocorticoids and stress. J. Neurosci. **11:** 583–599.

26. IMAKI, T., T. SHIBASAKI, M. HOTTA & D. DEMURA. 1992. Early induction of c-*fos* precedes increased expression of corticotropin-releasing factor messenger ribonucleic acid in the paraventricular nucleus after immobilization stress. Endocrinology **131:** 240–246.

27. RIVEST, S., S. LEE, C. RIVIER & D. RICHARD. 1992. Expression of *FOS* and CRF mRNA in the brain of female rats subjected to single or repeated running sessions. Proceeding of the 22nd Annual Meeting of the Society for Neuroscience. Vol. **18(1):** 194. Anaheim, CA.

28. RIVEST, S. & C. RIVIER. 1991. Influence of the paraventricular nucleus of the hypothalamus in the alteration of neuroendocrine functions induced by intermittent footshock or interleukin. Endocrinology **129:** 2049–2057.

29. SWANSON, L. W. 1991. Biochemical switching in hypothalamic circuits mediating responses to stress. *In* Progress in Brain Research. G. Holstege, Ed. Vol. **87:** 181–200. Elsevier Science Publishers B. V. Amsterdam.

30. MCDONALD, A. J. 1988. Projections of the intermediate subdivision of the central amygdaloid nucleus to the bed nucleus of the stria terminalis and medial diencephalon. Neurosci. Lett. **85:** 285–290.

31. SWANSON, L. W., P. E. SAWCHENKO, J. RIVIER & W. W. VALE. 1983. Organization of ovine corticotropin releasing factor (CRF)-immunoactive cells and fibers in the rat brain: An immunohistochemical study. Neuroendocrinology **36:** 165–186.

32. PETRAGLIA, F., W. VALE & C. RIVIER. 1986. Opioids act centrally to modulate stress-induced decrease in luteinizing hormone in the rat. Endocrinology **119:** 2445–2450.

33. WEINER, R. I., P. R. FINDELL & C. KORDON. 1988. Role of classic and peptide neuromodulators in the neuroendocrine regulation of LH and prolactin. *In* The Physiology of Reproduction. E. Knobil & J. Neil, Eds. Vol. 1:1235–1281. Raven Press. New York, NY.

34. SARKAR, D. & S. YEN. 1985. Hyperprolactinemia decreases the luteinizing hormone-releasing hormone concentration in pituitary portal plasma: A possible role for β-endorphin as mediator. Endocrinology **116:** 2080–2084.

35. CHING, M. 1983. Morphine suppresses the proestrus surge of GnRH in pituitary portal plasma of rats. Endocrinology **112:** 2209–2211.

36. KESNER, J., J. M. KAUFMAN, R. C. WILSON, G. KURODA & E. KNOBIL. 1986. The effect of morphine on the electrophysiological activity of the hypothalamic luteinizing hormone-releasing hormone pulse generator in the rhesus monkey. Endocrinology **43:** 686–688.

37. RASMUSSEN, D. D., M. GAMBACCIANI, W. SWARTZ, V. S. TUEROS & S. S. C. YEN. 1989. Pulsatile gonadotropin-releasing hormone release from the human mediobasal hypothalamus *in vitro:* Opiate receptor-mediated suppression. Neuroendocrinology **49:** 150–156.

38. DROUVA, S. V., J. EPELBAUM, L. TAPIA-ARANCIBIA, E. LAPLANTE & C. KORDON. 1981. Opiate receptors modulate LHRH and SRIF release from mediobasal hypothalamic neurons. Neuroendocrinology **32:** 163–167.

39. CHEN, W. P., J. W. WITKIN & A. J. SILVERMAN. 1989. Beta-endorphin and gonadotropin-releasing hormone synaptic input to gonadotropin-releasing hormone neurosecretory cells in the male rat. J. Comp. Neurol. **286:** 85–95.

40. CHEN, W.-P., J. W. WITKIN & A.-J. SILVERMAN. 1990. Sexual dimorphism in the synaptic input to gonadotropin releasing hormone neurons. Endocrinology **126:** 695–702.

41. LERANTH, C., N. J. MACLUSKY, M. SHANABROUGH & F. NAFTOLIN. 1988. Immunohistochemical evidence for synaptic connections between proopiomenalocortin-immunoreactive axons and LH-RH neurons in the preoptic area of the rat. Brain Res. **449:** 167–176.

42. BRUHN, T. O., R. E. SUTTON, C. RIVIER & W. VALE. 1984. Corticotropin-releasing factor regulates proopiomelanocortin messenger ribonucleic acid levels *in vivo.* Neuroendocrinology **39:** 170–177.

43. RIVIER, C., M. BROWNSTEIN, J. SPIESS, J. RIVIER & W. VALE. 1982. *In vivo* CRF-induced secretion of ACTH, β-endorphin and corticosterone. Endocrinology **110:** 272–278.

44. VALE, W., J. SPIESS, C. RIVIER & J. RIVIER. 1981. Characterization of a 41-residue ovine hypothalamic peptide that stimulates secretion of corticotropin and β-endorphin. Science **213:** 1394–1397.

45. NIKOLARAKIS, K. E., O. F. X. ALMEIDA & A. HERZ. 1986. Stimulation of hypothalamic β-endorphin and dynorphin release by corticotropin-releasing factor (in vitro). Brain Res. **399:** 152–155.

46. DESOUZA, E. B. & T. R. INSEL. 1990. Corticotropin-releasing factor (CRF) receptors in the rat central nervous system: Autoradiographic localization studies. *In* Corticotropin-Releasing Factor: Basic and Clinical Studies of a Neuropeptide. E. B. DeSouza & C. B. Nemeroff, Eds.: 69 90. CRC Press, Inc. Boca Raton, FL.

47. MORGAN, J. I. & T. CURRAN. 1991. Stimulus-transcription coupling in the nervous system: Involvement of the inductible proto-oncogenes fos and jun. Annu. Rev. Neurosci. **14:** 421–451.

48. O'LEARY, A. 1990. Stress, emotion, and human immune function. Psychol. Bull. **108**: 363–376.
49. RABIN, B. S., J. E. CUNNICK & D. T. LYSLE. 1990. Stress-induced alteration of immune function. Prog. NeuroEndocrinImmunol. **3**: 116–125.
50. DINARELLO, C. A. 1989. Interleukin-1 and its biologically related cytokines. Adv. Immunol. **44**: 153–161.
51. RIVEST, S., G. TORRES & C. RIVIER. 1992. Differential effects of central and peripheral injection of interleukin-1β on brain c-*fos* expression and neuroendocrine functions. Brain Res. **587**: 13–23.
52. SAPOLSKY, R., C. RIVIER, G. YAMAMOTO, P. PLOTSKY & W. VALE. 1987. Interleukin-1 stimulates the secretion of hypothalamic corticotropin-releasing factor. Science **238**: 522–524.
53. BERKENBOSCH, F., J. V. OERS, A. D. REY, F. TILDERS & H. BESEDOVSKY. 1987. Corticotropin-releasing factor producing neurons in the rat activated by interleukin-1. Science **238**: 524–526.
54. BARBANEL, G., G. IXART, A. SZAFARCZYK, F. MALAVAL & I. ASSENMACHER. 1990. Intrahypothalamic infusion of interleukin-1β increases the release of corticotropin-releasing hormone (CRH 41) and adrenocorticotropic hormone (ACTH) in free-moving rats bearing a push-pull cannula in the median eminence. Brain Res. **516**: 31–56.
55. SUDA, T., F. TOZAWA, T. USHIYAMA, T. SUMITOMO, M. YAMADA & H. DEMURA. 1990. Interleukin-1 stimulates corticotropin-releasing factor gene expression in rat hypothalamus. Endocrinology **126**: 1223–1228.
56. NAVARRA, P., S. TSAGARAKIS, M. S. FARIA, L. H. REES, G. M. BESSER & A. B. GROSSMAN. 1991. Interleukin-1 and -6 stimulate the release of corticotropin-releasing hormone-41 from rat hypothalamus *in vitro* via the eicosanoid cyclooxygenase pathway. Endocrinology **128**: 37–44.
57. TSAGARAKIS, S., G. GILLIES, L. H. REES, M. BESSER & A. GROSSMAN. 1989. Interleukin-1 directly stimulates the release of corticotrophin-releasing factor from rat hypothalamus. Neuroendocrinology **49**: 98–101.
58. SOLOMON, G. F. 1969. Stress and antibody response in rats. Int. Arch. Allergy **35**: 97–108.
59. KOENIG, J. I. 1991. Presence of cytokines in the hypothalamic-pituitary axis. Prog. NeuroEndocrinImmunol. **4**: 143–153.
60. BUSBRIDGE, N. J. & A. B. GROSSMAN. 1991. Stress and the single cytokine: Interleukin modulation of the pituitary-adrenal axis. Mol. Cell. Endocrinol. **82**: C209–C214.
61. FONTANA, A., F. KRISTENSE, R. DUBS, D. GEMSA & E. WEBER. 1982. Production of prostaglandins E and an interleukin-1 like factor by cultured astrocytes and C glioma cells. J. Immunol. **129**: 2413–2419.
62. FONTANA, A., E. WEBER & J. M. DAYER. 1984. Synthesis of interleukin-1/endogenous pyrogen in the brain of endotoxin-treated mice: A step in fever induction? J. Immunol. **133**: 1696–1698.
63. BREDER, C. D., C. A. DINARELLO & C. B. SAPER. 1988. Interleukin-1 immunoreactive innervation in the human hypothalamus. Science **240**: 321–324.
64. LECHAN, R. M., R. TONI, B. D. CLARK, J. G. CANNON, A. R. SHAW, C. A. DINARELLO & S. REICHLIN. 1990. Immunoreactive interleukin-1β localisation in the rat forebrain. Brain Res. **514**: 135–140.
65. RETTORI, V., W. L. DEES, J. K. HINEY, L. MILENKOVIC & S. M. MCCANN. 1992. Interleukin-1 alpha (IL-1α)-immunoreactive neurons in the hypothalamus of the rat are increased after lipopolysaccharide (LPS) injection. Proceedings of the 74th Annual Meeting of the Endocrine Society. Vol. **1**: 185. San Antonio, Texas.
66. MINAMI, M., Y. KURAISHI, T. YAMAGUCHI, S. NAKAI, Y. HIRAI & M. SATOH. 1991. Immobilization stress induces interleukin-1β mRNA in the rat hypothalamus. Neurosci. Lett. **123**: 254–256.
67. BAN, E., F. HAOUR & R. LENSTRA. 1992. Brain interleukin 1 gene expression induced by peripheral lipopolysaccharide administration. Cytokine **4**: 48–54.
68. EBISUI, O., J. FUKATA, T. TOMINAGA, N. MURAKAMI, H. KOBAYASHI, H. SEGAWA, S. MURO, Y. NAITO, Y. MASUI, T. NISHIDA & H. IMURA. 1992. Roles of interleukin-1α

and β in endotoxin-induced suppression of plasma gonadotropin levels in rats. Endocrinology **130**: 3307–3313.

69. RIVEST, S. & C. RIVIER. 1993. Centrally injected interleukin-1β inhibits the hypothalamic LHRH secretion and circulating LH levels via prostaglandins in rats. J. Neuroendocrinol. In press.

70. CHARPENET, G., Y. TACHÉ, M. G. FOREST, F. HAOUR, J. M. SAEZ, M. BERNIER, J. R. DUCHARME & R. COLLU. 1981. Effects of chronic intermittent immobilization stress on rat testicular androgenic function. Endocrinology **109**: 1254–1258.

71. NORMAN, R. L. & C. J. SMITH. 1992. Restraint inhibits luteinizing hormone and testosterone secretion in intact male rhesus macaques: Effects of concurrent naloxone administration. Neuroendocrinology **55**: 405–415.

72. RIVIER, C., W. VALE & M. BROWN. 1989. In the rat, interleukin-1α and β stimulate ACTH and catecholamine release. Endocrinology **125**: 3096–3102.

73. RIVIER, C. & W. VALE. 1990. Cytokines act within the brain to inhibit LH secretion and ovulation in the rat. Endocrinology **127**: 849–856.

74. RIVIER, C. & W. VALE. 1989. In the rat, interleukin-1α acts at the level of the brain and the gonads to interfere with gonadotropin and sex steroid secretion. Endocrinology **124**: 2105–2109.

75. GONG, J., X. ZHANG, B. Q. JIN & C. S. HUANG. 1991. Activation of corticotropin-releasing factor-containing neurons in the paraventricular nucleus of the hypothalamus by interleukin-1 in the rat. Neurosci. Lett. **132**: 151–154.

76. KALRA, P. S., M. FUENTES, A. SAHU & S. P. KALRA. 1990. Endogenous opioid peptides mediate the interleukin-1-induced inhibition of the release of luteinizing hormone (LH)-releasing hormone and LH. Endocrinology **127**: 2381–2386.

77. RETTORI, V., M. F. GIMENO, A. KARARA, M. C. GONZALEZ & S. M. MCCANN. 1991. Interleukin-1α inhibits prostanglandins E2 release to suppress pulsatile release of luteinizing hormone but not follicle-stimulating hormone. Proc. Natl. Acad. Sci. USA **88**: 2763–2767.

78. HEIJNEN, C. J., A. KAVELAARS & R. E. BALLIEUX. 1991. Beta-endorphin—cytokine and neuropeptide. Immunol. Rev. **119**: 41–63.

79. CARR, D. B., R. BERGLAND, A. HAMILTON, H. BLUME, M. KASTING, M. ARNOLD & J. B. MARTIN. 1982. Endotoxin-stimulated opioid peptide secretion: Two secretory pools and feedback control *in vivo*. Science **217**: 845–847.

80. KALRA, S. P. & P. S. KALRA. 1983. Neural regulation of luteinizing hormone secretion in the rat. Endocr. Rev. **4**: 311–351.

81. MEZEY, E., J. Z. KISS, G. P. MUELLER, R. ESKAY, T. L. O'DONOHUE & M. PALKOVITS. 1985. Distribution of the pro-opiomelacortin derived peptides, adrenocorticotrope hormone, alpha-melanocyte-stimulating hormone and β-endorphin (ACTH, alpha-MSH, β-END) in the rat hypothalamus. Brain Res. **328**: 341–347.

82. THIND, K. K. & P. C. GOLDSMITH. 1988. Infundibular gonadotropin-releasing hormone neurons are inhibited by direct opioid and autoregulatory synapses in juvenile monkeys. Neuroendocrinology **47**: 203–216.

83. KATSUURA, G., P. E. GOTTSCHALL, R. R. DAHL & A. ARIMURA. 1989. Interleukin-1β increases prostaglandin E2 in rat astrocyte cultures: Modulating effect of neuropeptides. Endocrinology **124**: 3125–3127.

84. ERTEL, W., M. H. MORRISON, P. WANG, Z. F. BA, A. AYALA & I. H. CHAUDRY. 1992. The complex pattern of cytokines in sepsis—Association between prostaglandins, cachectin, and interleukins. Ann. Surg. **214**: 141–148.

85. OJEDA, S. R., A. NEGRO-VILAR & S. M. MCCANN. 1979. Release of prostaglandins by hypothalamic tissue: Evidence for their involvement in catecholamine-induced luteinizing hormone-releasing hormone release. Endocrinology **104**: 617–624.

86. DUNN, A. J. 1990. Interleukin-1 as stimulator of hormone secretion. Prog. NeuroEndocrinImmunol. **3**: 26–34.

87. KINOSHITA, F., Y. NAKAI, H. KATAKAMI, H. IMURA, T. SHIMIZU & O. HAYAISHI. 1982. Suppressive effect of prostaglandin (PG)D2 on pulsatile luteinizing hormone release in concious castrated rats. Endocrinology **110**: 2207–2209.

88. VAN DAM, A. M., M. BROUNS, S. LOUISSE & F. BERKENBOSCH. 1992. Appearance of

interleukin-1 in macrophages and in ramified microglia in the brain of endotoxin-treated rats: A pathway for the induction of non-specific symptoms of sickness? Brain Res. **588:** 291–296.

89. HIGGINS, G. A. & J. A. OLSCHOWKA. 1991. Induction of interleukin-1β mRNA in adult rat brain. Mol. Brain Res. **9:** 143–148.

90. BRISTOW, A. F., K. MOSLEY & S. POOLE. 1991. Interleukin-1β production in vivo and in vitro in rats and mice measured using specific immunoradiometric assays. J. Mol. Endocrinol. **7:** 1–7.

91. RIVIER, C. 1989. Role of endotoxin and interleukin-1 in modulating ACTH, LH and sex steroid secretion. *In* Circulating Regulatory Factors and Neuroendocrine Function. J. C. Porter & D. Jezova, Eds.: 295–301. Plenum Press. New York, NY.

92. RIVIER, C., R. CHIZZONITE & W. VALE. 1989. In the mouse, the activation of the hypothalamic-pituitary-adrenal axis by a lipopolysaccharide (endotoxin) is mediated through interleukin-1. Endocrinology **125:** 2800–2805.

93. ZOELLER, R. T. & W. S. YOUNG. 1988. Changes in cellular levels of messenger ribonucleic acid encoding gonadotropin-releasing hormone in the anterior hypothalamus of female rats during the estrus cycle. Endocrinology **123:** 1688–1689.

94. PETERSEN, S. L., C. CHEUK, R. D. HARTMAN & C. BARRACLOUGH. 1989. Medial preoptic microimplants of the antiestrogen, keoxifene, affect luteinizing hormone-releasing hormone mRNA levels, median eminence luteinizing hormone-releasing hormone concentrations and luteinizing hormone release in ovariectomized, estrogen-treated rats. J. Neuroendocrinol. **1:** 279–283.

95. CHIU, R., W. J. BOYLE, J. MEEK, T. SMEAL, T. HUNTER & M. KARIN. 1988. The c-*fos* protein interacts with c-*jun*/AP-1 to stimulate transcription of AP-1 responsive genes. Cell **54:** 541–552.

96. TURNER, R. & R. TJIAN. 1989. Leucine repeats and an adjacent DNA binding domain mediate the formation of functional cFos-cJun heterodimers. Science **243:** 1689–1694.

97. SHENG, M. & M. E. GREENBERG. 1990. The regulation and function of c-*fos* and other immediate early genes in the nervous system. Neuron **4:** 477–495.

98. DRAISCI, G. & M. IADAROLA. 1989. Temporal analysis of increases in c-fos preprodynorphin and pre-proenkephalin mRNAs in rat spinal cord. Mol. Brain Res. **6:** 31–37.

99. MACCONNIE, S. E., A. BARKAN, R. M. LAMPMAN, A. SHORK & I. Z. BEITINS. 1986. Decreased hypothalamic gonadotropin-releasing hormone secretion in male marathon runners. N. Engl. J. Med. **315:** 411–417.

100. BARRON, J. L., T. D. NOAKES, W. LEVY, C. SMITH & R. P. MILLAR. 1985. Hypothalamic dysfunction in overtrained athletes. J. Clin. Endocrinol. & Metab. **60:** 803–806.

101. LINNELL, S. L., J. M. STAGER, P. W. BLUE, N. OYSTER & D. ROBERTSHAW. 1984. Bone mineral content and menstrual regularity in female runners. Med. Sci. Sports Exercise **16:** 343–348.

102. LINDSAY, R. D., D. M. HART, J. M. AITKEN, E. B. MACDONALD, J. ANDERSON & A. C. CLARKE. 1976. Long-term prevention of post-menopausal osteoporosis by oestrogen: Evidence for an increased bone mass after delayed onset of oestrogen treatment. Lancet **1:** 1038–1041.

103. SCHWARTZ, J. A., B. SHERMAN & R. MARTIN. 1983. Bone density in amenorrheic women with and without hyperprolactinemia. J. Clin. Endocrinol. & Metab. **56:** 1120–1123.

The Role of Limbic and Hypothalamic Corticotropin-Releasing Factor in Behavioral Responses to Stress

FRÉDÉRIQUE MENZAGHI, STEPHEN C. HEINRICHS,
EMILIO MERLO PICH, FRIEDBERT WEISS,
AND GEORGE F. KOOB[a]

The Scripps Research Institute
Department of Neuropharmacology, CVN7
10666 North Torrey Pines Road
La Jolla, California 92037

Stress is classically defined as a nonspecific response to any demand (usually noxious) upon the body[1] and is accompanied by various physiological changes including activation of the pituitary-adrenal axis. This activation is dependent upon hypothalamic releasing hormones such as corticotropin-releasing factor (CRF) that regulate the secretion of adrenocorticotropic hormone (ACTH) from the pituitary. The endocrine action of ACTH in turn stimulates the release of adrenal steroid hormones which have widespread systemic effects on metabolic and immunologic variables. Because these events represent appropriate biological responses to stress,[2] hypothalamo-pituitary-adrenal activation has been extensively quantified experimentally in order to infer the presence and intensity of stress in an affected organism.

Later theorists emphasized the potency of psychological stimuli in inducing a stress response.[3] Indeed, common physiological stressors such as exercise and hunger do not activate the pituitary-adrenal axis when they are presented in a way that eliminates the perception of fear or conflict.[4] The salience of psychological variables suggests that there is a neurobiological substrate that interprets alerting or threatening cognitive stimuli and consequently stimulates the appropriate physiological stress response. This substrate has been hypothesized to be the brain system classically involved in the processing of emotion—the limbic system. Thus, stressors that disturb psychological homeostasis activate the pituitary-adrenal system via limbic inputs to the hypothalamus.[5,6] Although such stress-induced activation is largely dependent on the neuroendocrine action of hypothalamic CRF, the concurrent stimulation of CRF activity outside of the hypothalamo-pituitary axis (HPA) which accompanies increased emotionality suggests a direct neurotropic role for CRF in coordinating separate behavioral or autonomic responses to stress.

CRF AS NEUROTRANSMITTER IN THE CENTRAL NERVOUS SYSTEM

CRF immunoreactivity has been localized in the central nervous system both in the hypothalamus and in extrahypothalamic structures.[7] Notable are CRF-stained cells and fibers in the paraventricular nucleus (PVN) of the hypothalamus, the

---

[a]Corresponding author.

central nucleus of the amygdala (CeA), the bed nucleus of the stria terminalis, the substantia innominata, the region of the locus coeruleus and parabrachialis nucleus. *In situ* hybridization techniques have confirmed the presence of CRF mRNA in cells containing CRF-like immunoreactivity in most of these brain structures.[8] Other studies have described the presence of high-affinity binding sites for ^{125}I-CRF in various brain structures with a particularly marked distribution in the cerebral cortex, the amygdaloid nuclei, and the PVN.[9]

A variety of stressors alter CRF concentrations, receptors, and messenger RNA levels in discrete brain regions, and not only in populations of hypothalamic CRF neurons. As expected, given the hypophysiotropic role of CRF in the hypothalamus, stressors such as cold swim, physical restraint or ether inhalation induce an immediate release of CRF into the pituitary portal system and an increase in synthesis of CRF within the PVN.[10] Furthermore, measurement of CRF content or synthesis in extrahypothalamic brain structures of rats exposed to acute and chronic stressors reveals selective increases or decreases in CRF levels within the locus coeruleus, Barrington's nucleus, and olfactory bulb depending on the nature and duration of the stressor.[11,12] More importantly, the majority of discrete brain regions in which CRF neurons can be visualized under basal conditions do not exhibit alterations in CRF concentrations following exposure to a stressor.[10] These results provide evidence for regional differences in the regulation of CRF by stress.

The evidence for modified CRF release after exposure to a stressor has been recently supported in our laboratory using intracranial microdialysis in freely moving rats.[13] CRF release monitored through a dialysis probe inserted into the mediobasal hypothalamus of awake rats increased significantly over basal levels after exposure to immobilization or osmotic stress (FIG. 1). Further, plasma ACTH and corticosterone levels paralleled the fluctuating levels of CRF measured in dialysate. These data confirm previous results obtained by measuring CRF concentrations in the portal blood of anesthetized rats,[14] and in push-pull perfusates of freely moving rats.[15]

BEHAVIORAL EFFECTS OF CRF

Direct administration of CRF into the central nervous system produces a dose-dependent behavioral activation.[16,17] CRF administered intracerebroventricularly (i.c.v.) increases locomotor activity, rearing, and grooming when rats are tested in a familiar environment. This activation is not observed after systemic administration of CRF and is not blocked by hypophysectomy or pretreatment with dexamethasone, suggesting that this effect of CRF is mediated by actions in the central nervous system independent of the pituitary-adrenal axis.

The profile of the behavioral actions of exogenously administered CRF changes dramatically when the animals are exposed to a stressor. The same i.c.v. doses that produced behavioral activation in a familiar environment suppress exploration of a novel, presumably stressful environment. Rodents pretreated with CRF show behavioral inhibition in an open field, in a multicompartment chamber, and in an elevated plus-maze. CRF also enhances the behavioral reactivity of animals subjected to noxious stimuli or aversive psychological states induced by acoustic startle, conditioned fear in an operant suppression paradigm, and shock-induced freezing. Thus, behavioral activation produced by exogenously administered CRF in unstressed animals is transformed into a behaviorally inhibiting effect of CRF under stressful conditions.

Support for a role of brain CRF in behavioral responses to stress comes from studies using a CRF antagonist. α-Helical CRF$_{9-41}$, a competitive antagonist for the brain CRF receptors, reverses the behavioral effect of exogenously administered CRF and has some antistress actions in non-CRF-treated animals. In a recent study, the CRF antagonist administered i.c.v. reversed the decrease in exploration of the open arms of an elevated plus-maze caused by exposure to a social stressor.[18]

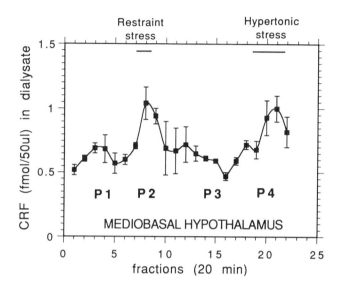

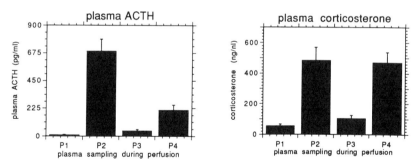

FIGURE 1. Effects of restraint stress and hypertonic saline stress on CRF levels in dialysate collected from mediobasal hypothalamus of awake, freely moving rats ($n = 5$) (*upper panel*). P1, P2, P3, and P4 indicate the time of blood sampling from an indwelling intracardiac catheter for plasma ACTH and corticosterone measurements ($n = 5$) (*lower panels*).

Further, i.c.v. administration of this CRF antagonist attenuates the behavioral reactivity to a wide range of stressors including physical restraint, electric shock, acoustic startle, and drug withdrawal symptoms. Thus, the effects of CRF antagonist observed after i.c.v. administration are suggestive of enhanced CRF activity during stress, but do not provide anatomical specificity for these effects.

LOCAL BRAIN SITES FOR THE BEHAVIORAL EFFECTS OF CRF

Direct administration of CRF into local brain areas of the rat produces a dose-dependent pattern of behavioral effects that is homologous to that observed after i.c.v. administration. The locus coeruleus is particularly sensitive to the suppression of exploratory behavior produced by central administration of CRF.[19] A locomotor-activating effect of CRF is exerted in the region of the substantia innominata[20] and the ventral tegmental area,[21] whereas a decrement in open-field exploration is produced by injection of CRF into the amygdala.[22] In addition, the PVN is a sensitive substrate for the anorexic effect of CRF.[23] A series of studies designed to evaluate the involvement of CRF neurons in the PVN and the CeA are in progress in our laboratory. These two structures are included by Nauta[24] in the "extended limbic system" and are thought to be involved in neuroendocrine and autonomic regulatory functions.

Paraventricular Nucleus of the Hypothalamus

The dense representation of CRF neurons in the PVN serves a classic hypophysiotropic function in the stimulatory control of ACTH release. In addition, subpopulations of CRF immunoreactive neurons have been shown to project to autonomic structures in the brain stem and spinal cord.[8] In support of a functional role for this CRF pathway, Brown and Fisher[25] injected CRF into 48 different brain sites and observed a robust autonomic CRF response at several hypothalamic sites, especially after administration of CRF into the PVN. Further, intra-PVN injection of CRF increases gastric secretory volume.[26] These results suggest that CRF acts within the PVN to elicit a stress-like pattern of autonomic nervous outflow and cardiovascular changes. At the behavioral level, local administration of CRF into the PVN has been shown to induce dose-dependent locomotor-activating and anxiogenic effects.[27] Thus, a comprehensive pattern of endocrine, autonomic, and behavioral activation appears to be exerted by CRF systems within the PVN.

In order to further test the involvement of PVN CRF systems in the response to stress, a novel technique of immunotargeting of cellular toxins to CRF neurons[28] has been used to produce lesions of the CRF system of the PVN. The immunotargeting of toxins is a well-known technique used for killing tumor cells in the treatment of cancer[29] and has only recently evolved into a technique for inducing neurotoxic lesions in the central nervous system.[30] In a typical experiment, a mixture of ricin A chain toxin, an inhibitor of protein synthesis, and of IgG2a monoclonal antibody to CRF (CRF-mAb) is injected in rat brain structures containing CRF neurons. This isotype (IgG2a) of CRF-mAb permits the activation of the endogenous complement pathways that results in the passage of exogenous unconjugated toxins across the membrane of targeted neurons.[31,32] In this way, toxins such as ricin A chain, which do not cross cell membranes, may passively penetrate some CRF neurons of the hypothalamus via complement-induced porosities in the membrane and produce subsequent cellular damage of CRF-targeted neurons.[33] Consequently, a specific decrease of CRF content in the site of injection and in some sites of projection is observed (FIG. 2). Using this procedure, long-term disturbances of the pituitary-adrenal axis have been described in response to ether stress, adrenalectomy or circadian rhythmicity two to four weeks after immunotargeting of rat PVN neurons with CRF-mAb and toxins.[35–37]

In a recent study, CRF-mAb–targeted toxin administered into the PVN reversed the decrease in exploration of the open arms of an elevated plus-maze caused by exposure to a social stressor.[38] CRF-mAb/toxin-treated rats were placed for 5 minutes on the plus-maze after being subjected to social defeat and after 30 minutes of social threat by a resident rat. Social defeat and social threat were produced by allowing the resident to attack the intruder. When the resident attack resulted in biting or when the intruder assumed a defensive supine posture, the intruder was

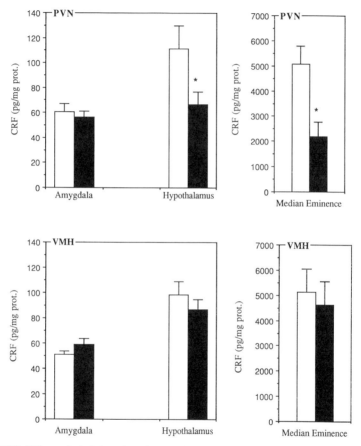

FIGURE 2. Effects of administration of monoclonal antibody to CRF and toxins (*solid bars*) or a nonspecific immunoglobulin and toxins (*open bars*) as controls on CRF content in various brain areas. Rats were sacrificed two weeks after simultaneous injection into the PVN or the VMH of CRF-mAb/toxins or nsp IgG/toxins. Each group contained 6–12 rats. *$p < 0.05$, nsp IgG/toxins. (Menzaghi *et al.*[34] Reproduced, with permission, from *Brain Research.*)

placed in a protective wire mesh enclosure, where intraspecific aggression occurred without physical contact or injury. Socially defeated rats were placed on the elevated plus-maze two weeks after intra-PVN administration of CRF-mAb and toxins. The effect of CRF-mAb and toxins on social stress-induced emotionality was paralleled by a significant decrease of CRF content in the hypothalamus and median eminence, and a decrease of ACTH and corticosterone responses to stress.[38] These data suggest the possible involvement of CRF neurons within the PVN in mediating not only endocrine responses, but also behavioral responses to stress.

The PVN is also involved in the regulation of food intake because bilateral electrolytic lesions of the PVN induce persistent hyperphagia and exaggerated weight gain.[39] CRF is particularly effective in decreasing food intake when injected into the PVN.[23] This effect may not depend on hypophysiotropic CRF neurons that project from the PVN to the median eminence, but may reflect actions of PVN projections to brainstem autonomic systems involved in appetite regulation.[40,41]

The hypothesis that endogenous CRF has an inhibitory action on food intake was recently tested using brain microinjections of α-helical CRF_{9-41}. Pretreatment with α-helical CRF_{9-41} either i.c.v. or directly into the PVN enhanced the ability of neuropeptide Y (NPY) administered into the same locus to stimulate feeding.[42,43] α-Helical CRF_{9-41} injected into the ventromedial hypothalamic nucleus (VMH) or the CeA did not affect the food intake induced by NPY administration into the VMH or the CeA, respectively (FIG. 3). Enhancement of NPY orexigenic effects was also observed two weeks after immunotargeting of CRF neurons in the PVN using local administration of CRF-mAb and toxins.[34] As shown in FIGURE 4, the selective inactivation of CRF neurons in the PVN, but not VMH or CeA, significantly enhanced the hyperphagia induced by NPY in these same brain sites, respectively. These results are in agreement with previous reports of antistress effect of α-helical CRF_{9-41} in reversing the anorexia produced by restraint stress.[44] In addition, food intake occurring in response to a physiological stressor such as nutritional imbalance may be constrained by anorexic actions of endogenous CRF systems.[45,46] Thus, CRF neurons of the PVN may serve to limit food intake when an element of risk intrudes upon established feeding patterns of animals forced by biological need to consume novel foodstuffs or to consume food under stressful conditions.

Central Nucleus of Amygdala

Amygdalofugal pathways have been well documented to participate in autonomic, endocrine, and behavioral responses to stress.[47] Electrical stimulation of the CeA increases respiration and cardiac output and produces affective behavioral responses;[47] lesions to the CeA block the elevation in ACTH caused by immobilization stress[5] and block corticosterone responses to "psychological" stressors.[6] CRF neurons densely innervate the CeA, and injection of CRF into this region increases locomotor activity in a familiar environment[20] and reduces exploratory behavior in an unfamiliar open field.[22]

In a recent study designed to test the role of CRF systems in the CeA in coordinating behavioral and endocrine responses to stress, α-helical CRF_{9-41} administered into the CeA reversed the decrease in exploration of the open arms of an elevated plus-maze caused by exposure to a social stressor.[18] Socially defeated rats placed on the elevated plus-maze showed a suppression of time spent on the open arms that was reversed by α-helical CRF_{9-41} injected bilaterally into the CeA (FIG. 5). The dose of CRF antagonist required to reverse stress-induced suppression of behavior in the plus-maze test of emotionality was 100 times lower with intracerebral injections into the CeA than that effective by the i.c.v. route.[18] This same dose of α-helical CRF_{9-41} injected into the CeA failed to reverse the short-term increase in ACTH and corticosterone (15 min) observed after exposure to the social stressor, suggesting that the behavioral effect observed is independent of the activation of the pituitary adrenal axis.[18] Consistent with this observation, intravenous administration of an antibody to CRF sufficient to block the ACTH and corticosterone response to

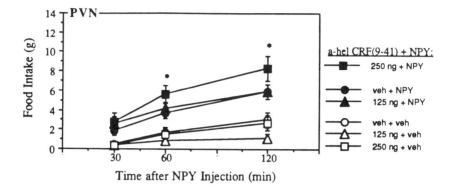

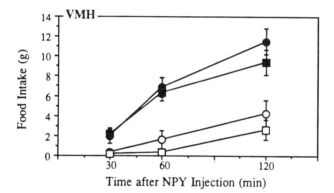

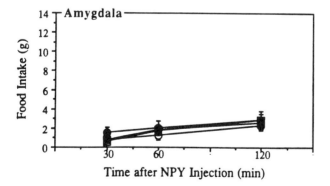

FIGURE 3. Effect of bilateral administration of alpha-helical CRF antagonist within different brain areas on neuropeptide Y (NPY)-induced food intake. NPY (500 ng) was administered 15 minutes after the injection of α-helical CRF_{9-41} (125 or 250 ng) or vehicle into the same nucleus. Cumulative food intake was measured at three different time points after the injection of NPY. Each group contained 7–8 rats. *$p < 0.05$, vehicle + NPY group. (Heinrichs et al.[43] Reproduced, with permission, from *Brain Research*.)

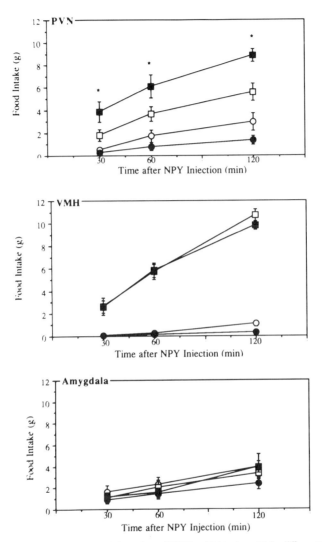

FIGURE 4. Effect of bilateral administration of CRF-mAb/toxins within different brain areas on neuropeptide Y (NPY)-induced food intake. NPY was administered two weeks after the injection of monoclonal antibody to CRF (mAb) or nonspecific IgG (nsp) and toxins into the same nucleus. Cumulative food intake was measured at three different time points after the injection of NPY. Each group contained 8–10 rats. *Filled squares,* mAb/NPY; *open squares,* nsp/NPY; *open circles,* nsp/veh; *filled circles,* mAb/veh. *$p < 0.05$, nsp/NPY. (Menzaghi *et al.*[34] Reproduced, with permission, from *Brain Research.*)

the social stressor did not affect the behavioral response on the plus-maze.[48] Moreover, CRF-mAb and toxins administered within the CeA two weeks before social stress blocked the anxiogenic effects of stress on open-arm exploration in the plus-maze, but not the ACTH response to stress (unpublished observations). One possible conclusion is that the efferent connection between the CeA and the HPA is not directly dependent on a CRF pathway. Finally, results from microdialysis studies show also a stress-induced increase in the release of CRF from the rat amygdala[49] providing additional evidence for a possible neurotropic role of CRF within the central nervous system outside of the hypothalamic-pituitary connection.

SUMMARY AND CONCLUSIONS

CRF in the central nervous system appears to have activating properties on behavior and to coordinate behavioral responses to stress. These behavioral effects of CRF appear to be independent of the pituitary-adrenal axis and can be reversed by a CRF antagonist, α-helical CRF_{9-41}. The CRF antagonist reverses not only decreases in behavior associated with stress, but also increases in behavior associated with stress, thus suggesting that the role of CRF is stress dependent and not intrinsic to a given behavioral response. Further, microinjection of α-helical CRF_{9-41} and immunotargeting of CRF neurons in separate brain compartments reveal a link between the anatomical sites that contain CRF and the nature of the behavioral response to stress that can be modified by suppression of endogenous CRF activity therein. Hence, consistent with the dual role of other hypothalamic-releasing factors in integrating hormonal and neural mechanisms by acting both as secretagogues for anterior pituitary hormones and as extrapituitary peptide neurotransmitters, CRF

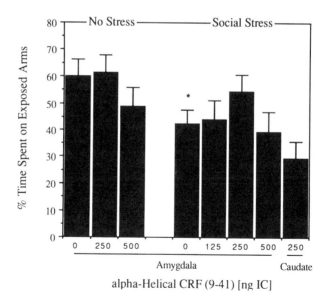

FIGURE 5. Time on exposed maze arms for subjects either taken directly from the home cage (No Stress) and infused with 0, 250 or 500 ng doses of α-helical CRF_{9-41} bilaterally into the central nucleus of the amygdala or defeated socially and exposed to conspecific aggression for 30 minutes (Social Stress) and infused with 0, 125, 250 or 500 ng doses of α-helical CRF_{9-41} bilaterally into the central nucleus of the amygdala. Each group contained 10–13 rats. $*p < 0.05$, vehicle-treated control group. (Heinrichs et al.[18] Reproduced, with permission, from *Brain Research*.)

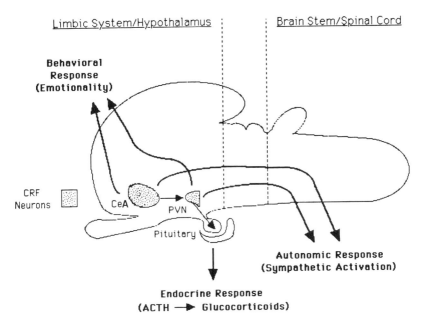

FIGURE 6. Schematic diagram depicting limbic and hypothalamic structures which coordinate the behavioral, endocrine, and autonomic responses to stress. PVN, paraventricular nucleus of the hypothalamus; CeA, central nucleus of the amygdala. (Adapted from Nauta.[24])

may coordinate coping responses to stress at several bodily levels (FIG. 6). Moreover, dysfunction in such a fundamental homeostatic system may be the key to a variety of pathophysiological conditions including mental disorders.

REFERENCES

1. SELYE, H. 1936. A syndrome produced by diverse noxious agents. Nature **32:** 138.
2. MUNCK, A. S., P. M. GUYRE & N. J. HOLBROOK. 1984. Physiological functions of glucocorticoids in stress and their relation to pharmacological action. Endocr. Rev. **5:** 25–44.
3. BURCHFIELD, S. 1979. The stress responses: A new perspective. Psychosom. Med. **41:** 661–672.
4. MASON, J. W. 1971. A re-evaluation of the concept of "non-specificity" in stress specificity in stress theory. J. Psychiatr. Res. **8:** 323–333.
5. BEAULIEU, S., T. DI PAOLO & N. BARDEN. 1986. Control of ACTH secretion by the central nucleus of the amygdala: Implication of the serotoninergic system and its relevance to glucocorticoid delayed negative feedback mechanism. Neuroendocrinology **44:** 247–254.
6. VAN DE KAR, L. D., R. A. PEICHOWSHI, P. A. RITTENHOUSE & T. S. GRAY. 1991. Amygdaloid lesions: Differential effect of conditioned stress and immobilization-induced increases in corticosterone and renin secretion. Neuroendocrinology **54:** 89–95.
7. SWANSON, L. W., P. E. SAWCHENKO, J. RIVIER & W. VALE. 1983. The organization of ovine corticotropin-releasing factor (CRF) immunoreactive cells and fibres in the rat brain: An immunohistochemical study. Neuroendocrinology **36:** 165–186.
8. SAWCHENKO, P. E. 1987. Evidence for differential regulation of corticotropin-releasing

factor and vasopressin immunoreactivities in parvocellular neurosecretory and auto-nomic-related projections of the paraventricular nucleus. Brain Res. **437:** 253–263.

9. DE SOUZA, E. B. 1987. Corticotropin-releasing factor receptors in the rat central nervous system: Characterization and regional distribution. J. Neurosci. **7:** 88–100.

10. CHAPPELL, P. B., M. A. SMITH, C. D. KILTS, G. BISSETTE, J. RITCHIE, C. ANDERSON & C. B. NEMEROFF. 1986. Alterations in corticotropin-releasing factor-like immunoreactivity in discrete rat brain regions after acute and chronic stress. J. Neurosci. **6:** 2908–2914.

11. VALENTINO, R. J. & R. G. WEHBY. 1988. Corticotropin-releasing factor: Evidence for a neurotransmitter role in the locus coeruleus during hemodynamic stress. Neuroendocrinology **48(6):** 674–677.

12. IMAKI, T., J. L. NAHAN, C. RIVIER, P. E. SAWCHENKO & W. VALE. 1991. Differential regulation of corticotropin-releasing factor mRNA in rat brain regions by glucocorti-coids and stress. J. Neurosci. **11:** 585–599.

13. MERLO PICH, E., G. F. KOOB, M. HEILIG, F. MENZAGHI, W. VALE & F. WEISS. 1993. Corticotropin releasing factor release from the mediobasal hypothalamus of the rat as measured by microdialysis. Neuroscience **55(3):** 695–707.

14. PLOTSKY, P. M. & W. W. VALE. 1984. Hemorrhage-induced secretion of corticotropin-releasing factor-like immunoreactivity into the rat hypophysial portal circulation and its inhibition by glucocorticoid. Endocrinology **114:** 164–169.

15. IXART, G., G. BARBANEL, B. CONTE-DEVOLX, M. GRINO, C. OLIVER & I. ASSENMACHER. 1987. Evidence for basal and stress-induced release of corticotropin-releasing factor in the push-pull cannulated median eminence of conscious free-moving rat. Neurosci. Lett. **74:** 85–89.

16. DUNN, A. J. & C. W. BERRIDGE. 1990. Physiological and behavioral responses to corticotropin-releasing factor administration: Is CRF a mediator of anxiety or stress responses? Brain Res. Rev. **15:** 71–100.

17. KOOB, G. F., S. C. HEINRICHS, E. MERLO-PICH, F. MENZAGHI, H. BALDWIN, K. MICZEK & K. T. BRITTON. 1993. The role of corticotropin-releasing factor in behavioural re-sponses to stress. *In* Corticotropin-Releasing Factor: Basic and Clinical Studies of a Neuropeptide. E. B. De Souza & C. B. Nemeroff, Eds.: 277–295. CRC Press. Boca Raton, FL.

18. HEINRICHS, S. C., E. M. PICH, K. MICZEK, K. T. BRITTON & G. F. KOOB. 1992. Corticotropin-releasing factor antagonist reduces emotionality in socially defeated rats via direct neurotropic action. Brain Res. **581:** 190–197.

19. BUTLER, P. D., J. M. WEISS, J. C. STOUT & C. R. NEMEROFF. 1990. Corticotropin-releasing factor produces fear-enhancing and behavioral activating effects following infusion into the locus coeruleus. J. Neurosci. **10:** 176–183.

20. TAZI, A., N. R. SWERDLOW, M. LE MOAL, J. RIVIER, W. VALE & G. F. KOOB. 1987. Behavioral activation of CRF: Evidence for the involvement of the ventral forebrain. Life Sci. **41:** 41–49.

21. KALIVAS, P. W., P. DUFFY & L. G. LATIMER. 1987. Neurochemical and behavioral effects of corticotropin-releasing factor in the ventral tegmental area of the rat. J. Pharmacol. Exp. Ther. **242:** 757–763.

22. LIANG, K. C. & E. H. Y. LEE. 1988. Intra-amygdala injections of corticotropin-releasing factor facilitate inhibitory avoidance learning and reduce exploratory behavior in rats. Psychopharmacology **96:** 232–236.

23. KRAHN, D. D., B. A. GOSNELL, A. S. LEVINE & J. E. MORLEY. 1988. Behavioral effects of corticotropin-releasing factor: Localization and characterization of central effects. Brain Res. **443:** 63–69.

24. NAUTA, W. J. H. 1986. Affect and motivation: the limbic system. *In* Fundamental Neuroanatomy.: 120–131. John Freeman & Co. New York, NY.

25. BROWN, M. & L. A. FISHER. 1990. Regulation of the autonomic nervous system by corticotropin-releasing factor. *In* Corticotropin-Releasing Factor: Basic and Clinical Studies of a Neuropeptide. E. B. De Souza & C. B. Nemeroff, Eds.: 291–307. CRC Press. Boca Raton, FL.

26. GUNION, M. W. & Y. TACHÉ. 1987. Intrahypothalamic microinfusion of corticotropin-

releasing factor inhibits gastric acid secretion but increases secretion volume in rats. Brain Res. **411:** 156–161.

27. MÖNNIKES, H., I. HEYMANN-MÖNNIKES & Y. TACHÉ. 1992. CRF in the paraventricular nucleus of the hypothalamus induces dose-related behavioral profile in rats. Brain Res. **574:** 70–76.

28. BURLET, A. J., F. MENZAGHI, F. J. H. TILDERS, J. W. A. M. VAN OERS, J. P. NICOLAS & C. R. BURLET. 1990. Uptake of monoclonal antibody to corticotropin-releasing factor (CRF) into rat hypothalamic neurons. Brain Res. **517:** 283–293.

29. PASTAN, I. & D. FITZGERALD. 1991. Recombinant toxins for cancer treatment. Science **254:** 1173–1177.

30. WILEY, R. G. 1992. Neural lesioning with ribosome-inactivating proteins: Suicide transport and immunolesioning. TINS **15:** 286–290.

31. SCHUPF, N. & C. A. WILLIAMS. 1987. Psychopharmacological activity of immune complexes in rat brain is complement dependent. J. Neuroimmunol. **13:** 293–303.

32. PODACK, E. R. & J. TSCHOPP. 1984. Membrane attack by complement. Mol. Immunol. **21:** 589–604.

33. MENZAGHI, F., A. BURLET, J. W. A. M. VAN OERS, G. BARBANEL, F. J. H. TILDERS, J. P. NICOLAS & C. BURLET. 1992. A new perspective for the study of central neuronal network implicated in stress. *In* Stress: Neuroendocrine and Molecular Approaches. R. Kvetnansky, R. McCarty & J. Axelrod, Eds.: 439–448. Gordon and Breach Science. New York, NY.

34. MENZAGHI, F., S. C. HEINRICHS, E. MERLO PICH, F. J. H. TILDERS, & G. F. KOOB. 1993. Functional impairment of hypothalamic corticotropin releasing factor neurons with immunotargeted toxins enhances food intake induced by neuropeptide Y. Brain Res. **618:** 76–82.

35. MENZAGHI, F., A. BURLET, J. W. A. M. VAN OERS, F. J. H. TILDERS, J. P. NICOLAS & C. BURLET. 1991. Long-term inhibition of stress-induced adrenocorticotropin release by intracerebral administration of a monoclonal antibody to rat corticotropin-releasing factor together with ricin A chain and monensin. J. Neuroendocrinology **3:** 469–475.

36. MENZAGHI, F., A. BURLET, M. CHAPLEUR, J. P. NICOLAS & C. BURLET. 1992. Alteration of pituitary-adrenal responses to adrenalectomy by the immunological targeting of CRF neurons. Neurosci. Lett. **135:** 49–52.

37. MENZAGHI, F., A. BURLET, M. CHAPLEUR, J. VAN OERS, F. J. H. TILDERS, J. P. NICOLAS & C. BURLET. Immunotoxic disturbances of corticotropin releasing factor neurons of the paraventricular nuclei differentially alter the stress and circadian responses of the rat hypothalamo-pituitary-adrenal axis. Submitted.

38. MENZAGHI, F., S. C. HEINRICHS, E. MERLO PICH, F. J. H. TILDERS & G. F. KOOB. 1992. Attenuation of endocrine and behavioral responses to social conflict stress in rats by microinjection of cytotoxic antibody to corticotropin releasing factor and ricin A chain toxin within the paraventricular nuclei. Soc. Neurosci. Abstr. **18:** 535.

39. WEINGARTEN, H. P., P. CHANG & T. J. MCDONALD. 1985. Comparison of the metabolic and behavioral disturbances following paraventricular- and ventromedial-hypothalamic lesions. Brain Res. Bull. **14:** 551–559.

40. GRAY, T. S. & D. J. MAGNUSON. 1987. Neuropeptide neuronal efferents from the bed nucleus of the stria terminalis and central amygdaloid nucleus to the dorsal vagal complex in the rat. J. Comp. Neurol. **262:** 365–374.

41. KIRCHGESSNER, A. N. & A. SCLAFANI. 1988. Histochemical identification of a PVN-hindbrain feeding pathway. Physiol. Behav. **42:** 529–543.

42. HEINRICHS, S. C., B. J. COLE, E. MERLO PICH, F. MENZAGHI, G. F. KOOB & R. L. HAUGER. 1992. Endogenous corticotropin-releasing factor modulates feeding induced by neuropeptide Y or a tail-pinch stressor. Peptides **13:** 879–884.

43. HEINRICHS, S. C., F. MENZAGHI, E. MERLO PICH, R. L. HAUGER & G. F. KOOB. 1993. Corticotropin-releasing factor in the paraventricular nucleus modulates feeding induced by neuropeptide Y. Brain Res. **611:** 18–24.

44. KRAHN, D. D., B. A. GOSNELL, M. GRACE & A. S. LEVINE. 1986. CRF antagonist partially reverses CRF- and stress-induced effects on feeding. Brain Res. Bull. **17:** 285–289.

45. WIDMAIER, E. P., P. M. PLOTSKY, S. W. SUTTON & W. VALE. 1988. Regulation of corticotropin-releasing factor secretion *in vitro* by glucose. Am. J. Physiol. **255:** 287–292.
46. HEINRICHS, S. C. & G. F. KOOB. 1992. Corticotropin-releasing factor modulates dietary preference in nutritionally and physically stressed rats. Psychopharmacology **109:** 177–184.
47. GRAY, T. S. 1990. The organization and possible function of amygdaloid corticotropin-releasing factor pathways. *In* Corticotropin-Releasing Factor: Basic and Clinical Studies of a Neuropeptide. E. B. De Souza & C. B. Nemeroff, Eds.: 53–68. CRC Press. Boca Raton, FL.
48. MERLO PICH, E., S. C. HEINRICHS, C. RIVIER, K. A. MICZEK, D. A. FISHER & G. F. KOOB. 1993. Blockade of pituitary-adrenal axis activation induced by peripheral immunoneutralization of corticotropin-releasing factor does not affect the behavioral response to social defeat stress in rats. Psychoneuroendocrinology. In press.
49. MERLO PICH, E., G. F. KOOB, S. C. SATTLER, F. MENZAGHI, M. HEILIG, S. C. HEINRICHS, W. W. VALE & F. WEISS. 1992. Stress-induced release of corticotropin releasing factor in the amygdala measured by *in vivo* microdialysis. Soc. Neurosci. Abstr. **18:** 535.

Involvement of Corticotropin-Releasing Factor in the Control of Food Intake and Energy Expenditure

DENIS RICHARD

Département de Physiologie
Faculté de Médecine, Université Laval
Québec G1K 7P4, Canada

Corticotropin-releasing factor (CRF) is a 41-residue peptide characterized from ovine and rat hypothalami by Vale *et al.* in 1981[1] and Spiess *et al.* in 1983.[2] In rats, CRF is contained in neurons that are widely distributed throughout the brain, with one of the most noticeable clusters of these cells found in the medial parvocellular division of the paraventricular nucleus (PVN) of the hypothalamus.[3–7] The CRF-containing cell bodies in the medial parvocellular division of the PVN, whose fibers abundantly project to the neurohemal zone of the median eminence, are dominantly involved in the control of the pituitary-adrenal axis, which represents the primary role of CRF.[8,9] Within and outside the PVN, there are also CRF-containing cell perikarya, not involved in the pituitary function, which project to neuronal structures that modulate behavioral and autonomic functions.[3–7] Outside the PVN, CRF-containing cell bodies implicated in the behavioral and autonomic regulations are found in the diencephalon, where the medial preoptic area (MPOA) comprises the second largest CRF-containing cell groups in the hypothalamus after the PVN. Particularly dense clusters of CRF-containing cell bodies are also found in the telencephalon, located in the bed nucleus of the stria terminalis (BNST) and the central nucleus of the amygdala (CeA). Finally, in the brain stem, populations of CRF-containing cell perikarya are found in the periaqueductal gray (PAG), the locus coeruleus (LC), the parabrachial nucleus (PBN), the nucleus of the solitary tract (NST), and the dorsal motor nucleus of the vagus (DMV).

In recent years, the effects of CRF on behavioral and autonomic functions have aroused as much interest as the role CRF is exerting on the pituitary secretion of ACTH or other proopiomelanocortin (POMC) products.[10–25] Among the most outlined pituitary-unrelated actions of CRF is its influence on energy balance; in small laboratory animals, CRF treatment blunts energy storage (energy balance) by concomitantly reducing energy intake and augmenting energy expenditure.

The effect of CRF on food intake has been extensively reviewed[10,16,20–22,26–29] in recent years. However, possibly because of the complexity of the mechanisms involved in the control of food intake, the understanding of the mechanisms involved in the anorectic action of CRF is still partly obscure. Nonetheless, two neuropeptides have been identified as mediators of the anorectic action of CRF. Somatostatin has been reported to reverse the CRF-dependent suppressing effect of restraint stress on food intake,[30] and oxytocin antagonists have been shown to prevent the anorectic effect of central injection of CRF.[31] It is noteworthy that CRF treatment induces, concurrently with a reduction in food intake, an increase in the activity of the sympathetic nervous system (SNS),[11–13,18,23] a finding that suggests that the anorectic effect of CRF may be mediated, as it is for its thermogenic effect (see below), by central control over the autonomic nervous system (ANS). This suggestion is supported by the experimental demonstration that the ganglionic blockade with chlorisondamine[32] or surgical adrenal demedullation[33] attenuates the anorectic effect of CRF.

In contrast with its action on energy intake, the effect of CRF on energy expenditure has been addressed rather scantily. Nonetheless, sound evidence exists that CRF stimulates energy expenditure in small laboratory animals by activating brown adipose tissue (BAT).[14,29,34,35] In small rodents, BAT has been undeniably recognized as the main peripheral site of cold-induced thermogenesis,[36–38] and considered as the thermogenic effector of diet-induced thermogenesis (DIT). In small mammals, DIT represents a useful energy-buffering process which allows energy dissipation in response to overfeeding.[39–44] BAT has an enormous thermogenic potential because of the presence of a unique protein in its mitochondrial inner membrane, making up a proton conductance pathway that uncouples ATP synthesis from the oxidation of energy substrates.[45–50] Because fatty acid oxidation in BAT is not under the respiratory constraint imposed by the intracellular accumulation of ATP, it can occur at an accelerated rate, thereby producing a large quantity of heat. BAT is richly innervated by nerve terminals of the SNS, whose activation in response to cold or overfeeding triggers thermogenesis.[51–55] CRF stimulates SNS activity in various tissues,[11–13,15,18,23,56–58] including BAT.[14,59–62] The mechanisms underlying the effects of CRF on SNS are not known but evidence for the involvement of POMC products in these effects has been recently provided.[63] Treatment with either an antibody for α-melanocyte-stimulating hormone (α-MSH) or with the β-endorphin antagonist naloxone attenuated the thermogenic effect of CRF.[63] Very recently, lipocortin 1 has been identified as a mediator of the CRF-dependent thermogenic effects of certain cytokines.[64] Lipocortin-1 attenuates the thermogenic effects of interleukin (IL)-1α, IL-1β, IL-6, IL-8, and CRF.

INVOLVEMENT OF CRF IN THE REGULATION OF ENERGY BALANCE IN EXPERIMENTALLY OBESE ANIMALS

The sustained interest in the involvement of CRF in the regulation of energy balance has been driven by experiments designed to assess the effects of bilateral adrenalectomy (ADX) on body weight, body fat or energy gain in various animal models of obesity. From these investigations, it has emerged that bilateral ADX prevents, attenuates or reverses the development of obesity in genetically obese mutants, such as the ob/ob mouse[65–67] and the fa/fa rat (Zucker "fatty" rat);[68–71] in animals with obesity-inducing brain alterations, such as the electrolytic lesion of the ventromedial nucleus of the hypothalamus (VMH),[72] the electrolytic lesion of the PVN,[72] the gold-thioglucose lesion of the VMH,[73] the chemical lesion of the hypothalamus with glutamate,[74] and in chemically and surgically castrated female rats.[75,76] It is worthwhile mentioning that bilateral ADX also prevents, attenuates or reverses most of the metabolic abnormalities associated with obesity. ADX alters the regulation of energy balance in obese animals not only through a reduction of energy intake but also through a stimulation of energy expenditure. Pair-feeding studies have shown that obese animals with intact adrenals, on a level of energy intake comparable to that of obese adrenalectomized rats, deposit energy with more efficiency than do obese adrenalectomized rats.[69] Many authors have provided evidence that BAT is stimulated following ADX;[61,66,77–85] ADX restores BAT SNS activity to normal levels in obese laboratory animals.

The observation that ADX, which promotes the synthesis and release of CRF, prevents, attenuates or reverses most forms of animal obesity relates the development of obesity to a reduction in the central CRF-ergic activity. This inference is further supported by experiments that show that the central administration of CRF prevents weight gain in Zucker rats, with little effect in lean animals;[86] that the effects of the type II glucocorticoid receptor antagonist RU38486, which prevents obesity in fa/fa rats,[87] are blocked by a CRF antagonist;[60] and that a deficit exists in the hypophyseal-portal plasma CRF in fa/fa rats.[88]

The mechanisms governing the reduction in CRF-ergic activity in obese animals are still unclear. Evidence is nonetheless accumulating which tends to link this reduction to an amplified retroinhibitory action of the glucocorticoids in obese animals. In fact, normal[87,89] to high[90] levels of corticosterone have been reported in obese laboratory rodents, which seem far more sensitive to the action of the glucocorticoids.[91,92] An increased sensitivity to glucocorticoids might be attributable to an augmented function of glucocorticoid type I (mineralocorticoid) and type II (glucocorticoid) receptors in the hypothalamus and hippocampus of obese rats. This suggestion is supported by the observation that the development of obesity in the Zucker rat is prevented by treatment with the glucocorticoid receptor antagonist RU 38486.[87] Increases in the number of type I and type II glucocorticoid receptors and in the activities of two glucocorticoid-sensitive enzymes, glycerol-3-phosphate dehydrogenase and glutamine synthetase,[89,93] have been reported in the Zucker rat, whereas reduced glucocorticoid receptor binding activities have been noted in obese (ob/ob)[94] and diabetic (mdb/mdb)[95] mice.

FIGURE 1 hypothetically illustrates the regulation of energy balance in intact and adrenalectomized obese animals. Essentially, ADX might exert its effects in the regulation of energy balance by enhancing CRF tone, whose reduction in obese animals would cause obesity through an increase in food intake and a reduction of energy expenditure. The effect of a reduction in the CRF tone in the regulation of energy balance of obese animals could express itself as follows. In intact animals, the potent retroinhibitory signal from the circulating glucocorticoids might weaken the capacity of the CRF system to oppose the enlargement of energy stores either by directly inhibiting the central effectors of feeding and stimulating SNS-mediated BAT thermogenesis, or by overriding other systems that could stimulate energy intake and reduce energy expenditure in obese animals. The neuropeptide Y (NPY) system represents one of these peptidergic systems suspected of playing a genuine role in the regulation of energy balance;[96] in contrast to the effects of CRF, NPY promotes energy storage through concomitantly increasing energy intake and reducing energy expenditure.[97] The NPY-ergic activity is enhanced in obese laboratory animals, possibly because of either the weakness of the inhibitory signals from the brain (CRF system) and its periphery, or the inability of the NPY system to respond to peripheral inhibitory signals. As suggested by parabiotic studies,[98] either the absence of peripheral signals, the intensity of which might be determined by the energy stores, or the inability of the central systems (CRF or NPY) to recognize these circulating signals could be fundamental in the alteration in energy balance in animal obesity.

The sites of action of a potentially CRF-mediated effect of ADX in the regulation of energy balance in obese animals are not known. The PVN, because of its high density of CRF-containing cell bodies and because of the effects of its lesions on energy balance,[99–101] has been regarded as the most likely site of action of CRF in the regulation of energy balance. However, although the PVN has been proposed as the main structure for the anorectic effects of CRF,[102] it has not proved to be essential in the regulation of energy balance in obese animals; bilateral PVN lesions do not prevent the effects of ADX in obesity.[72] In addition, the role of PVN as a site for the action of CRF on thermogenesis has been recently questioned because an injection

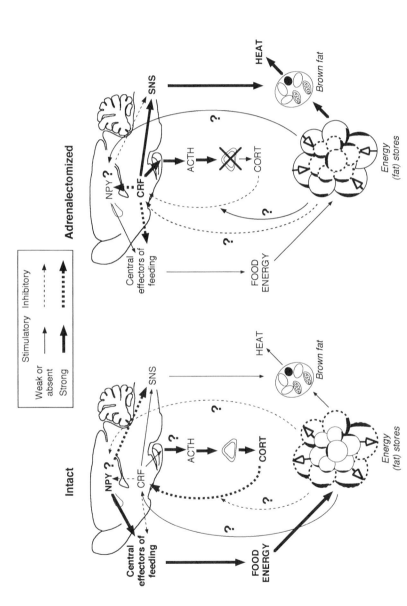

FIGURE 1. Hypothetical representation of the regulation of energy balance in intact and adrenalectomized obese laboratory animals (see text for details).

of CRF into the PVN does not increase the firing rate of the SNS nerves stimulating BAT thermogenesis.[62] Similar to PVN lesions, VMH lesions do not hinder the effects of ADX in obese rats. It therefore appears that VMH is not an essential structure in the effect of CRF on energy balance.[72] Interestingly, injection of CRF in the MPOA led to a 150% increase in the firing rate of the SNS fibers innervating BAT,[62] thus supporting a role for this region in the CRF action on energy expenditure. In further support of MPOA as a site of CRF action are the observations that chronic infusions of CRF in MPOA produce dramatic loss of body weight in rats (Rivest and Rivier, unpublished results). Finally, it is obvious that many other sites could be involved in the effects of CRF in the regulation of energy balance; CRF cell bodies and terminals and CRF receptors are found in numerous brain regions that may also influence feeding and thermogenesis.

Although undoubtedly of importance, the CRF system is likely not the only system involved in the alteration of the regulation of energy balance that leads to obesity in laboratory animals. As suggested elsewhere[103] the fact that ADX prevents, reverses or attenuates most forms of obesity in laboratory rodents does not warrant an exclusive role for CRF in the regulation of energy balance in obese animals. The possibility that ADX may, independently of its effect on the CRF system, affect other peptidergic and aminergic systems involved in the regulation of energy balance of obese animals cannot be ruled out.

INVOLVEMENT OF CRF IN THE EFFECTS OF EXERCISE IN THE REGULATION OF ENERGY BALANCE

It has been known for years that exercise, an experimental treatment known to stimulate the hypothalamo-pituitary-adrenal (HPA) axis, produces gender-dependent effects on energy balance in rats.[104-110] With no apparent effects in female animals, exercise markedly influences energy balance in males, in which it blunts fat and protein tissue growth. Exercise brings about effects on energy balance primarily by reducing energy intake; no convincing evidence exists that exercise affects energy balance by generating adaptations promoting energy expenditure.[106,109,110] Some studies have suggested that exercise may stimulate energy expenditure in rats by stimulating SNS-mediated BAT thermogenesis.[111-114] However, the evidence for a stimulating effect of exercise on BAT is far from definitive.[115-117] It is worth pointing out that the reported increases in BAT thermogenesis in response to exercise emerged from experiments involving swimming exercise, which are liable to cause cold-specific adaptations.[118,119] In contrast to activating BAT, exercise would, in some circumstances, diminish the metabolic activity of this tissue. During acute cold-exposure, for instance, exercise has been reported to suppress cold-induced thermogenesis[116] through a specific reduction in BAT SNS activity.[120]

The postulating of the mediating role of CRF in the influence of exercise on energy balance occurred when the effects of CRF on energy intake were delineated. Similar to exercise, CRF is a potent anorectic agent,[10,16,20,21] capable of reproducing the gender-dependent effects of exercise on energy balance.[121] The involvement of CRF in the anorectic effect of exercise was confirmed with the use of the CRF antagonist α-helical CRF$_{9-41}$, which, as it did in a restraint stress,[30,122] prevented the anorectic effect of an acute bout of exercise.[123] Interestingly, treadmill running, which undeniably stimulates CRF synthesis in rats,[124] does not, in contrast to a central injection of CRF, influence energy expenditure[111-114] by affecting BAT thermogenesis.[115-117] The increase in heat production induced by muscular activity appears to switch off BAT thermogenesis during exercise, that is, at a time when CRF will have been able to exert a stimulating effect on BAT thermogenesis.

The recent suggestion[125] that acute, but not chronic exercise affects the regulation of energy balance is noteworthy, and conforms with the idea that CRF mediates the effect of exercise on energy balance. As with CRF, the anorectic action of exercise is of short duration,[123] that is, strong immediately after an exercise session and vanishing gradually after the end of the exercise. Interestingly, soon after the cessation of an exercise-training program, chronically exercised rats began to gain weight at an accelerated pace, catching up with their growth retardation.[126] The rapid energy gain of the carcass after the cessation of an exercise-training program seems due to an increase in energy intake relative to the metabolic body size.[126] It appears that the regular exercise sessions that stimulate CRF-ergic activity are required for exercise to induce a negative energy balance. It is also probable that the long-term influence of exercise tends to oppose its CRF-related acute influence by stimulating energy storage through promoting energy intake. This probability is worth considering because chronic exercise, similar to food restriction, seems to stimulate the orexigenic NPY-ergic system,[96] whose activation promotes energy storage.[97] The stimulation of the NPY tone in response to exercise would be generated by the low levels of insulin led to by chronic exercise;[127-129] low levels of insulin could be the signal by which the NPY system is informed of energy deficits.[96,130,131] Acute exercise, like CRF, might override the orexigenic effects of NPY.

FIGURE 2A is a hypothetical representation of the effects of exercise in the regulation of energy balance. The increase in the CRF-ergic activity induced by exercise would retard energy deposition through a decrease in energy intake and an increase in muscle energy expenditure. The heat produced by muscles would inhibit the stimulating effects of CRF on SNS-mediated BAT thermogenesis. The enhanced CRF-ergic activity induced by acute exercise could directly inhibit the central effectors of feeding, thereby outweighing possible peripheral inhibitory signals on the CRF system associated with the reduction of the energy stores. In addition, the enhanced CRF-ergic activity induced by exercise could override peptidergic systems such as the NPY system, which may stimulate energy intake and reduce energy expenditure, and whose activity is enhanced by an energy deficit such as that induced by exercise.

The sites of action of CRF in the regulation of energy balance have not been determined. The PVN does not appear to be essential for the anorectic action of exercise because PVN lesions do not prevent the reduction in food intake induced by exercise. As revealed by a recent report on the postexercise mapping of the CRF mRNA,[124] numerous brain structures comprise CRF-containing cell bodies or terminals that are stimulated during exercise and may be involved as well in the regulation of energy balance.

INVOLVEMENT OF CRF IN THE EFFECTS OF ESTROGENS IN THE REGULATION OF ENERGY BALANCE

It is largely recognized that estrogens affect energy balance in laboratory rodents[132-134] as well as in other species.[135,136] The effects of estrogens appear to be primarily due to the effects of the steroid on food intake; estrogens have not so far been convincingly shown to promote energy expenditure through stimulating BAT thermogenesis.[137-139] Estrogens exert anorectic effects in rodents[132-134] as well as in other species.[135,136] Reduced intakes of food have been observed after the preovula-

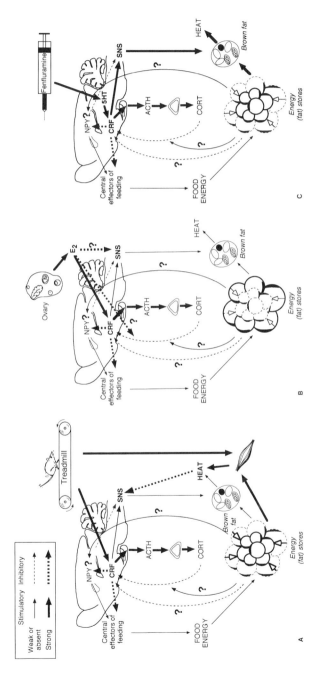

FIGURE 2. Hypothetical representation of CRF mediation of the effects of exercise, estrogens, and 5-hydroxytryptamine on energy balance (see text for details).

tory surge of estradiol (E_2),[134–136,140,141] which occurs either at proestrus or at the end of the follicular phase, depending on the species. In addition, the anorectic effects of estrogens have also been emphasized in ovariectomized animals, in which E_2 replacement therapies prevent the orexigenic effect of estrogen removal.[135,136,142]

In rats, estrogens, in parallel to their effects on energy balance, stimulate the HPA axis[143] (Dagnault and Richard, unpublished results), and indications that CRF may mediate the effects of estrogens on energy balance have emerged from the demonstrations that bilateral ADX significantly attenuates the effects of ovariectomy on body weight and energy gain.[75,76] These studies indicate that estrogen removal, which enhances energy deposition primarily by increasing energy intake,[134,137] appears to produce its action by reducing the CRF tone in the brain. Supporting this hypothesis are recent data that extended the involvement of CRF to the anorexia caused by E_2 (Dagnault et al., unpublished data.) The effect of E_2 on food intake was prevented by concomitantly treating chemically ovariectomized rats with E_2 and the CRF antagonist α-helical $CRF_{9–41}$. As is the case for exercise, estrogens bring about the stimulation of the CRF-ergic activity without stimulating BAT thermogenesis[137–139] and by hindering cold-induced thermogenesis.[138]

FIGURE 2B hypothetically illustrates the effects of estrogens in the regulation of energy balance. The increase in the CRF-ergic activity induced by estrogens would retard energy deposition through a decrease in energy intake not compensated by an decrease energy expenditure. For unknown reasons, estrogens would tend to inhibit the stimulating effects of CRF on SNS-mediated BAT thermogenesis. As with exercise, the enhanced CRF-ergic activity induced by estrogens could directly inhibit the central effectors of feeding, thereby offsetting possible peripheral inhibitory signals on the CRF system related to the reduction of the energy reserves. In addition, the enhanced CRF tone resulting from estrogens could counteract other systems such as the NPY system, which might, as previously mentioned, stimulate energy intake and reduce energy expenditure, and whose activity is stimulated by energy deficits.

The brain sites of action of estrogens on energy balance are unclear. It has been recently suggested that an E_2 treatment may induce a functional loss in the ability of glucocorticoid receptors to autoregulate. This loss could lead to a stimulation of CRF activity, which could in turn translate into an increase in the plasma concentrations of ACTH and corticosterone. In this regard, it has been recently reported that CRF mRNA is elevated in the parvocellular portion of the PVN on the afternoon of proestrus[144] coincidentally with the proestrus peak of E_2. The proestrus peak of E_2 is known to induce, together with a gonadotropin-releasing hormone (GnRH)-dependent surge of gonadotropins, a noticeable reduction in food intake.[134,140,141] PVN has been suggested as a potential site for the anorectic effects of E_2.[145,146] However, PVN lesions do not prevent the long-term effects of E_2 on energy gain, intake, and expenditure in ovariectomized rats (Dagnault and Richard, unpublished data). The exact mechanisms by which E_2 inhibits food intake through a CRF-modulated process need further characterization.

CRF MEDIATION OF THE EFFECTS OF SEROTONIN ON ENERGY BALANCE

The 5-hydroxytryptamine (5-HT) system, which is one of the most prominent neurotransmitter systems in the brain,[147,148] is thought to play an important role in the regulation of energy balance. The action of 5-HT has been particularly emphasized in studies addressing the effects of the 5-HT agonist, fenfluramine, on energy balance. Fenfluramine, either in its D,L-racemic or its D-enantiomer form, has been tested for many years in the treatment of obesity.[149-153] Fenfluramine is a 5-HT indirect agonist that increases 5-HT availability at the nerve terminals by promoting its release and blocking its reuptake. This agent modulates energy balance through effects exerted both on energy intake and energy expenditure. Specifically, treatment with 5-HT agonists promotes satiation[154] and modifies the choice of food[155] while enhancing energy expenditure by activating SNS-mediated BAT thermogenesis.[156,157]

Concurrent to its action on energy balance, fenfluramine influences the HPA axis.[158,159] In fact, acute treatment with fenfluramine increases plasma corticosterone[160-161] and adrenocorticotropic hormone (ACTH) while concomitantly decreasing the hypothalamic CRF content.[159] Evidence for the involvement of CRF in the effects of fenfluramine on energy balance has been recently provided by investigators,[162] who, using a CRF antibody, were able to attenuate the effects of fenfluramine on oxygen consumption and food intake.

FIGURE 2C is a hypothetical representation of the effects of fenfluramine in the regulation of energy balance. The increase in the CRF-ergic activity induced by fenfluramine would retard energy deposition through a decrease in energy intake and an increase in energy expenditure. The enhanced CRF-ergic activity induced by fenfluramine could directly inhibit the central effectors of feeding and stimulate SNS-mediated BAT thermogenesis, thereby counterbalancing possible peripheral inhibitory signals on the CRF system determined by the reduction of the energy stores. As in the case for exercise and estrogens, the enhanced CRF-ergic activity induced by fenfluramine could override peptidergic systems such as the NPY system, which, as mentioned above, may stimulate energy intake and reduce energy expenditure, and whose activity is enhanced by energy losses.

The mechanisms and sites of action of fenfluramine in its CRF-mediated effects in the regulation of energy balance are poorly understood. The fenfluramine-inducible *fos*-like immunoreactivity (F-LI) in the CRF-containing neurons of the parvocellular division of the PVN[163] supports the presence of CRF–5-HT communications in the PVN and therefore points to a neuroanatomical site for the central action of 5-HT-ergic agonists on both the HPA axis and the regulation of energy balance. CRF-containing neurons projecting from the PVN receive input from 5-HT neurons originating from the B7, B8, and B9 divisions of the mesencephalic raphe nuclei.[147,148,164,165] Such CRF–5-HT communications may be involved in the HPA activation[166,167] and changes in energy balance[16,162] associated to stressing stimuli[168] because both CRF-ergic and 5-HT-ergic neurons appear to be stimulated under stressing conditions. Interestingly, fenfluramine also brings about an increase in F-LI into the CeA.[163] The contribution of CeA in the regulation of energy balance has not been fully explored but some recent studies provide evidence for a role of this brain structure in the control of food intake.[169,170] Interestingly, CeA seems necessary for the acquisition of a learned taste aversion,[171] a phenomenon which could likely be brought about by a high dose of fenfluramine. The observation, however, that F-LI in CeA and CRF-like immunoreactivity are not colocalized within the same neurons tends not to support a role for CeA as a brain site for CRF–5-HT communications.

FURTHER CRF INVOLVEMENTS IN THE REGULATION OF ENERGY BALANCE

CRF mediations in the regulation of energy balance can be extended further. Evidence that shows that CRF mediates the effects of certain cytokines on energy metabolism is rapidly accumulating.[172,173] Cytokines are peptides secreted by cells of the immune system, which, together with inducing fever, alter the regulation of energy balance. Central treatment with IL-1α, IL-1β, IL-6, IL-8, or tumor necrosis factor-α (TNF-α) increases energy expenditure and decreases energy intake. Similar to the increase in metabolic rate caused by either cold or overfeeding, the pyrogenic response to interleukins seems dependent on the SNS-mediated process of BAT thermogenesis. Interestingly, the CRF mediation of the effects of cytokines on BAT thermogenesis seems to pertain to IL-1β, IL-6, and IL-8, but not to IL-1α. The effects of IL-1 on food intake have also been reported to be dependent on CRF.[174] Recently, CRF has been shown to mediate the effects of caffeine on food intake (Racotta *et al.,* unpublished data). Finally, although there has been no evidence yet for CRF mediation in the suppressing effects of cholecystokinin (CCK) on food intake, evidence exists that an intraperitoneal injection of CCK activates c-*fos* expression in CRF neurons.[175] It is tempting to suggest a CRF-mediation in the effects of CCK on food intake, but this mediation has yet to be demonstrated.

CONCLUSION

The mediating role of CRF in the regulation of energy balance has been emphasized in various investigations including those designed to assess the effects of ADX in obese laboratory animals and those aimed at understanding the effects of exercise, estrogens, and serotonin in the regulation of energy balance. In all these investigations CRF has emerged as being involved in the control of energy intake and energy expenditure. The mechanisms of action and the brain sites involved in the effects of CRF in the regulation of energy balance remain obscure. POMC products, oxytocin, and somatostatin have all been proposed as mediators of the CRF action on energy balance. The PVN, which contains the highest hypothalamic concentration of CRF, has been the most often suggested potential site for the action of CRF on energy metabolism. This suggestion has, however, been disputed by experiments in which PVN lesions were shown not to prevent either exercise- and estrogen-induced anorexia or the antiobesity effects of ADX in obese animals. Numerous hypothalamic and extrahypothalamic areas that contain noticeable populations of CRF-containing cell bodies and terminals, such as the MPOA, the BNST, the CeA, PAG, the LC, the PBN, the NST, and the DMV, have to be considered as potential sites for the effects of CRF on energy balance.

ACKNOWLEDGMENTS

The author gratefully thanks Drs. Y. Deshaies and Michel Cabanac for their helpful comments on the manuscript.

REFERENCES

1. VALE, W., J. SPIESS, C. RIVIER & J. RIVIER. 1981. Characterization of a 41-residue ovine hypothalamic peptide that stimulates secretion of corticotropin and beta-endorphin. Science **213:** 1394–1397.
2. SPIESS, J., J. RIVIER & W. VALE. 1983. Sequence analysis of rat hypothalamic corticotropin-releasing factor with the o-phthalaldehyde strategy. Biochemistry **22:** 4341–4346.

3. SAWCHENKO, P. E. & L. W. SWANSON. 1985. Localization, colocalization, and plasticity of corticotropin-releasing factor immunoreactivity in rat brain. Fed. Proc. **44:** 221–227.

4. PALKOVITS, M., M. J. BROWNSTEIN & W. VALE. 1985. Distribution of corticotropin-releasing factor in rat brain. Fed. Proc. **44:** 215–219.

5. SAWCHENKO, P. E. & L. W. SWANSON. 1990. Organization of CRF immunoreactive cells and fibers in the rat brain: Immunohistochemical studies. *In* Corticotropin-Releasing Factor: Basic and Clinical Studies of a Neuropeptide. E. B. De Souza & C. B. Nemeroff, Eds.: 30–51. CRC Press. Boca Raton, FL.

6. SWANSON, L. W. 1991. Biochemical switching in hypothalamic circuits mediating responses to stress. *In* Progress in Brain Research, Vol. 8. G. Holstege, Ed.: 181–200. Elsevier Science. New York, NY.

7. PETRUSZ, P. & I. MERCHENTHALER. 1992. The corticotropin-releasing factor system. *In* Neuroendocrinology. C. B. Nemeroff, Ed.: 129–183. CRC Press. Boca Raton, FL.

8. ANTONI, F. A. 1986. Hypothalamic control of adrenocorticotropin secretion: Advances since the discovery of 41-residue corticotropin-releasing factor. Endocr. Rev. **7:** 351–378.

9. HARBUZ, M. S. & S. L. LIGHTMAN. 1992. Review—stress and the hypothalamo-pituitary-adrenal axis—acute, chronic and immunological activation. J. Endocrinol. **134:** 327–339.

10. MORLEY, J. E. 1989. Appetite regulation: The role of peptides and hormones. Annu. Rev. Nutr. **9:** 201–227.

11. FISHER, L. A., J. RIVIER, C. RIVIER, J. SPIESS, W. VALE & M. R. BROWN. 1982. Corticotropin-releasing factor (CRF): Central effects on mean arterial pressure and heart rate in rats. Endocrinology **110:** 2222–2224.

12. BROWN, M. R., L. A. FISHER, J. SPIESS, C. RIVIER, J. RIVIER & W. VALE. 1982. Corticotropin-releasing factor: Actions on the sympathetic nervous system and metabolism. Endocrinology **111:** 928–931.

13. BROWN, M. R. & L. A. FISHER. 1985. Corticotropin-releasing factor: Effects on the autonomic nervous system and visceral systems. Fed. Proc. **44:** 243–248.

14. ROTHWELL, N. J. 1990. Central effects of CRF on metabolism and energy balance. Neurosci. Biobehav. Rev. **14:** 263–271.

15. FISHER, L. A. & M. R. BROWN. 1991. Central regulation of stress responses—Regulation of the autonomic nervous system and visceral function by corticotrophin releasing factor-41. Clin. Endocrinol. Metab. **5:** 35–50.

16. MORLEY, J. E. & A. S. LEVINE. 1990. Corticotropin-releasing factor and ingestive behaviors. *In* Corticotropin-Releasing Factor Basic and Clinical Studies of a Neuropeptide. E. B. De Souza & C. B. Nemeroff, Eds.: 267–274. CRC Press. Boca Raton, FL.

17. KOOB, G. F. & K. T. BRITTON. 1990. Behavioral effects of corticotropin-releasing factor. *In* Corticotropin-Releasing Factor: Basic and Clinical Studies of a Neuropeptide. E. B. De Souza & C. B. Nemeroff, Eds.: 253–265. CRC Press. Boca Raton, FL.

18. BROWN, M. R. & L. A. FISHER. 1990. Regulation of the autonomic nervous system by corticotropin-releasing factor. *In* Corticotropin-Releasing Factor: Basic and Clinical Studies of a Neuropeptide. E. B. De Souza & C. B. Nemeroff, Eds.: 291–298. CRC Press. Boca Raton, FL.

19. OWENS, M. J. & C. B. NEMEROFF. 1991. Physiology and pharmacology of corticotropin-releasing factor. Pharmacol. Rev. **43:** 425–473.

20. BECK, B. 1992. Cholecystokinin, neurotensin and corticotropin-releasing factor—3 important anorexic peptides. Ann. Endocrinol. **53:** 44–56.

21. GLOWA, J. R., J. E. BARRETT, J. RUSSELL & P. W. GOLD. 1992. Effects of corticotropin releasing hormone on appetitive behaviors. Peptides **13:** 609–621.

22. LEVINE, A. S. & C. J. BILLINGTON. 1991. Stress, peptides, and regulation of ingestive behavior. *In* Stress, Neuropeptides, and Systemic Disease. J. A. McCubbin, P. G. Kaufmann & C. B. Nemeroff, Eds.: 327–339. Academic Press. San Diego, CA.

23. BROWN, M. R. 1991. Neuropeptide-mediated regulation of the neuroendocrine and autonomic response to stress. *In* Stress, Neuropeptides, and Systemic Disease. J. A.

McCubbin, P. G. Kaufmann & C. B. Nemeroff, Eds.: 73–93. Academic Press. San Diego, CA.

24. KOOB, G. F. 1992. The behavioral neuroendocrinology of corticotropin-releasing factor, growth hormone-releasing factor, somatostatin, and gonadotropin-releasing hormone. *In* Neuroendocrinology. C. B. Nemeroff, Ed.: 353–364. CRC Press. Boca Raton, FL.

25. COLE, B. J. & G. F. KOOB. 1991. Corticotropin-releasing factor, stress, and animal behavior. *In* Stress, Neuropeptides, and Systemic Disease. J. A. McCubbin, P. G. Kaufmann & C. B. Nemeroff, Eds.: 119–148. Academic Press. San Diego, CA.

26. LEVINE, A. S., J. E. MORLEY, B. A. GOSNELL, C. J. BILLINGTON & D. D. KRAHN. 1986. Neuropeptides as regulators of consummatory behaviors. J. Nutr. **116:** 2067–2077.

27. BURLET, C. 1988. Stress et comportement alimentaire. Ann. Endocrinol. **49:** 141–145.

28. MORLEY, J. E., A. S. LEVINE, B. A. GOSNELL & D. D. KRAHN. 1985. Peptides as central regulators of feeding. Brain Res. Bull. **14:** 511–519.

29. BRAY, G. A. 1992. Peptides affect the intake of specific nutrients and the sympathetic nervous system. Am. J. Clin. Nutr. **55:** S265–S271.

30. SHIBASAKI, T., N. YAMAUCHI, Y. KATO, A. MASUDA, T. IMAKI, M. HOTTA, H. DEMURA, H. OONO, N. LING & K. SHIZUME. 1988. Involvement of corticotropin-releasing factor in restraint stress-induced anorexia and reversion of the anorexia by somatostatin in the rat. Life Sci. **43:** 1103–1110.

31. OLSON, B. R., M. D. DRUTAROSKY, E. M. STRICKER & J. G. VERBALIS. 1991. Brain oxytocin receptors mediate corticotropin-releasing hormone-induced anorexia. Am. J. Physiol. **260:** R448–R452.

32. BRITTON, D. R. & E. INDYK. 1989. Effects of ganglionic blocking agent on behavioral responses to centrally administered CRF. Brain Res. **478:** 205–210.

33. GOSNELL, B. A., J. E. MORLEY & A. S. LEVINE. 1983. Adrenal modulation of the inhibitory effect of corticotropin releasing factor on feeding. Peptides **4:** 807–812.

34. LEFEUVRE, R. A., N. J. ROTHWELL & M. J. STOCK. 1987. Activation of brown fat thermogenesis in response to central injection of corticotropin releasing hormone in the rat. Neuropharmacology **26:** 1217–1221.

35. LEFEUVRE, R. A., N. J. ROTHWELL & A. WHITE. 1989. A comparison of the thermogenic effects of CRF, sauvagine and urotensin-I in the Rat. Horm. Metab. Res. **21:** 525–526.

36. FOSTER, D. O. 1984. Quantitative contribution of brown adipose tissue thermogenesis to overall metabolism. Can. J. Biochem. Cell Biol. **62:** 618–622.

37. FOSTER, D. O. & M. L. FRYDMAN. 1978. Nonshivering thermogenesis in the rat. II. Measurements of blood flow with microspheres point to brown adipose tissue as the dominant site of the calorigenesis induced by noradrenaline. Can. J. Physiol. Pharmacol. **56:** 110–122.

38. FOSTER, D. O. & M. L. FRYDMAN. 1979. Tissue distribution of cold-induced thermogenesis in conscious warm- or cold-acclimated rats reevaluated from changes in tissue blood flow: The dominant role of brown adipose tissue in the replacement of shivering by nonshivering thermogenesis. Can. J. Physiol. Pharmacol. **57:** 257–270.

39. TRAYHURN, P. & W. P. T. JAMES. 1981. Thermogenesis: Dietary and non-shivering aspects. *In* The Body Weight Regulatory System: Normal and Disturbed Mechanisms. L. A. Cioffi, W. P. T. James & T. B. Van Itallie, Eds.: 97–105. Raven Press. New York, NY.

40. ROTHWELL, N. J. & M. J. STOCK. 1983. Luxuskonsumption, diet-induced thermogenesis and brown fat: The case in favour. Clin. Sci. **64:** 19–23.

41. SEYDOUX, J. 1983. Recent evidence for the involvement of brown adipose tissue in body weight regulation. Diabetes & Metab. **9:** 141–147.

42. HIMMS-HAGEN, J. 1984. Thermogenesis in brown adipose tissue as an energy buffer. N. Engl. J. Med. **311:** 1549–1558.

43. HIMMS-HAGEN, J. 1984. Brown adipose tissue thermogenesis, energy balance, and obesity. Can. J. Biochem. Cell Biol. **62:** 610–617.

44. ROTHWELL, N. J. & M. J. STOCK. 1986. Brown adipose tissue and diet-induced thermogenesis. *In* Brown Adipose Tissue. P. Trayhurn & D. G. Nicholls, Eds.: 269–298. Edward Arnold. London.

45. RICQUIER, D., L. CASTEILLA & F. BOUILLAUD. 1991. Molecular studies of the uncoupling protein. FASEB J. **5:** 2237–2242.

46. HIMMSHAGEN, J. 1990. Brown adipose tissue thermogenesis—Interdisciplinary studies. FASEB J. **4:** 2890–2898.

47. RICQUIER, D., B. L. CASTEILLA, A-M. CASSARD, S. RAIMBAULT, S. KLAUS, O. CHAMPIGNY & E. HENTZ. 1990. The uncoupling protein of brown adipose tissue: Physiological and molecular aspects. *In* Obesity: Towards a Molecular Approach. G. A. Bray, D. Ricquier & B. M. Spiegelman, Eds.: 107–116. Wiley-Liss. New York, NY.

48. NICHOLLS, D., S. CUNNINGHAM & H. WIESINGER. 1986. Mechanisms of thermogenesis in brown adipose tissue. Biochem. Soc. Trans. **14:** 223–226.

49. NICHOLLS, D. G. & R. M. LOCKE. 1984. Thermogenic mechanisms in brown fat. Physiol. Rev. **64:** 1–64.

50. HIMMS-HAGEN, J. 1992. Brown adipose tissue metabolism. *In* Obesity. P. Bjorntorp & B. N. Brodoff, Eds.: 15–34. J. B. Lippincott Company. Philadelphia, PA.

51. LEBLANC, J., P. DIAMOND, M. A. GRIGGIO, A. NADEAU & D. RICHARD. 1992. Control of cephalic thermogenic phase of feeding. *In* Obesity in Europe 91. G. Ailhaud, B. Guy-Grand, M. Lafontan & D. Ricquier, Eds.: 241–247. John Libbey. London.

52. LANDSBERG, L. & J. B. YOUNG. 1987. Autonomic regulation of thermogenesis. *In* Mammalian Thermogenesis. L. Girardier & M. J. Stock, Eds.: 99–140. Chapman and Hall. London.

53. GIRARDIER, L. & J. SEYDOUX. 1986. Neural control of brown adipose tissue. *In* Brown Adipose Tissue. P. Trayhurn & D. G. Nicholls, Eds.: 122–151. Edward Arnold. London.

54. LANDSBERG, L. & J. B. YOUNG. 1984. The role of the sympathoadrenal system in modulating energy expenditure. Clin. Endocrinol. Metab. **13:** 475–499.

55. ROTHWELL, N. J. & M. J. STOCK. 1982. Neural regulation of thermogenesis. Trends Neurosci. **5:** 124–126.

56. ENGELAND, W. C., M. P. LILLY, T. O. BRUHN & D. S. GANN. 1987. Comparison of corticotropin-releasing factor and acetylcholine on catecholamine secretion in dogs. Am. J. Physiol. **253:** R209–R215.

57. KREGEL, K. C., J. M. OVERTON, D. R. SEALS, C. M. TIPTON & L. A. FISHER. 1990. Cardiovascular responses to exercise in the rat—Role of corticotropin-releasing factor. J. Appl. Physiol. **68:** 561–567.

58. IRWIN, M., R. HAUGER & M. BROWN. 1992. Central corticotropin-releasing hormone activates the sympathetic nervous system and reduces immune function—Increased responsivity of the aged rat. Endocrinology **131:** 1047–1053.

59. ARASE, K., N. S. SHARGILL & G. A. BRAY. 1989. Effects of corticotropin releasing factor on genetically obese (fatty) rats. Physiol. Behav. **45:** 565–570.

60. HARDWICK, A. J., E. A. LINTON & N. J. ROTHWELL. 1989. Thermogenic effects of the antiglucocorticoid RU-486 in the rat: Involvement of corticotropin-releasing factor and sympathetic activation of brown adipose tissue. Endocrinology **124(4):** 1684–1688.

61. HOLT, S. J. & D. A. YORK. 1989. The effects of adrenalectomy, corticotropin releasing factor and vasopressin on the sympathetic firing rate of nerves to interscapular brown adipose tissue in the Zucker rat. Physiol. Behav. **45:** 1123–1129.

62. EGAWA, M., H. YOSHIMATSU & G. A. BRAY. 1990. Preoptic area injection of corticotropin-releasing hormone stimulates sympathetic activity. Am. J. Physiol. **259:** R799–R806.

63. ROTHWELL, N. J., A. HARDWICK, R. A. LEFEUVRE, S. R. CROSBY & A. WHITE. 1991. Central actions of CRF on thermogenesis are mediated by proopiomelanocortin products. Brain Res. **541:** 89–92.

64. STRIJBOS, P. J., A. J. HARDWICK, J. K. RELTON, F. CAREY & N. J. ROTHWELL. 1992. Inhibition of central actions of cytokines on fever and thermogenesis by lipocortin-1 involves CRF. Am. J. Physiol. **263:** E632–E636.

65. SOLOMON, J. & J. MAYER. 1973. The effect of adrenalectomy on the development of the obese-hyperglycemic syndrome in ob/ob mice. Endocrinology **93:** 510–513.

66. VANDER TUIG, J. G., K. OHSHIMA, T. YOSHIDA, D. R. ROMSOS & G. A. BRAY. 1984.

Adrenalectomy increases norepinephrine turnover in brown adipose tissue of obese (ob/ob) mice. Life Sci. **34:** 1423–1432.

67. ROMSOS, D. R. 1991. Energy balance: Role of adrenal gland secretions. *In* Proceedings of the 14th International Congress of Nutrition. K. W. Young, L. Y. Cha, L. K. Yull, J. J. Soon & K. S. He, Eds.: 129–132. Seoul.

68. BRAY, G. A., J. S. STERN & T. W. CASTONGUAY. 1992. Effect of adrenalectomy and high-fat diet on the fatty Zucker rat. Am. J. Physiol. **262:** E32–E39.

69. FLETCHER, J. M. & N. McKENZIE. 1988. The effects of dietary fat content on the growth and body composition of lean and genetically obese Zucker rats adrenalectomized before weaning. Br. J. Nutr. **60:** 563–569.

70. YORK, D. A. & V. GODBOLE. 1979. Effect of adrenalectomy on obese "fatty" rats. Horm. Metab. Res. **11:** 646.

71. YUKIMURA, Y., G. A. BRAY & A. R. WOLFSEN. 1978. Some effects of adrenalectomy in the fatty rat. Endocrinology **103:** 1924–1928.

72. TOKUNAGA, K., M. FUKUSHIMA, J. R. LUPIEN, G. A. BRAY, J. W. KEMNITZ & R. SCHEMMEL. 1989. Effects of food restriction and adrenalectomy in rats with Vmh or Pvh lesions. Physiol. Behav. **45:** 1131–1137.

73. DEBONS, A. F., E. SICLARI, K. C. DAS & B. FUHR. 1982. Gold thioglucose-induced hypothalamic damage, hyperphagia, and obesity: Dependence on the adrenal gland. Endocrinology **110:** 2024–2029.

74. TOKUYAMA, K. & J. HIMMSHAGEN. 1989. Adrenalectomy prevents obesity in glutamate-treated mice. Am. J. Physiol. **257:** E139–E144.

75. OUERGHI, D., S. RIVEST & D. RICHARD. 1992. Adrenalectomy attenuates the effect of chemical castration on energy balance in rats. J. Nutr. **122:** 369–373.

76. MOOK, D. G., N. J. KENNEDY, S. ROBERTS, A. I. NUSSBAUM & W. I. RODIER III. 1972. Ovarian-adrenal interactions in regulation of body weight by female rats. J. Comp. Physiol. Psychol. **81:** 198–211.

77. HOLT, S. J. & D. A. YORK. 1984. Effect of adrenalectomy on brown adipose tissue of obese (ob/ob) mice. Horm. Metab. Res. **16:** 378–379.

78. ROTHWELL, N. J., M. J. STOCK & D. A. YORK. 1984. Effects of adrenalectomy on energy balance, diet-induced thermogenesis and brown adipose tissue in adult cafeteria-fed rats. Comp. Biochem. Physiol. A **78A:** 565–569.

79. MARCHINGTON, D., N. J. ROTHWELL, M. J. STOCK & D. A. YORK. 1986. Thermogenesis and sympathetic activity in BAT of overfed rats after adrenalectomy. Am. J. Physiol. **250:** E362–E366.

80. WICKLER, S. J., B. A. HORWITZ & J. S. STERN. 1986. Blood flow to brown fat in lean and obese adrenalectomized Zucker rats. Am. J. Physiol. **251:** R851–R858.

81. ROTHWELL, N. J. & M. J. STOCK. 1986. Energy balance and brown fat activity in adrenalectomized male, female, and castrated male rats. Metabolism **35:** 657–660.

82. HOLT, S. & D. A. YORK. 1982. The effect of adrenalectomy on GDP binding to brown-adipose tissue mitochondria of obese rats. Biochem. J. **208:** 819–822.

83. SHARGILL, N. S., J. R. LUPIEN & G. A. BRAY. 1989. Adrenalectomy in genetically obese Ob/Ob and Db/Db mice increases the proton conductance pathway. Horm. Metab. Res. **21:** 463–467.

84. SEYDOUX, J., R. H. BENZI, M. SHIBATA & L. GIRARDIER. 1990. Underlying mechanisms of atrophic state of brown adipose tissue in obese Zucker rats. Am. J. Physiol. **259:** R61–R69.

85. YORK, D. A., S. J. HOLT & D. MARCHINGTON. 1985. Regulation of brown adipose tissue thermogenesis by corticosterone in obese fa/fa rats. Int. J. Obes. **9:** 89–95.

86. ROHNER-JEANRENAUD, F., C. D. WALKER, R. GRECO-PEROTTO & B. JEANRENAUD. 1989. Central corticotropin-releasing factor administration prevents the excessive body weight gain of genetically obese (fa/fa) rats. Endocrinology **124:** 733–739.

87. LANGLEY, S. C. & D. A. YORK. 1990. Effects of antiglucocorticoid RU 486 on development of obesity in obese fa/fa Zucker rats. Am. J. Physiol. **259:** R539–R544.

88. PLOTSKY, P. M., K. V. THRIVIKRAMAN, A. G. WATTS & R. L. HAUGER. 1992. Hypothalamic-pituitary-adrenal axis function in the Zucker obese rat. Endocrinology **130:** 1931–1941.

89. LANGLEY, S. C. & D. A. YORK. 1992. Glucocorticoid receptor numbers in the brain and liver of the obese Zucker rat. Int. J. Obes. **16:** 135–143.

90. CUNNINGHAM, J. J., J. CALLES-ESCANDON, F. GARRIDO, D. B. CARR & H. H. BODE. 1986. Hypercorticosteronuria and diminished pituitary responsiveness to corticotropin-releasing factor in obese Zucker rats. Endocrinology **118:** 98–101.

91. TOKUYAMA, K. & J. HIMMS-HAGEN. 1987. Increased sensitivity of the genetically obese mouse to corticosterone. Am. J. Physiol. **252:** E202–E208.

92. FREEDMAN, M. R., B. A. HORWITZ & J. S. STERN. 1986. Effect of adrenalectomy and glucocorticoid replacement on development of obesity. Am. J. Physiol. **250:** R595–R607.

93. LANGLEY, S. C. & D. A. YORK. 1990. Increased type-II glucocorticoid-receptor numbers and glucocorticoid-sensitive enzyme activities in the brain of the obese Zucker rat. Brain Res. **533:** 268–274.

94. TSAI, H. J. & D. R. ROMSOS. 1991. Glucocorticoid and mineralocorticoid receptor-binding characteristics in obese (ob/ob) mice. Am. J. Physiol. **261:** E495–E499.

95. WEBB, M. L., J. J. FLYNN, T. J. SCHMIDT, D. L. MARGULES & G. LITWACK. 1986. Decreased glucocorticoid binding and receptor activation in brain of genetically diabetic (mdb/mdb) mice. J. Steroid Biochem. **25:** 649–657.

96. WILLIAMS, G., P. E. MCKIBBIN & H. D. MCCARTHY. 1991. Hypothalamic regulatory peptides and the regulation of food intake and energy balance—Signals or noise. Proc. Nutr. Soc. **50:** 527–544.

97. BILLINGTON, C. J. & A. S. LEVINE. 1992. Hypothalamic neuropeptide Y regulation of feeding and energy metabolism. Curr. Opinion Neurobiol. **2:** 847–851.

98. COLEMAN, D. L. 1978. Obese and diabetes: Two mutant genes causing diabetes-obesity syndromes in mice. Diabetologia **14:** 141–148.

99. TOKUNAGA, K., M. FUKUSHIMA, J. W. KEMNITZ & G. A. BRAY. 1986. Comparison of ventromedial and paraventricular lesions in rats that become obese. Am. J. Physiol. **251:** R1221–R1227.

100. FUKUSHIMA, M., K. TOKUNAGA, J. LUPIEN, J. W. KEMNITZ & G. A. BRAY. 1990. Dynamic and static phases of obesity following lesions in PVN and VMH. Am. J. Physiol. **253:** R523–R529.

101. WEINGARTEN, H. P., P. CHANG & T. J. MCDONALD. 1985. Comparison of the metabolic and behavioral disturbances following paraventricular- and ventromedial-hypothalamic lesions. Brain Res. Bull. **14:** 551–559.

102. KRAHN, D. D., B. A. GOSNELL, A. S. LEVINE & J. E. MORLEY. 1988. Behavioral effects of corticotropin-releasing factor: Localization and characterization of central effects. Brain Res. **443:** 63–69.

103. YORK, D. 1992. Genetics models of animal obesity. *In* Obesity. P. Bjorntorp & B. N. Brodoff, Eds.: 233–240. J. B. Lippincott Company. Philadelphia, PA.

104. BJORNTORP, P. A. 1989. Sex differences in the regulation of energy balance with exercise. Am. J. Clin. Nutr. **49:** 958–961.

105. OSCAI, L. B. 1973. The role of exercise in weight control. *In* Exercise and Sport Sciences Reviews. J. H. Wilmore, Ed.: 103–123. Academic Press. New York, NY.

106. RICHARD, D. 1989. Influence of exercise training on energy balance. *In* Proceedings of the 14th Congress of Nutrition. K. W. Young, L. Y. Cha, L. K. Yull, J. J. Soon & K. S. He, Eds.: 121–124. The 14th ICN Organizing Committee. Seoul.

107. NIKOLETSEAS, M. M. 1980. Food intake in the exercising rat: A brief review. Neurosci. Biobehav. Rev. **4:** 265–267.

108. NANCE, D. M., B. BROMLEY, R. J. BARNARD & R. A. GORSKI. 1977. Sexually dimorphic effects of forced exercise on food intake and body weight in the rat. Physiol. Behav. **19:** 155–158.

109. RICHARD, D. & J. ARNOLD. 1987. Influence of exercise training in the regulation of energy balance. J. Obesity Weight Regul. **6:** 212–224.

110. RICHARD, D. & S. RIVEST. 1989. The role of exercise in thermogenesis and energy balance. Can. J. Physiol. Pharmacol. **67:** 402–409.

111. HILL, J. O., J. R. DAVIS & A. R. TAGLIAFERRO. 1983. Effects of diet and exercise training on thermogenesis in adult female rats. Physiol. Behav. **31:** 133–135.

112. HIRATA, K. 1982. Enhanced calorigenesis in brown adipose tissue in physically trained rats. Jpn. J. Physiol. **32:** 647–653.
113. HIRATA, K. 1982. Blood flow to brown adipose tissue and norepinephrine-induced calorigenesis in physically trained rats. Jpn. J. Physiol. **32:** 279–291.
114. HILL, J. O., J. R. DAVIS, A. R. TAGLIAFERRO & J. STEWART. 1984. Dietary obesity and exercise in young rats. Physiol. Behav. **33:** 321–328.
115. WICKLER, S. J., J. S. STERN, Z. GLICK & B. A. HORWITZ. 1987. Thermogenic capacity and brown fat in rats exercise-trained by running. Metabolism **36:** 76–81.
116. ARNOLD, J., J. LEBLANC, J. CÔTÉ, J. LALONDE & D. RICHARD. 1986. Exercise suppression of thermoregulatory thermogenesis in warm- and cold-acclimated rats. Can. J. Physiol. Pharmacol. **64:** 922–926.
117. BELL, R. R., T. J. MCGILL, P. W. DIGBY & S. A. BENNETT. 1984. Effects of dietary protein and exercise on brown adipose tissue and energy balance in experimental animals. J. Nutr. **114:** 1900–1908.
118. HARRI, M., T. DANNENBERG, R. OKSANEN-ROSSI, E. HOHTOLA & U. SUNDIN. 1984. Related and unrelated changes in response to exercise and cold in rats: A reevaluation. J. Appl. Physiol. **57:** 1489–1497.
119. HARRI, M. & P. KUUSELA. 1986. Is swimming exercise or cold exposure for rats? Acta Physiol. Scand. **126:** 189–197.
120. RICHARD, D., A. LABRIE & S. RIVEST. 1992. Tissue specificity of SNS response to exercise in mice exposed to low temperatures. Am. J. Physiol. **262:** R921–R925.
121. RIVEST, S. & D. RICHARD. 1989. The effects of corticotropin-releasing factor on energy balance in rats are sex-dependent. Am. J. Physiol. **257:** R1417–R1422.
122. KRAHN, D. D., B. A. GOSNELL, M. GRACE & A. S. LEVINE. 1986. CRF antagonist partially reverses CRF- and stress-induced effect on feeding. Brain Res. Bull. **17:** 285–289.
123. RIVEST, S. & D. RICHARD. 1990. Involvement of corticotropin-releasing factor in the anorexia induced by exercise. Brain Res. Bull. **25:** 169–172.
124. RIVEST, S., S. LEE, C. RIVIER & D. RICHARD. 1992. Expression of *FOS* and CRF mRNA in the brain of female rats subjected to single or repeated running sessions. Soc. Neurosci. Abstr. **18:** 194.
125. CABANAC, M. & J. MORRISSETTE. 1992. Acute, but not chronic, exercise lowers the body weight set-point in male rats. Physiol. Behav. **52:** 1173–1177.
126. ARNOLD, J. & D. RICHARD. 1987. Detraining of exercise-trained rats: Effects on energetic efficiency and brown adipose tissue thermogenesis. Br. J. Nutr. **57:** 363–370.
127. RICHARD, D. & J. LEBLANC. 1980. Effects of physical training and food restriction on insulin secretion and glucose tolerance in male and female rats. Am. J. Clin. Nutr. **33:** 2588–2594.
128. GALBO, H., C. J. HEDESKOV, K. CAPITO & J. VINTEN. 1981. The effect of physical training on insulin secretion of rat pancreatic islets. Acta Physiol. Scand. **111:** 75–79.
129. RICHARD, D., A. TREMBLAY & J. LEBLANC. 1982. Diminished insulin secretion in exercised-trained rats. Proc. Annu. Meet. Can. Fed. Biol. Soc. **25:** 145.
130. SCHWARTZ, M. W., A. J. SIPOLS, J. L. MARKS, G. SANACORA, J. D. WHITE, A. SCHEURINK, S. E. KAHN, D. G. BASKIN, S. C. WOODS, D. P. FIGLEWICZ & D. PORTE. 1992. Inhibition of Hypothalamic Neuropeptide-Y Gene Expression by Insulin. Endocrinology **130:** 3608–3616.
131. SCHWARTZ, M. W., D. P. FIGLEWICZ, D. G. BASKIN, S. C. WOODS & D. PORTE. 1992. Insulin in the brain—A hormonal regulator of energy balance. Endocr. Rev. **13:** 387–414.
132. WADE, G. N. & J. M. GRAY. 1979. Gonadal effects on food intake and adiposity: A metabolic hypothesis. Physiol. Behav. **22:** 583–593.
133. WADE, G. N. 1976. Sex hormones, regulatory behaviors, and body weight. *In* Advances in the Study of Behavior. J. S. Rosenblatt, R. A. Hinde, E. Show & C. G. Beer, Eds.: 201–279. Academic Press. New York, NY.
134. WADE, G. N., J. M. GRAY & T. J. BARTNESS. 1985. Gonadal influences on adiposity. Int. J. Obes. **9:** 83–92.
135. KEMNITZ, J. W., J. R. GIBBER, K. A. LINDSAY & S. G. EISELE. 1989. Effects of ovarian

hormones and eating behaviors, body weight, and glucoregulation in rhesus monkeys. Horm. Behav. **23:** 235–250.

136. CZAJA, J. A. & R. W. GOY. 1975. Ovarian hormones and food intake in female guinea pigs and rhesus monkeys. Horm. Behav. **6:** 329–349.

137. RICHARD, D. 1986. Effects of ovarian hormones on energy balance and brown adipose tissue thermogenesis. Am. J. Physiol. **250:** R245–R249.

138. PUERTA, M. L., M. P. NAVA, M. ABELENDA & A. FERNANDEZ. 1990. Inactivation of brown adipose tissue thermogenesis by oestradiol treatment in cold-acclimated rats. Pflugers Arch. Eur. J. Physiol. **416:** 659–662.

139. ROCHON, L. & D. RICHARD. 1986. Effects of estradiol and exercise on energy balance and brown adipose tissue in rats. Proc. Annu. Can. Sports Sci. **19:** 2P.

140. TARTTELIN, M. F. & R. A. GORSKI. 1971. Variations in food and water intake in the normal and acyclic female rat. Physiol. Behav. **7:** 847–852.

141. HAAR, M. B. T. 1972. Circadian and estrual rhythms in food intake in the rat. Horm. Behav. **3:** 213–219.

142. LANDAU, T. & I. ZUCKER. 1976. Estrogenic regulation of body weight in the female rat. Horm. Behav. **7:** 29–39.

143. BUCKINGHAM, J. C., K. D. DOHLER & C. A. WILSON. 1978. Activity of the pituitary-adrenocortical system and thyroid gland during the oestrous cycle of the rat. J. Endocrinol. **78:** 359–366.

144. BOHLER, H. C. L., R. T. ZOELLER, J. C. KING, B. S. RUBIN, R. WEBER & G. R. MERRIAM. 1990. Corticotropin releasing hormone messenger RNA is elevated on the afternoon of proestrus in the parvocellular paraventricular nuclei of the female rat. Mol. Brain Res. **8:** 259–262.

145. BUTERA, P. C. & R. J. BEIKIRCH. 1989. Central implants of diluted estradiol—independent effects on ingestive and reproductive behaviors of ovariectomized rats. Brain Res. **491:** 266–273.

146. BUTERA, P. C., D. M. WILLARD & S. A. RAYMOND. 1992. Effects of PVN lesions on the responsiveness of female rats to estradiol. Brain Res. **576:** 304–310.

147. HILLEGAART, V. 1991. Functional topography of brain serotonergic pathways in the rat. Acta Physiol. Scand. **142:** 1–54.

148. JACOBS, B. L. & E. C. AZMITIA. 1992. Structure and function of the brain serotonin system. Physiol. Rev. **72:** 165–229.

149. SAMANIN, R. & S. GARATTINI. 1989. Serotonin and the pharmacology of eating disorders. Ann. N.Y. Acad. Sci. **575:** 194–207.

150. BLUNDELL, J. E. & A. J. HILL. 1987. Serotoninergic modulation of the pattern of eating and the profile of hunger-satiety in humans. Int. J. Obes. **11:** 141–155.

151. GUYGRAND, B., G. CREPALDI, P. LEFEBVRE, M. APFELBAUM, A. GRIES & P. TURNER. 1989. International trial of long-term dexfenfluramine in obesity. Lancet **2:** 1142–1145.

152. GARATTINI, S., T. MENNINI & R. SAMANIN. 1989. Reduction of food intake by manipulation of central serotonin—Current experimental results. Br. J. Psychiatry **155:** 41–51.

153. ROWLAND, N. E. & J. CARLTON. 1986. Neurobiology of an anorectic drug: Fenfluramine. Prog. Neurobiol. **27:** 13–62.

154. BLUNDELL, J. E., A. J. HILL & T. C. KIRHAM. 1987. Dextrofenfluramine and eating behaviour in animals: Action on food selection, motivation and body weight. *In* Body Weight Control. The Physiology, Clinical Treatment and Prevention of Obesity. A. E. Bender & L. J. Brookes, Eds.: 233–239. Churchill Livingstone. London.

155. BLUNDELL, J. E. & A. J. HILL. 1989. Do serotoninergic drugs decrease energy intake by reducing fat or carbohydrate intake? Effect of d-fenfluramine with supplemented weight-increasing diets. Pharmacol. Biochem. Behav. **31:** 773–778.

156. ROTHWELL, N. J. & M. J. STOCK. 1987. Effect of diet and fenfluramine on thermogenesis in the rat: Possible involvement of serotonergic mechanisms. Int. J. Obes. **11:** 319–324.

157. LUPIEN, J. R. & G. A. BRAY. 1986. Effects of fenfluramine on GDP-binding to brown adipose tissue mitochondria. Pharmacol. Biochem. Behav. **23:** 509–513.

158. FULLER, R. W. 1990. Serotonin receptors and neuroendocrine responses. Neuropsychopharmacology **3:** 495–502.

159. APPEL, N. M., M. J. OWENS, S. CULP, R. ZACZEK, J. F. CONTRERA, G. BISSETTE, C. B. NEMEROFF & E. B. DESOUZA. 1991. Role for brain corticotropin-releasing factor in the weight-reducing effects of chronic fenfluramine treatment in rats. Endocrinology **128:** 3237–3246.

160. FULLER, R. W. & H. D. SNODDY. 1980. Effect of serotonin-releasing drugs on serum corticosterone concentration in rats. Neuroendocrinology **31:** 96–100.

161. MCELROY, J. F., J. M. MILLER & J. S. MEYER. 1984. Fenfluramine, p-chloroamphetamine and p-fluoroamphetamine stimulation of pituitary-adrenocortical activity in rat: Evidence for differences in site and mechanism of action. J. Pharmacol. Exp. Ther. **228:** 593–599.

162. LEFEUVRE, R. A., L. AISENTHAL & N. J. ROTHWELL. 1991. Involvement of corticotrophin-releasing factor (CRF) in the thermogenic and anorexic actions of serotonin (5-HT) and related compounds. Brain Res. **555:** 245–250.

163. RICHARD, D., S. RIVEST & C. RIVIER. 1992. The 5-hydroxytryptamine agonist fenfluramine increases Fos-like immunoreactivity in the brain. Brain Res. **594:** 131–137.

164. MA, Q. P., G. F. YIN, M. K. AI & J. S. HAN. 1991. Serotoninergic projections from the nucleus raphe dorsalis to the amygdala in the rat. Neurosci. Lett. **134:** 21–24.

165. SAWCHENKO, P. E., L. W. SWANSON, H. W. M. STEINBUSCH & A. A. J. VERHOFSTAD. 1983. The distribution and cells of origin of serotoninergic inputs to the paraventricular and supraoptic nuclei of the rat. Brain Res. **277:** 355–360.

166. CHAOULOFF, F., D. LAUDE, B. SERRURRIER, D. MERINO, Y. GUEZENNEC & J. L. ELGHOZI. 1987. Brain serotonin response to exercise in the rat: The influence of training duration. Biog. Amines **4:** 99–106.

167. HARBUZ, M. S. & S. L. LIGHTMAN. 1989. Responses of hypothalamic and pituitary messenger RNA to physical and psychological stress in the rat. J. Endocrinol. **122:** 705–711.

168. CHAOULOFF, F. 1989. Physical exercise and brain monoamines—A review. Acta Physiol. Scand. **137:** 1–13.

169. KYRKOULI, S. E., B. G. STANLEY, R. D. SEIRAFI & S. F. LEIBOWITZ. 1990. Stimulation of feeding by galanin—Anatomical localization and behavioral specificity of this peptide's Effects in the Brain. Peptides **11:** 995–1001.

170. WYRWICKA, W., Ed. 1979. Brain and Feeding Behavior. Charles C. Thomas. Springfield, IL.

171. BORSINI, F. & E. T. ROLLS. 1984. Role of adrenaline and serotonin in the basolateral region of the amygdala in food preferences and learned taste aversions in the rat. Physiol. Behav. **33:** 37–43.

172. ROTHWELL, N. J. 1992. Hypothalamus and thermogenesis. *In* Energy Metabolism. Tissue Determinants and Cellular Corollaries. J. M. Kinney & H. N. Tucker, Eds.: 229–245. Raven Press. New York, NY.

173. ROTHWELL, N. J. 1991. Functions and mechanisms of interleukin-1 in the brain. Trends Pharmacol. Sci. **12:** 430–436.

174. UEHARA, A., C. SEKUYA, Y. TAKASAKI, M. NAMIKI & A. ARMURA. 1989. Anorexia induced by interleukin 1: Involvement of corticotropin-releasing factor. Am. J. Physiol. **257:** R616–R617.

175. OLSON, B. R., G. E. HOFFMAN, A. F. SVED, E. M. STRICKER & J. G. VERBALIS. 1992. Cholecystokinin induces c-fos expression in hypothalamic oxytocinergic neurons projecting to the dorsal vagal complex. Brain Res. **569:** 238–248.

The Locus Coeruleus as a Site for Integrating Corticotropin-Releasing Factor and Noradrenergic Mediation of Stress Responses[a]

RITA J. VALENTINO,[b] STEPHEN L. FOOTE,[c]
AND MICHELLE E. PAGE[b]

[b]Department of Mental Health Sciences
Hahnemann University
Philadelphia, Pennsylvania 19102-1192

[c]Department of Psychiatry
University of California, San Diego
La Jolla, California 92093

This review describes the results of studies designed to test the hypothesis that corticotropin-releasing factor (CRF) serves as a neurotransmitter in the locus coeruleus (LC) during stress, and discusses potential implications of CRF neurotransmission in the LC. The isolation and characterization of the 41-amino-acid peptide, CRF, by Vale and colleagues[1] was the result of experiments designed to determine how the cascade of endocrine responses to stress is initiated. The anatomic studies that followed revealed a distribution of CRF in the central nervous system (CNS) that far exceeded the necessary anatomic substrate for its role in adrenocorticotropin (ACTH) release.[2–4] Specifically, numerous CRF-containing cell groups were visualized in the brain outside of the hypothalamic-pituitary axis, and CRF-immunoreactive (CRF-IR) fibers were visualized in nuclei that were not directly involved with endocrine aspects of stress responses. At the same time, several studies reported that intracerebroventricular (i.c.v.) administration of CRF, in doses that elicited ACTH release, also altered cardiovascular function,[5,6] gastrointestinal function,[7,8] and behavior,[9–12] and that these effects could be produced in hypophysectomized or adrenalectomized animals[13,14] demonstrating that they were not dependent on CRF endocrine activity. Thus, these findings implicated extrahypophyseal CRF in behavioral and autonomic aspects of stress responses. The development of a CRF antagonist,[15] α-helical CRF$_{9-41}$, provided a tool to test the function of endogenous CRF in nonendocrine aspects of stress responses. Studies demonstrating that α-helical CRF$_{9-41}$ prevented many stress-elicited responses including cardiovascular effects,[16] gastrointestinal changes,[17,18] and several behavioral responses[19–21] strongly implied an involvement of CRF in these effects. These studies suggested that CRF may have a global role in the stress response, whereby it serves as a neurotransmitter in regions outside of the hypothalamic-pituitary axis to mediate behavioral and/or autonomic responses to stress, in addition to participating as a neurohormone in hypophyseal circuits to initiate the cascade of endocrine effects that have been the hallmark of

[a]This work was supported by Public Health Service grants MH 40008, MH 00840, and MH 42796.

stress. This hypothesis is intriguing because it offers a mechanism by which diverse challenges could elicit relatively comparable effects on diverse physiologic systems.

In spite of this substantial evidence for the role of CRF as neurotransmitter, the criteria that must be met to verify this role in a specific nucleus have yet to be satisfied. The major brain noradrenergic nucleus, the locus coeruleus, is one site for which certain of the criteria for CRF neurotransmission have been met.

INVOLVEMENT OF THE LOCUS COERULEUS IN STRESS

Activation of the LC noradrenergic system was implicated in stress long before the isolation and characterization of CRF, by neurochemical studies that demonstrated that stress increased norepinephrine turnover in brain regions (i.e, the cortex and hippocampus), for which the LC is the sole source of norepinephrine.[22-24] This scenario has been supported more recently by microdialysis studies demonstrating increased norepinephrine in extracellular fluid in hippocampus during stress[25] and by increased expression of tyrosine hydroxylase in the LC of stressed rats.[26] Electrophysiologic studies have supported the idea that the LC is activated by stressors. Thus, in anesthetized rats, footshock[27] and several physiologic challenges (i.e., hypotension,[28] hypoxia,[29] visceral stimulation[30]) increase spontaneous discharge rates of LC neurons. In unanesthetized cats, physiologic challenges as well as environmental stressors increase LC discharge rate.[31-34]

Although LC activation appears to be an integral component of stress, the circuitry underlying this activation has not been elucidated, nor has the function of LC activation in stress been determined. Anatomic and physiologic studies have revealed an excitatory amino acid afferent to the LC from the nucleus paragigantocellularis (PGi) in the ventrolateral medulla.[35,36] This input is one potential means by which stressors could activate the LC. However, immunohistochemical studies indicate that the LC and its pericoerulear dendritic zone receive innervation from other neurotransmitters, including acetylcholine and serotonin, and numerous peptides, including substance P and enkephalin.[37-40] Shortly after the isolation of CRF, immunohistochemical studies suggested that this neurohormone is also present in axons innervating the LC.[2-4] Based on the role of CRF in stress and the finding of CRF-IR fibers in the LC, the hypothesis that CRF could serve as a neurotransmitter in the LC to activate these noradrenergic neurons during stress was investigated.

DISTRIBUTION OF CRF CELLS AND FIBERS
IN THE LOCUS COERULEUS REGION

Many of the initial immunohistochemical studies of the distribution of CRF cells and fibers throughout the rat CNS indicated that the LC contained CRF-IR fibers.[2-4] Some studies suggested the presence of CRF-IR neurons within the LC.[3,4] A detailed study of CRF-IR in the LC region revealed moderate CRF-IR fibers throughout the rostral-caudal levels of the LC, and these were more dense in the medial pericoerulear band between the LC and ventricle where numerous LC dendrites extend[41] (FIG. 1). At more rostral levels, a dense region of CRF-IR fibers was visualized just ventral and lateral to the LC in a region between the LC and the mesencephalic nucleus of the trigeminus. Double-labeling studies that visualized tyrosine hydroxylase immunoreactivity (TH-IR) and CRF-IR showed that the region of CRF-IR fibers overlapped with TH-IR neurons and processes which were probably both dendrites and axons.[41]

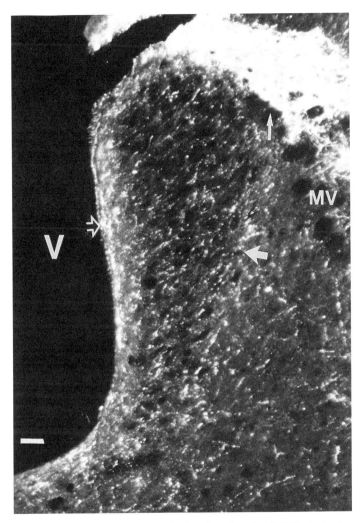

FIGURE 1. CRF-IR in the locus coeruleus (LC) region of rat. Brightfield photomicrograph of a 30-μm coronal section at the level of mid-LC (*filled arrow*). Note CRF-IR fibers in LC and in the medial pericoerulear band adjacent to the ventricle (*open arrow*). Additionally, CRF-IR fibers are particularly dense in the parabrachial nucleus (*vertical filled arrow*). *Abbreviations:* MV, mesencephalic nucleus of the trigeminus; V, ventricle. Calibration bar = 50 μm.

CRF-IR neurons were visualized in pericoerulear regions both lateral and medial to the LC. These CRF-IR neurons were not TH-IR. Additionally, numerous CRF-IR neurons were visualized in the region corresponding to Barrington's nucleus ventromedial to the rostral pole of the LC. These neurons overlapped with TH-IR processes, suggesting reciprocal communications between this CRF-containing nucleus and the noradrenergic LC.[41] CRF-IR fibers have also been visualized in monkey[42] and human LC.[43] The CRF innervation of monkey LC appears to be more dense than that in rats. Although the results of these studies suggest that CRF innervates LC neurons of different species, this has yet to be confirmed at the ultrastructural level.

To provide additional information about the sources of CRF-IR fibers in the LC region, injections of a retrograde tract tracer (wheat germ agglutinin conjugated to inactivated horseradish peroxidase coupled to gold particles) were made into the LC, and sections were visualized for the tracer and for CRF-IR.[41] As previously reported,[44] retrogradely labeled neurons were numerous in the nucleus PGi and the nucleus prepositus hypoglossi (PrH). Both of these regions also contained CRF-IR neurons.[41] Approximately 10% of the retrogradely labeled neurons in PGi were CRF-IR, implicating this nucleus as one source of CRF-IR fibers in LC.[41] In contrast, no double-labeled neurons were observed in the PrH. In the PrH, CRF-IR neurons appeared to be a distinct population of cells lying lateral to the retrogradely labeled neurons. Occassional double-labeled neurons were visualized in the dorsal cap of the paraventricular nucleus of the hypothalamus.[41] Other potential sources of CRF-IR fibers in the LC included CRF-IR neurons in pericoerulear regions and Barrington's nucleus.[41] However, it has been difficult to confirm whether these neurons project to LC using retrograde tracing studies because of their close proximity to the LC.

Neurochemical findings suggest that CRF levels in LC are stress sensitive.[45] Thus, both acute and chronic stress have been demonstrated to increase CRF levels in micropunches of LC as measured by radioimmunoassay. Interestingly, the increase in CRF levels associated with acute stress was specific to the LC region and not observed in numerous other brain sites. It is not clear, however, whether increased CRF levels in LC during stress are indicative of enhanced CRF processing or decreased CRF release. Acute stress has also been shown to selectively increase CRF mRNA expression in the nearby Barrington's nucleus.[46] It is possible that enhanced CRF levels in micropunches of the LC region after acute stress are partly due to some contamination by CRF from Barrington's nucleus.

In addition to the presence of CRF-IR fibers in the LC, specific binding sites for CRF would be predicted in this region if CRF serves as a neurotransmitter in the LC. This has now been confirmed using autoradiography.[47]

CRF EFFECTS ON ELECTROPHYSIOLOGIC ACTIVITY OF THE LOCUS COERULEUS

If CRF acts as a neurotransmitter to enhance LC discharge rates, exogenous CRF should activate these neurons. CRF effects on LC discharge characteristics have been described in both anesthetized[48,49] and unanesthetized rats.[50] Central administration of CRF in the lateral ventricle in doses that mimic autonomic and behavioral aspects of stress increases LC spontaneous discharge rates in a dose-dependent manner.[48,50] The effect produced by CRF is greater in unanesthetized rats, as demonstrated by a shift to the left in the CRF dose-response curve.[50] Interestingly, in unanesthetized rats, the increase in LC discharge rate is greater at 40 minutes than at 5 minutes after injection.[50] This is in contrast to CRF effects in anesthetized rats which remain unchanged up to 40 minutes after administration. The mechanism for this amplified CRF effect on LC discharge rates of unanesthetized rats with time is unknown. However, it is consistent with the time course of some behavioral effects of CRF. For example, CRF potentiation of a fear-elicited startle response peaks 1–2 hours after injection.[51]

The activating effects of CRF on LC neurons are structurally specific, such that analogues of CRF (i.e., Ala¹⁴CRF and the free acid analogue, CRF-OH) that do not mimic other aspects of stress responses do not increase the LC spontaneous discharge rate after central administration.[48,49] Moreover, the effect is regionally specific so that direct microinjection of CRF onto LC cells, but not onto cerebellar neurons or neurons of the mesencephalic nucleus of the trigeminus, increases the discharge rate.[48] Interestingly, preliminary findings indicate that direct application of CRF onto neurons of the parabrachial nucleus activates these cells, suggesting that this nucleus may also be a target for CRF neurotransmission.[48]

CRF also disrupts the pattern of LC discharge in response to phasic sensory stimuli[49,50] (FIG. 2). Short-duration sensory stimuli such as the presentation of a

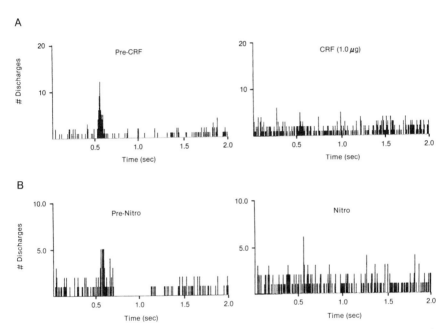

FIGURE 2. CRF and hypotensive stress disrupt response of locus coeruleus to repeated footshock. Shown are peristimulus time histograms (PSTHs) from two individual halothane-anesthetized rats (**A** and **B**) generated during repeated trials of footshock (1.3 mA, 0.5 ms, 0.1 Hz; 50 trials). The stimulus was presented at 0.5 s; bin width = 8 ms. (**A**) PSTHs generated from the same rat before (Pre-CRF) and after (CRF) i.c.v. administration of 1.0 μg CRF. (**B**) PSTHs generated from a rat before (Pre-Nitro) and during (Nitro) infusion of nitroprusside. Note that both CRF and nitroprusside increase unstimulated discharge and decrease discharge evoked by the footshock. (Valentino & Wehby.[54] Reproduced, with permission, from *Neuroendocrinology*.)

0.5-ms footshock to anesthetized rats or a 20-ms tone to unanesthetized rats produces a period of greatly elevated LC discharge (80–100-ms duration) followed by a longer period of inhibited activity. This pattern is disrupted in a dose-dependent manner by centrally administered CRF, such that unstimulated discharge during trials of repeated sensory stimulation is increased and evoked activity is either decreased or unchanged. The net effect of CRF on this response is to decrease the ratio of evoked-to-tonic discharge rate (i.e., the signal-to-noise ratio). This effect occurs in both anesthetized rats where the stimulus is footshock[49] and in unanesthe-tized rats where the stimulus is auditory.[50] The responsiveness of LC neurons to phasic sensory stimulation has been a basis of the hypothesized function of the LC in arousal and attention.[52] However, it is not known how the response is translated to norepinephrine release in LC target regions or to an effect on target-cell activity, making it difficult to interpret the effect of a disruption of the response by CRF. In general, the effect of CRF appears to be a persistent activation of LC such that short-lived stimuli, which may be of little importance, do not affect discharge rate.

EFFECTS OF PHYSIOLOGIC CHALLENGES ON ELECTROPHYSIOLOGIC ACTIVITY OF THE LOCUS COERULEUS

Another important criterion that must be met to establish a putative neurotrans-mitter role for CRF in the LC requires that stimulation of CRF neurons projecting to the LC mimic the effects of exogenous CRF, and these effects be prevented by a CRF antagonist. This criterion has been difficult to fulfill because the CRF afferents to the LC were unknown until recently. Moreover, an important source of these afferents may be from pericoerulear CRF neurons which make this a technically difficult criterion to test with presently available tools. One way to indirectly test this criterion is to compare the effects of stressors on the LC discharge to those of exogenous CRF and to determine their sensitivity to CRF antagonists. These experiments have used the physiologic challenges of hypotension and bladder distention as stressors.

Hypotension elicited by intravenous (i.v.) infusion of nitroprusside (10 μg in 30 μL/min for 15 min) has been shown to elicit CRF release into the hypophyseal portal system.[53] This infusion decreases mean arterial blood pressure of anesthetized rats by approximately 50% and simultaneously increases the LC discharge rate by approximately 30%.[54] There appears to be a strong inverse temporal correlation between mean arterial blood pressure and LC discharge rate throughout nitroprus-side infusion and after termination of the infusion. Thus, blood pressure recovers and remains elevated above pre-nitroprusside levels for 6–9 minutes after termina-tion of the infusion, and the LC discharge rate decreases to below pre-nitroprusside rates for the same time after infusion. In unanesthetized rats, the same dose of nitroprusside has little effect on either blood pressure or LC discharge rate, supporting the idea that LC activation is the result of hypotension rather than some other effect of nitroprusside.[55] In these rats a higher concentration of nitroprusside (30 μg in 30 μL/min for 15 min) is necessary to decrease blood pressure by 50%, and this increases the LC discharge rates of unanesthetized rats by 200%.[55]

Like CRF, hypotensive stress disrupts LC responses to repeated sciatic nerve stimulation[54] (FIG. 2). Thus, when anesthetized rats are presented with a trial of repeated sciatic nerve stimulation during nitroprusside infusion, evoked discharge rate decreases and unstimulated discharge rate increases, that is, the signal-to-noise ratio is decreased. In fact, the pattern of responding is identical to that observed after CRF administration (see FIG. 2).

LC activation by hypotensive stress is prevented in rats administered α-helical CRF$_{9-41}$ i.c.v. (50 μg)[54] and in rats injected with α-helical CRF$_{9-41}$ directly into the LC (100–150 ng).[56] The CRF antagonist does not alter the magnitude or time course of hypotension associated with nitroprusside infusion.[54] In contrast, neither i.c.v. administration of the excitatory amino acid antagonist, kynurenic acid, nor injection of saline (100 nL) into the LC prevents activation by nitroprusside.[56] Moreover, systemic administration of dexamethasone (100 μg, i.m.) 6 hours prior to nitroprus-side infusion does not alter the response of LC neurons to hypotensive stress.[54] This pretreatment has been reported to prevent hypophyseal CRF release associated with hemodynamic stress.[57] Taken together, these results suggest that hypotensive stress elicited by i.v. infusion of nitroprusside activates the LC via CRF acting within the LC and that this CRF is not hypophyseal in origin.

In the studies cited above, the CRF antagonist did not affect spontaneous LC discharge or LC discharge evoked by repeated footshock. In contrast, i.c.v. administration of kynurenic acid in doses that did not affect LC activation by hypotensive stress completely prevented LC activation by footshock.[56] This confirms earlier work that demonstrated that LC activation by repeated footshock was mediated by excitatory amino acid afferents acting at non-NMDA receptors in the LC.[35,36]

Bladder distention via injection of 0.5 mL of saline into the bladder also increases the LC discharge rate[58] as previously reported.[30] Because Barrington's nucleus is a micturition center,[59] containing many CRF-IR neurons,[41] and is a possible source of LC afferents, it was predicted that, as for hypotensive stress, LC activation by bladder distention was mediated by direct CRF actions in the LC. However, this effect was not prevented by pretreatment with the CRF antagonist, but was prevented by i.c.v. injection of kynurenic acid and the non-NMDA antagonist, CNQX.[58] In addition, local LC injection of kynurenic acid greatly attenuated LC activation by bladder distention. Thus, the pharmacology of this effect appears to be similar to that of LC activation by footshock. However, it is possible that more potent CRF antagonists are necessary to prevent LC activation by bladder distention.

The series of experiments described above have provided information about the circuitry and neurotransmitters underlying LC activation by different stimuli (FIG. 3). LC activation by footshock has been well characterized by Ennis and Aston-Jones.[35,36] This effect requires an excitatory amino acid pathway from the nucleus PGi and activation of non-NMDA excitatory amino acid receptors in the LC. LC activation by bladder distention may utilize similar pathways because the pharmacology of the responses is similar. Experiments are in progress that involve reversibly inactivating the PGi with lidocaine to determine if this region is the source of excitatory amino acid afferents involved in LC activation by bladder distention. In contrast to footshock or bladder distention, hypotension activates the LC by CRF acting within the LC and does not require excitatory amino acid input. The CRF afferents mediating this response have yet to be elucidated. Nitroprusside infusion also activated PGi neurons.[59] It is tempting to speculate that the neurons in the PGi that are activated by nitroprusside infusion are CRF neurons that project to the LC, but this has yet to be determined. Other sources that could mediate this effect are CRF neurons in the dorsal cap of the paraventricular nucleus of the hypothalamus or pericoerulear CRF neurons, as mentioned above.

POTENTIAL FUNCTIONS OF CRF NEUROTRANSMISSION
IN THE LOCUS COERULEUS DURING STRESS

The functions ascribed to the LC have been based on (1) its divergent efferent projections, (2) its discharge characteristics, and (3) the effects of norepinephrine on target neurons. The LC gives rise to an extensive system of projections that innervates targets of very diverse functions.[60,61] Potentially, any stimulus that alters LC discharge can simultaneously affect activity in all of these functionally diverse targets. This structural characteristic places the LC in a position to simultaneously influence CNS targets that are involved in endocrine, autonomic, sensory, motor, and behavioral functions. Based on this characteristic alone, it is not surprising that the

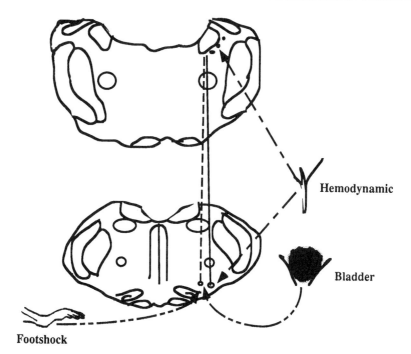

Footshock

FIGURE 3. Schematic representation of potential pathways by which footshock, bladder distention, and hypotensive stress may activate the locus coeruleus (LC). The dotted line from the nucleus paragigantocellularis (PGi) to the LC represents excitatory amino acid neurotransmission, and the solid line from the PGi to the LC represents CRF neurotransmission. Footshock activates the LC via excitatory amino acid afferents from the PGi. LC activation by bladder distention is sensitive to the same pharmacologic antagonists as LC activation by footshock, and therefore may utilize a similar pathway. LC activation by hypotensive stress requires CRF release in the LC. This may derive from CRF neurons in the PGi, pericoerulear sources, or the dorsal cap of the paraventricular nucleus of the hypothalamus as suggested by studies of CRF afferents to LC.[41]

LC has been implicated in syndromes that are characterized by multisystem events such as the opiate withdrawal syndrome,[62] anxiety,[63] and stress.

Studies comparing LC spontaneous discharge activity during different states of arousal have demonstrated that the mean discharge rate is state dependent, that is, higher with increased levels of arousal and vigilance and lower with decreasing levels of arousal.[64] Taken together with the finding that LC neurons are responsive to multimodal sensory stimuli,[65,66] these discharge characteristics suggest that LC activation is associated with arousal and attention to environmental stimuli. However, in order to assign some function to the LC in stress or other situations in which it is activated, it is necessary to predict the outcome of LC activation on activity of its target neurons. Numerous studies have demonstrated that electrical stimulation of the LC or application of the neurotransmitter, norepinephrine, onto LC target neurons enhances responses of these neurons to other neurotransmitters or synaptic inputs.[67–70] These effects have been relatively consistent regardless of the target region studied or whether the effects of LC stimulation or norepinephrine application were studied. Based on these observations, LC activation by stressors would be predicted to bias target cell activity towards processing information about the stressor. If this occurred simultaneously in brain regions involved in autonomic, behavioral, and motor functions, the end result could be an enhancement of processes that would counteract the stressor or maintain homeostasis. Although this is an attractive hypothesis, several gaps in the experimental evidence upon which it is based must be filled. For example, although substantial evidence exists for LC activation by stressors, few studies have demonstrated that this results in sufficient norepinephrine release in LC terminal regions to affect target cell activity. This is particularly important because many of the stressors studied, as well as exogenously administered CRF, produce only a moderate increase in the LC spontaneous discharge rate (at most, twofold). A recent study that has addressed this issue demonstrated that i.c.v. administration of CRF in doses that activate the LC increased norepinephrine overflow in prefrontal cortex measured by microdialysis.[71]

To begin to determine possible functions of LC activation during stress, a measure of overall forebrain activation, the electrocorticoencephalogram (EEG),

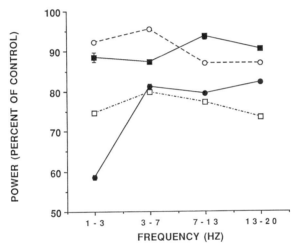

FIGURE 4. EEG activation elicited by hypotension stress is attenuated by local injection of clonidine or a CRF antagonist into the LC. The abscissa indicates frequency bands. The ordinate indicates the power in different frequency bands determined during nitroprusside infusion expressed as a percentage of the power determined in those frequency bands before administration of nitroprusside. Experiments were performed in halothane-anesthetized rats. Each point represents the mean determined in 10 rats administered nitroprusside only (*filled circles, solid line*), 5 rats injected bilaterally with clonidine (35–60 ng) directly into the LC (*open circles, dashed line*), 3 rats injected bilaterally with α-helical CRF$_{9-41}$ (100 ng) into the LC (*filled squares, solid line*), and 15 rats injected unilaterally (ipsilateral to the EEG recording electrode) with α-helical CRF$_{9-41}$ (*open squares, dotted line*). Nitroprusside decreased the power in all frequency bands, but had the greatest effect at lowest frequencies, indicative of increased EEG activity. Bilateral injection of clonidine inactivated the LC, prevented LC activation by nitroprusside, and prevented EEG activation by nitroprusside. Bilateral injection of α-helical CRF$_{9-41}$ prevented nitroprusside-induced LC activation and EEG activation. Unilateral injection of α-helical CRF$_{9-41}$ attenuated the decrease in the lowest frequency band produced by nitroprusside. Bars around symbols indicate mean ±1 SEM. Where not visible, the SEM bars lie within the symbols.

was used. Berridge and Foote[72] reported that selective LC activation in anesthetized rats with local injection of muscarinic agonists was associated with EEG activation recorded in the frontal cortex and hippocampus. Conversely, local selective inactivation of the LC by bilateral injections of clonidine decreased EEG frequency.[73] These studies suggested that LC discharge rates are closely linked to EEG measures and that enhanced levels of LC activity are sufficient to induce EEG activation. Consistent with these findings, LC activation in anesthetized rats during hemodynamic stress[56] or bladder distention[58] was also associated with EEG activation recorded from the frontal cortex and hippocampus. EEG activation during hemodynamic stress was prevented by bilateral inactivation of the LC with bilateral clonidine injection (FIG. 4). This injection prevented both LC and EEG activation by nitroprusside infusion. Bilateral injection of the CRF antagonist into the LC did not inactivate the LC, but did prevent LC activation by nitroprusside and also prevented EEG activation by nitroprusside (FIG. 4). These results raise several important points. First, they indicate that even the moderate increases in LC discharge (approximately 30%) associated with hemodynamic stress are sufficient to affect target cell activity. Second, they suggest that LC activation is necessary for the EEG activation associated with certain stressors. Finally, the results suggest that CRF may serve as a neurotransmitter in the LC during hemodynamic stress to increase or maintain arousal associated with this stressor. Interestingly, unilateral administration of α-helical CRF_{9-41} into the LC ipsilateral to the EEG recording electrodes attenuated, but did not completely prevent EEG activation associated with hemodynamic stress, suggesting that even the small percentage of LC axons that innervate the contralateral hemisphere may have an influence on cortical activity (FIG. 4).

Other findings suggest that even moderate increases in the LC discharge rate similar to those produced by CRF or physiologic challenges can have profound effects on tasks requiring focused attention.[74] For example, in monkeys trained to respond for juice after the presentation of an odd-ball (infrequent) stimulus, relatively small increases in the LC discharge rate (1 Hz) were associated with decreased fixation on visual stimuli and disruption of the task. Electrophysiologic findings suggest that increases in the LC discharge rate of this magnitude will also disrupt LC responses to phasic sensory stimuli, decreasing the signal-to-noise ratio.[49,50] It is possible that a behavioral consequence of this electrophysiologic effect of CRF is disruption of tasks requiring attention to selective short-duration stimuli. Thus, two consequences of CRF- or stress-elicited LC activation may be an increased level of arousal and decreased focused attention.

CLINICAL RELEVANCE OF CRF NEUROTRANSMISSION IN THE LOCUS COERULEUS

Recent neuroendocrine and clinical studies have led to the hypothesis that CRF may be hypersecreted in depression.[75-77] This is supported by findings of elevated CRF levels in the cerebrospinal fluid of depressed patients[78] and decreased CRF binding sites in the cortex of suicide victims.[79] Because CRF-IR fibers are found in biogenic amine nuclei, hypersecretion of CRF in these regions in depression could be the link between well-characterized neuroendocrine and biogenic amine abnormalities in this disease. Based on electrophysiologic findings,[48-50] increased CRF release in the LC would result in persistently elevated LC discharge rates and decreased responses to phasic sensory stimuli. This may be associated with the hyperarousal and inability to concentrate that is characteristic of certain depressions. If CRF effects on LC neurons are important in certain symptoms of depression, then antidepressants would be predicted to somehow interfere with CRF neurotransmission in the LC. The means by which antidepressants could achieve this end include: (1) pharmacologic antagonism of CRF in the LC; (2) functional or physiologic antagonism produced by effects on LC neurons that oppose those of CRF; or (3) attenuation of CRF release in the LC. To determine whether antidepressants could produce these effects the acute and chronic actions of four pharmacologically distinct antidepressants were investigated on the LC spontaneous discharge rate, LC sensory-evoked activity, LC activation by CRF, and LC activation by hemodynamic stress.[80–82] The four antidepressants included a norepinephrine reuptake inhibitor, desmethylimipramine; a serotonin reuptake inhibitor, sertraline; a monoamine oxidase inhibitor, phenelzine; and an atypical antidepressant, mianserin.

When acutely administered, the antidepressants had variable effects on LC spontaneous activity. Desmethylimipramine[80] and phenelzine[82] decreased the spontaneous discharge rate, mianserin[81] increased the discharge rate, and sertraline[80] had no effect. All drugs decreased the LC sensory-evoked discharge after acute administration, none altered LC activation by centrally administered CRF, and only mianserin decreased the LC discharge associated with hypotensive stress.[80–82] Because these drugs require chronic administration for clinical efficacy, their effects on the LC discharge after chronic administration are more relevant to the hypothesis. Chronic administration of either desmethylimipramine[80] or mianserin[81] greatly attenuated LC activation by hypotensive stress, but not by i.c.v. administered CRF. Because this activation requires CRF release in the LC, the results suggest that chronic administration of these antidepressants decreases stress-elicited CRF release in the LC and perhaps the hypersecretion of CRF that occurs in depression. In contrast, chronic administration of sertraline[80] and phenelzine[82] did not affect LC responses to hypotensive stress. However, these antidepressants altered LC responses to phasic sensory stimuli in a manner opposite to that of CRF after chronic administration, that is, they increased the signal-to-noise ratio of the LC sensory response.[80,82] The increased responsiveness of LC neurons in animals chronically administered sertraline or phenelzine may be sufficient to functionally antagonize effects of hypersecreted CRF on these neurons. Thus, four pharmacologically distinct antidepressants have the potential to interfere with CRF neurotransmission in the LC after chronic administration—desmethylimipramine and mianserin may attenuate CRF release, and sertraline and phenelzine may oppose the effects of CRF on LC neurons. Cocaine, a nonselective biogenic amine reuptake inhibitor that is not useful as an antidepressant, did not share any of these characteristics with the antidepressants after chronic administration.[82] These findings suggest that one common mechanism of antidepressant agents is to interfere with CRF neurotransmission in the LC, although the mechanism by which individual antidepressants acheive this end may differ.

SUMMARY

Anatomic and electrophysiologic studies have provided evidence that CRF meets some of the criteria as a neurotransmitter in the noradrenergic nucleus, the locus coeruleus (LC), although some of the criteria have yet to be satisfied. Thus, immunohistochemical findings suggest that CRF innervates the LC, but this must be confirmed at the ultrastructural level. CRF alters discharge activity of LC neurons and these effects are mimicked by some stressors. Moreover, the effects of hemodynamic stress on LC activity are prevented by a CRF antagonist. However, it has not been demonstrated that stimulation of CRF neurons that project to the LC activates the LC or that the effects of such stimulation are prevented by a CRF antagonist. The role of CRF in LC activation by stressors other than hemodynamic stress needs to be determined.

It could be predicted that the effects of CRF neurotransmission in the LC during stress would enhance information processing concerning the stressor or stimuli related to the stressor by LC target neurons. One consequence of this appears to be increased arousal. Although this may be adaptive in the response to an acute challenge, it could be predicted that chronic CRF release in the LC would result in persistently elevated LC discharge and norepinephrine release in targets. This could be associated with hyperarousal and loss of selective attention as occurs in certain psychiatric diseases. Manipulation of endogenous CRF systems may be a novel way in which to treat psychiatric diseases characterized by these maladaptive effects.

ACKNOWLEDGMENTS

The authors wish to thank Drs. Jean Rivier and Wylie Vale for generously providing CRF, α-helical CRF$_{9-41}$, and CRF antisera.

REFERENCES

1. VALE, W., J. SPIESS & C. RIVIER. 1981. Characterization of a 41-residue ovine hypothalamic peptide that stimulates secretion of corticotropin and beta-endorphin. Science 213: 1394–1397.
2. SWANSON, L. W., P. E. SAWCHENKO, J. RIVIER & W. VALE. 1983. Organization of ovine corticotropin-releasing factor immunoreactive cells and fibers in rat brain: An immunohistochemical study. Neuroendocrinology 36: 165–186.
3. SAKANAKA, M., T. SHIBASAKI & K. LEDERES. 1987. Corticotropin-releasing factor-like immunoreactivity in the rat brain as revealed by a modified cobalt-glucose oxide-diaminobenzidene method. J. Comp. Neurol. 260: 256–298.
4. CUMMINGS, S., R. ELDE, J. ELLS & A. LINDALL. 1983. Corticotropin-releasing factor immunoreactivity is widely distributed within the central nervous system of the rat: An immunohistochemical study. J. Neurosci. 3: 1355–1368.
5. BROWN, M. R. & L. A. FISHER. 1985. Corticotropin-releasing factor: Effects on the autonomic nervous systems and visceral systems. Fed. Proc. 44: 243–248.
6. FISHER, L. A., J. RIVIER, C. RIVIER, J. SPIESS, W. W. VALE & M. R. BROWN. 1982. Corticotropin-releasing factor (CRF): Central effects on mean arterial pressure and heart rate in rats. Endocrinology 110: 2222–2224.
7. TACHÉ, Y. & M. GUNION. 1985. Corticotropin-releasing factor: Central action to influence gastric secretion. Fed. Proc. 44: 255–258.
8. TACHÉ, Y., Y. GOTO, M. GUNION, W. VALE, J. RIVIER & M. BROWN. 1983. Inhibition of gastric acid secretion in rats by intracerebral injection of corticotropin-releasing factor (CRF). Science 222: 935–937.
9. SUTTON, R. E., G. F. KOOB, M. LEMOAL, J. RIVIER & W. VALE. 1982. Corticotropin-releasing factor produces behavioral activation in rats. Nature 297: 331–333.
10. BRITTON, D. R., G. F. KOOB, J. RIVIER & W. VALE. 1982. Intraventricular corticotropin-releasing factor enhances behavioral effects of novelty. Life Sci. 31: 363–367.
11. BRITTON, K., J. MORGAN, J. RIVIER, W. VALE & G. KOOB. 1985. Chlordiazepoxide attenuates CRF-induced response suppression in the conflict test. Psychopharmacology 86: 170–174.
12. KALIN, N. H. 1985. Behavioral effects of ovine corticotropin-releasing factor administered to rhesus monkeys. Fed. Proc. 44: 249–254.
13. EAVES, M., K. THATCHER-BRITTON, J. RIVIER, W. VALE & G. KOOB. 1985. Effects of

corticotropin-releasing factor on locomotor activity in hypophysectomized rats. Peptides **6:** 923–926.

14. FISHER, L. A., G. JESSEN & M. BROWN. 1983. Corticotropin-releasing factor (CRF): Mechanism to elevate mean arterial pressure and heart rate. Regul. Pept. **5:** 153–161.

15. RIVIER, J., C. RIVIER & W. VALE. 1984. Synthetic competitive antagonists of corticotropin releasing factor: Effect on ACTH secretion in the rat. Science **224:** 889–891.

16. BROWN, M. R., L. A. FISHER, V. WEBB, W. VALE & J. RIVIER. 1985. Corticotropin-releasing factor: A physiologic regulator of adrenal epinephrine secretion. Brain Res. **328:** 355–357.

17. STEPHENS, R. L., JR., H. YANG, J. RIVIER & Y. TACHÉ. 1988. Intracisternal injection of CRF antagonist blocks surgical stress-induced inhibition of gastric secretion in the rat. Peptides **9:** 1067–1070.

18. LENZ, H. J., A. RAEDLER, H. GETEN, W. VALE & J. RIVIER. 1988. Stress-induced gastrointestinal secretory and motor responses in rats are mediated by endogenous corticotropin-releasing factor. Gastroenterology **95:** 1510–1517.

19. TAZI, A., R. DANTZER, M. LEMOAL, J. RIVIER, W. VALE & G. F. KOOB. 1987. Corticotropin-releasing factor antagonist blocks stress-induced fighting in rats. Regul. Pept. **18:** 37–42.

20. KALIN, N. H., J. E. SHERMAN & L. K. TAKAHASHI. 1988. Antagonism of endogenous corticotropin-releasing hormone systems attenuates stress-induced freezing behaviors in rats. Brain Res. **457:** 130–135.

21. BRITTON, K. T., G. LEE, W. VALE, J. RIVIER & G. F. KOOB. 1986. Corticotropin-releasing factor (CRF) receptor antagonist blocks activating and "anxiogenic" actions of CRF in the rat. Brain Res. **369:** 303–306.

22. KORF, J., G. K. AGHAJANIAN & R. ROTH. 1973. Increased turnover of norepinephrine in the rat cerebral cortex during stress: Role of the locus coeruleus. Neuropharmacology **12:** 933–938.

23. CASSENS, G., G. ROFFMAN, A. KURUC, P. J. ORSULAK & J. J. SCHILDKRAUT. 1980. Alterations in brain norepinephrine metabolism induced by environmental stimuli previously paired with inescapable shock. Science **209:** 1138–1139.

24. THIERRY, A.-M., F. JAVOY, J. GLOWINSKI & S. S. KETY. 1968. Effects of stress on the metabolism of norepinephrine, dopamine and serotonin in the central nervous system of the rat: Modification of norpinephrine turnover. J. Pharmacol. Exp. Ther. **163:** 163–171.

25. ABERCROMBIE, E. D., R. W. KELLER & M. J. ZIGMOND. 1988. Characterization of hippocampal norepinephrine release as measured by microdialysis perfusion: Pharmacological and behavioral studies. Neuroscience **27:** 897–904.

26. MELIA, K. R. & R. S. DUMAN. 1991. Involvement of corticotropin-releasing factor in chronic stress regulation of the brain noradrenergic system. Proc. Natl. Acad. Sci. USA **88:** 8382–8386.

27. CEDARBAUM, J. M. & G. K. AGHAJANIAN. 1978. Activation of locus coeruleus neurons by peripheral stimuli: Modulation by a collateral inhibitory mechanism. Life Sci. **23:** 1383–1392.

28. ELAM, M., T. YAO, T. H. SVENSSON & P. THOREN. 1984. Regulation of locus coeruleus neurons and splanchnic, sympathetic nerves. Brain Res. **290:** 281–287.

29. ELAM, M., T. YAO, P. THOREN & T. H. SVENSSON. 1981. Hypercapnia and hypoxia: Chemoreceptor-mediated control of locus coeruleus neurons and splanchnic, sympathetic nerves. Brain Res. **222:** 373–381.

30. SVENSSON, T. H. 1987. Peripheral, autonomic regulation of locus coeruleus noradrenergic neurons in brain: Putative implications for psychiatry and psychopharmacology. Psychopharmacology **92:** 1–7.

31. ABERCROMBIE, E. D. & B. L. JACOBS. 1987. Single unit response of noradrenergic neurons in locus coeruleus of freely moving cats. I. Acutely presented stressful and nonstressful stimuli. J. Neurosci. **7:** 2837–2843.

32. ABERCROMBIE, E. D. & B. L. JACOBS. 1987. Single unit response of noradrenergic neurons in locus coeruleus of freely moving cats. II. Adaptation to chronically presented stressful stimuli. J. Neurosci. **7:** 2844–2848.

33. MORILAK, D. A., C. FORNAL & B. L. JACOBS. 1987. Effects of physiological manipulations

on locus coeruleus neuronal activity in freely moving cats. II. Glucoregulatory challenge. Brain Res. **422:** 17–23.

34. MORILAK, D. A., C. FORNAL & B. L. JACOBS. 1987. Effects of physiological manipulations on locus coeruleus neuronal activity in freely moving cats. I. Thermoregulatory challenge. Brain Res. **422:** 17–23.

35. ENNIS, M. & G. ASTON-JONES. 1988. Activation of locus coeruleus from nucleus paragigantocellularis: A new excitatory amino acid pathway in brain. J. Neurosci. **8:** 3644–3657.

36. ENNIS, M. & G. ASTON-JONES. 1986. A potent excitatory input to the nucleus locus coeruleus from the ventrolateral medulla. Neurosci. Lett. **71:** 299–305.

37. ALBANESE, A. & L. L. BUTCHER. 1980. Acetylcholinesterase and catecholamine distribution in the locus coeruleus of the rat. Brain Res. Bull. **5:** 127–134.

38. PICKEL, V. M., T. H. JOH & D. J. REIS. 1977. A serotonergic innervation of noradrenergic neurons in nucleus locus coeruleus: Demonstration by immunocytochemical localization of transmitter specific enzymes tyrosine and tryptophan hydroxylase. Brain Res. **131:** 197–214.

39. LJUNGDAHL, A., T. HOKFELT & G. NILSSON. 1978. Distribution of substance P-like immunoreactivity in the central nervous system of the rat. I. Cell bodies and nerve terminals. Neuroscience **3:** 861–943.

40. DROLET, G., E. J. VAN BOCKSTAELE & G. ASTON-JONES. 1992. Robust enkephalin innervation of the locus coeruleus from the rostral medulla. J. Neurosci. **12:** 3162–3174.

41. VALENTINO, R. J., M. PAGE, E. VAN BOCKSTAELE & G. ASTON-JONES. 1992. Corticotropin releasing factor innervation of the locus coeruleus region: Distribution of fibers and sources of input. Neuroscience **48:** 689–705.

42. FOOTE, S. L. & C. I. CHA. 1988. Distribution of corticotropin-releasing factor-like immunoreactivity in brainstem of two monkey species (*Saimiri sciureus* and *Macaca fascicularis*): An immunohistochemical study. J. Comp. Neurol. **276:** 239–264.

43. PAMMER, C., T. GORCS & M. PALKOVITS. 1990. Peptidergic innervation of the locus coeruleus cells in the human brain. Brain Res. **515:** 247–255.

44. ASTON-JONES, G., M. ENNIS, V. A. PIERIBONE, W. T. NICKELL & M. T. SHIPLEY. 1986. The brain nucleus locus coeruleus: Restricted afferent control of a broad efferent network. Science **234:** 734–737.

45. CHAPPELL, P. B., M. A. SMITH, C. D. KILTS, G. BISSETTE, J. RITCHIE, C. ANDERSON & C. B. NEMEROFF. 1986. Alterations in corticotropin-releasing factor-like immunoreactivity in discrete rat brain regions after acute and chronic stress. J. Neurosci. **6:** 2908–2914.

46. IMAKI, T., J.-L. NAHON, C. RIVIER, P. E. SAWCHENKO & W. VALE. 1991. Differential regulation of corticotropin-releasing factor mRNA in rat brain regions by glucocorticoids and stress. J. Neurosci. **11:** 585–599.

47. DESOUZA, E. B. 1987. Corticotropin-releasing factor receptors in the rat central nervous system: Characterization and regional distribution. J. Neurosci. **7:** 88–100.

48. VALENTINO, R. J., S. L. FOOTE & G. ASTON-JONES. 1983. Corticotropin-releasing factor activates noradrenergic neurons of the locus coeruleus. Brain Res. **270:** 363–367.

49. VALENTINO, R. & S. L. FOOTE. 1987. Corticotropin-releasing factor disrupts sensory responses of brain noradrenergic neurons. Neuroendocrinology **45:** 28–36.

50. VALENTINO, R. & S. L. FOOTE. 1988. Corticotropin-releasing hormone increases tonic but not sensory-evoked activity of noradrenergic locus coeruleus neurons in unanesthetized rats. J. Neurosci. **8:** 1016–1025.

51. LIANG, K. C., K. R. MELIA, M. J. D. MISERENDINO, W. A. FALLS, S. CAMPEAU & M. DAVIS. 1992. Corticotropin-releasing factor: Long-lasting facilitation of the acoustic startle reflex. J. Neurosci. **12:** 2303–2312.

52. FOOTE, S. L., F. E. BLOOM & G. ASTON-JONES. 1983. Nucleus locus coeruleus: New evidence of anatomical and physiological specificity. Physiol. Rev. **63:** 844–914.

53. PLOTSKY, P. M. 1987. Facilitation of immunoreactive corticotropin-releasing factor secretion into the hypophysial-portal circulation after activation of catecholaminergic pathways or central norepinephrine injection. Endocrinology **121:** 924–930.

54. VALENTINO, R. J. & R. G. WEHBY. 1988. Corticotropin-releasing factor: Evidence for a neurotransmitter role in the locus coeruleus during hemodynamic stress. Neuroendocrinology **48:** 674–677.

55. Curtis, A. L., G. Drolet & R. J. Valentino. 1993. Hemodynamic stress activates locus coeruleus neurons of unanesthetized rats. Brain Res. Bull. **31:** 737–744.
56. Valentino, R. J., M. E. Page & A. L. Curtis. 1991. Activation of noradrenergic locus coeruleus neurons by hemodynamic stress is due to local release of corticotropin-releasing factor. Brain Res. **555:** 25–34.
57. Plotsky, P. M. & W. Vale. 1984. Hemorrhage-induced secretion of corticotropin-releasing factor-like immunoreactivity into the rat hypophysial portal circulation and its inhibition by glucocorticoids. Endocrinology **114:** 164–170.
58. Page, M. E., H. Akaoka, G. Aston-Jones & R. J. Valentino. 1992. Bladder distention activates noradrenergic locus coeruleus neurons by an excitatory amino acid mechanism. Neuroscience **51:** 555–563.
59. Barrington, F. J. T. 1925. The effect of lesion of the hind- and mid-brain on micturition in the cat. Q. J. Exp. Physiol. **15:** 81–102.
60. Swanson, L. W. & B. K. Hartman. 1976. The central adrenergic system. An immunofluorescence study of the location of cell bodies and their efferent connections in the rat using dopamine-β-hydroxylase as a marker. J. Comp. Neurol. **163:** 467–506.
61. Grzanna, R. & M. E. Molliver. 1980. The locus coeruleus in the rat: An immunohistochemical delineation. Neuroscience **5:** 21–40.
62. Nestler, E. J. 1992. Molecular mechanisms of drug addiction. J. Neurosci. **12:** 2439–2450.
63. Redmond, D. E., Jr. & Y. H. Huang. 1979. Current concepts. 2. New evidence for a locus coeruleus-norepinephrine connection with anxiety. Life Sci. **25:** 2149–2162.
64. Aston-Jones, G. & F. E. Bloom. 1981. Activity of norepinephrine-containing locus coeruleus neurons in behaving rats anticipates fluctuations in the sleep-waking cycle. J. Neurosci. **1:** 876–886.
65. Foote, S. L., G. Aston-Jones & F. E. Bloom. 1980. Impulse activity of locus coeruleus neurons in awake rats and monkeys is a function of sensory stimulation and arousal. Proc. Natl. Acad. Sci. USA **77:** 3033–3037.
66. Aston-Jones, G. & F. E. Bloom. 1981. Norepinephrine-containing locus coeruleus neurons in behaving rats exhibit pronounced responses to non-noxious environmental stimuli. J. Neurosci. **1:** 887–900.
67. Waterhouse, B. D., H. C. Moises & D. J. Woodward. 1980. Noradrenergic modulation of somatosensory cortical neuronal responses to iontophoretically applied putative neurotransmitters. Exp. Neurol. **69:** 30–49.
68. Moises, H. C., B. D. Waterhouse & D. J. Woodward. 1981. Locus coeruleus stimulation potentiates Purkinje cell responses to afferent input: The climbing fiber system. Brain Res. **222:** 42–64.
69. Segal, M. & F. E. Bloom. 1976. The action of norepinephrine in the rat hippocampus. III. Hippocampal cellular responses to locus coeruleus stimulation in the awake rat. Brain Res. **107:** 499–511.
70. Moises, H. C., D. J. Woodward & B. J. Hoffer. 1979. Interaction of norepinephrine with cerebellar activity evoked by mossy and climbing fibers. Exp. Neurol. **64:** 493–515.
71. Lavicky, J. & A. Dunn. Corticotropin-releasing factor stimulates catecholamine release in hypothalamus and prefrontal cortex in freely moving rats as assessed by microdialysis. J. Neurochem. In press.
72. Berridge, C. W. & S. L. Foote. 1991. Effects of locus coerulues activation on electroencephalographic activity in the neocortex and hippocampus. J. Neurosci. **11:** 3135–3145.
73. Foote, S. L., M. E. Page, C. W. Berridge & R. J. Valentino. 1990. Effects of locus coeruleus inactivation on electroencephalographic (EEG) activity in neocortex and hippocampus. Soc. Neurosci. **16:** 1177.
74. Rajkowski, J., P. Kubiak & G. Aston-Jones. 1992. Activity of locus coeruleus (LC) neurons in behaving monkeys varies with changes in focused attention. Soc. Neurosci. Abstr. **18:** 538.
75. Lesch, K.-P., G. Laux, H. M. Schulte, H. Pfuller & H. Beckmann. 1988. Corticotropin and cortisol response to human CRH as a probe for HPA system integrity in major depressive disorder. Psychiatry Res. **24:** 25–34.
76. Gold, P. W., D. L. Loriaux, A. Roy, M. A. Kling, J. R. Calabrese, C. H. Kellner, L. K. Nieman, R. M. Post, D. Pickar, W. Gallucci, P. Avgerinos, S. Paul, E. H.

OLDFIELD, G. B. CUTLER, JR. & P. G. CHROUSOS. 1986. Responses to corticotropin-releasing hormone in the hypercortisolism of depression and Cushing's disease. N. Engl. J. Med. **314:** 1329–1342.

77. GOLD, P. W., F. K. GOODWIN & G. P. CHROUSOS. 1988. Clinical and biochemical manifestations of depression. N. Engl. J. Med. **319:** 413–420.

78. NEMEROFF, C. B., E. WIDERLOV, G. BISSETTE, H. WALLEUS, I. KARLSSON, K. EKLUND, C. D. KILTS, P. T. LOOSEN & W. VALE. 1984. Elevated concentrations of CSF corticotropin-releasing factor-like immunoreactivity in depressed patients. Science **226:** 1342–1344.

79. NEMEROFF, C. B., M. J. OWENS, G. BISSETTE, A. C. ANDORN & M. STANLEY. 1988. Reduced corticotropin releasing factor binding sites in the frontal cortex of suicide victims. Arch. Gen. Psychiatry **45:** 577–579.

80. VALENTINO, R., A. L. CURTIS, D. G. PARRIS & R. G. WEHBY. 1990. Antidepressant actions on brain noradrenergic neurons. J. Pharmacol. Exp. Ther. **253:** 833–840.

81. CURTIS, A. L. & R. VALENTINO. 1991. Acute and chronic effects of the atypical antidepressant, mianserin, on brain noradrenergic neurons. Psychopharmacology **103:** 330–338.

82. VALENTINO, R. & A. L. CURTIS. 1991. Antidepressant interactions with corticotropin-releasing factor in the noradrenergic nucleus locus coeruleus. Psychopharmacol. Bull. **27:** 263–269.

Role of Cytokines
in Infection-Induced Stress[a]

ADRIAN J. DUNN

Department of Pharmacology and Therapeutics
Louisiana State University Medical Center
P.O. Box 33932
Shreveport, Louisiana 71130-3932

Common experience suggests that infections can be stressful. It has been known for some time that infections are associated with activation of the hypothalamo-pituitary-adrenocortical (HPA) axis. In the 1950s it was shown that elevations of circulating glucocorticoids were associated with stimulation by endotoxin.[1] In 1969, Beisel and Rapoport reported that injection of mice with a large dose of *E. coli* caused a progressive increase in plasma corticosterone.[2] Such a treatment was considered to be stressful and therefore it was not surprising to observe activation of the HPA axis, which had by then been closely associated with stress. However, the mechanism was entirely unknown. The important clues derived from the work of Besedovsky in the early 1980s. Besedovsky showed that, when injected into rats, the supernatants of lymphocytes incubated *in vitro* with concanavalin A caused increases in plasma corticosterone. Similar data were later obtained with Newcastle disease virus (NDV).[3] Because the factor in the lymphocyte supernatants was heat labile, it was suspected to be a protein and attention was focused on the cytokines, chemical messengers secreted by lymphocytes. In a landmark paper, Besedovsky *et al.* injected recombinant human interleukin-1β (IL-1β) into mice and found that it caused increases in circulating concentrations of ACTH and corticosterone.[4] Thus it was suggested that IL-1 was the factor mediating the activation of the HPA axis. This suggestion was strengthened by the observation that treatment of the supernatants of stimulated cultured lymphocytes with an antibody to IL-1 could prevent the elevations of plasma corticosterone.[4] This paper will focus on our studies on the mechanism(s) by which the HPA axis is activated by immune stimuli.

Besedovsky had also made observations suggesting that hypothalamic norepinephrine (NE) metabolism was altered after immunization with sheep red blood cells.[5] We chose to study this further using HPLC with electrochemical detection to determine concentrations of catecholamines, indoleamines, and related compounds at various times after infection of mice with influenza virus.[6] Normally mice will succumb to the infection in 6–7 days. FIGURE 1 shows certain neurochemical and endocrine responses to this treatment. There was a progressive increase in the plasma concentrations of corticosterone following infection. No such changes were observed in the saline-infused mice. In parallel with the changes in plasma corticosterone were increases of 3-methoxy,4-hydroxyphenylethyleneglycol (MHPG), the major catabolite of NE, suggesting that increased quantities of this neurotransmitter were released. These changes are best expressed as MHPG:NE ratios which compensate for small variations in the dissection procedures, although the major changes were in MHPG. No consistent changes were observed in dopamine metabolism. The

[a]This research was supported by grants from the Office of Naval Research (N0001-4-85K-0300) and the National Institute of Mental Health (MH46261).

189

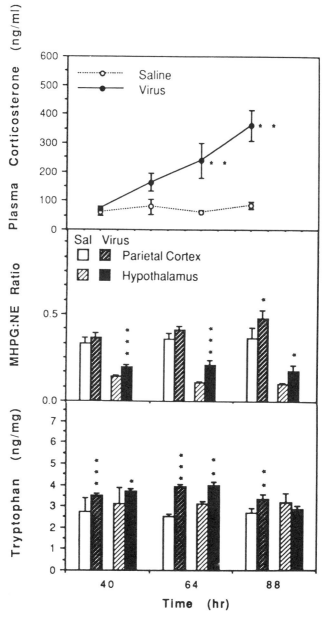

FIGURE 1. The effect of influenza virus infection on plasma corticosterone (*top panel*), brain norepinephrine (NE) metabolism (*middle panel*), and tryptophan (*lower panel*). Mice were lightly anesthetized and infused in the trachea with influenza virus (PR-8) or saline. Virus infection was verified in each animal by recovery of virus from the lungs. Plasma concentrations of corticosterone were determined by radioimmunoassay, and brain concentrations of MHPG, NE, and tryptophan were determined by HPLC. Asterisks indicate statistically significant differences between virus- and saline-infused mice. Data are from ref. 6.

changes in NE metabolism were greatest in the hypothalamus; similar changes in other brain regions were smaller, and not statistically significant until later times (FIG. 1). Free tryptophan was also increased, but, unlike the changes in MHPG, the increases in tryptophan were not regionally specific (FIG. 1).

We then studied IL-1 to determine whether the IL-1-induced activation of the HPA axis[4] was accompanied by neurochemical changes similar to those observed during influenza virus infection. Intraperitoneal (i.p.) injection of human IL-1α or -β caused a dose-dependent increase in plasma corticosterone, with statistical significance normally occurring with 4–10 ng. In parallel with this endocrine effect were dose-dependent increases in MHPG:NE ratios, and in tryptophan (FIG. 2). As in the influenza virus-infected mice, the proportional increase in MHPG was greatest in the hypothalamus; however, that for tryptophan was not regionally specific. Moreover, there were no significant changes in dopamine metabolism as indicated by concentrations of dopamine, 3,4-dihydroxyphenylacetic acid (DOPAC) or homovanillic acid (HVA). 5-hydroxyindoleacetic acid (5-HIAA) concentrations were increased in a pattern similar to that of tryptophan. Similar data were obtained with IL-1α, although only one dose was included in this particular experiment. Thus the pattern of the response to IL-1α or IL-1β was remarkably similar to that observed during influenza virus infection. The close parallel between the HPA activation and the changes in hypothalamic NE metabolism, coupled with the known involvement of NE in the regulation of corticotropin-releasing factor (CRF) secretion,[7] suggested that hypothalamic NE might be instrumental in the activation of the HPA axis.

Our working hypothesis (FIG. 3) is based on that proposed by Besedovsky et al.[4] T cells present the antigen to macrophages, resulting in the synthesis and secretion of IL-1. Then in some way not yet defined, the IL-1 activates the noradrenergic projections to the paraventricular nucleus (PVN) of the hypothalamus, causing activation of the CRF-containing neurons, resulting in secretion of CRF into the portal blood in the hypothalamic median eminence. The CRF is carried in the portal vessels to the anterior pituitary gland where it stimulates the secretion of ACTH, which ultimately stimulates the adrenal cortex to release glucocorticosteroids. The glucocorticosteroids provide negative feedback to the immune system, limiting the production of IL-1 and probably other cytokines.[4]

THE SITE OF ACTION OF IL-1

The site of action of IL-1 to increase plasma corticosterone has been controversial. Theoretically, IL-1 could act directly on the adrenal cortex, the pituitary, the hypothalamus, or any site connected to these structures. The literature contains evidence for each of these possibilities.

Adrenal Cortex

Although the increase of plasma ACTH in parallel with that in corticosterone suggests that the changes in corticosterone depend upon ACTH secretion (ref. 4 and others), several studies have suggested a direct adrenocortical action of IL-1.[8–10] However, several other studies have failed to find any effect of IL-1 on adrenal corticosterone secretion.[11 13] In each of the positive studies, the doses of IL-1 have been very high, and, in most, the tissues were preincubated for long periods of time in vitro.[9,10] Endocrinologists know well that such nonphysiological treatments can

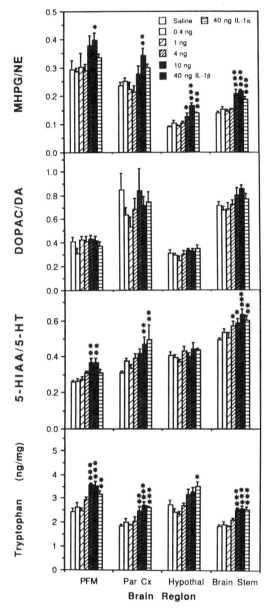

FIGURE 2. The effect of administration of IL-1 on brain catecholamines and tryptophan. Mice were injected intraperitoneally with recombinant human IL-1β (0, 0.4, 1, 4, 10, and 40 ng) or IL-1α (40 ng). Concentrations of MHPG, NE, DOPAC, DA, 5-HIAA, 5-HT, and tryptophan in medial prefrontal cortex (PFM), parietal cortex (Par Cx), hypothalamus (Hypothal), and brain stem were determined 2 hours later. Asterisks indicate statistically significant differences from the saline (zero IL-1β) group. Data from ref. 25.

change the sensitivity of tissues to secretagogues. Definitive evidence can only be derived *in vivo*. FIGURE 4 shows that hypophysectomized mice that have been rigorously tested for the completeness of the removal of the corticotropic tissue from the sella tursica showed no significant changes in plasma corticosterone after either intravenous (i.v.) or i.p. administration of IL-1. These results agree with those of

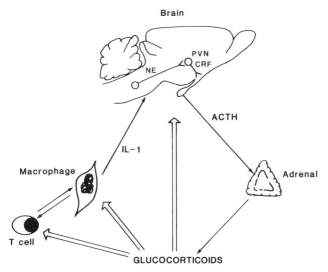

FIGURE 3. Schematic diagram of the working hypothesis for the activation of the HPA axis by IL-1.

other studies in rats.[11,14] They suggest strongly that the pituitary is required for the adrenocortical response of adult mice to IL-1 injected by either route. They also indicate that any direct adrenocortical effect of IL-1 is insignificant in adult male mice. Similar results were obtained after injection of either NDV or lipopolysaccha-

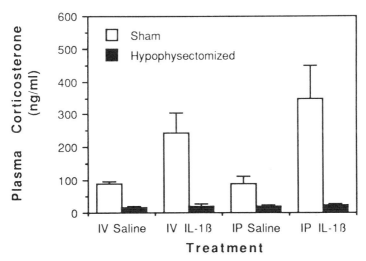

FIGURE 4. The effect of hypophysectomy on the plasma corticosterone response to IL-1. Recombinant human IL-1β (100 ng) was injected i.v. or i.p. and plasma corticosterone determined 45 minutes (i.v.) or 2 hours (i.p.) later. IL-1 significantly elevated plasma corticosterone in sham-operated mice, but no significant changes occurred in hypophysectomized mice.

ride (LPS); both resulted in a substantial increase in plasma corticosterone, whereas no such increase was observed in the hypophysectomized animals. The increase in hypothalamic MHPG that occurred after administration of IL-1, NDV or LPS was not prevented by hypophysectomy (data not shown). Interestingly, animals that had been operated upon to remove the pituitary but were removed from the hypophysectomized group because they showed an increase in plasma corticosterone after

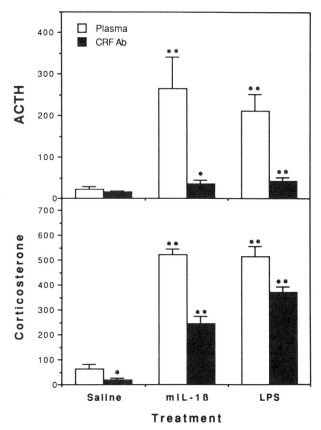

FIGURE 5. The effect of CRF antibody on plasma ACTH and corticosterone responses IL-1 and LPS. Mice were injected i.p. with 0.25 mL of CRF antibody or sheep plasma 1 hour before saline, murine IL-1β (mIL-1β: 100 ng), or LPS (5 μg). Plasma ACTH and corticosterone were elevated by both treatments in mice pretreated with sheep plasma or CRF antibody, but the latter significantly attenuated both responses to mIL-1β or LPS.

restraint (suggesting that the hypophysectomy was incomplete) frequently exhibited responses to IL-1, NDV, and LPS.

Pituitary

Following an initial report,[15] several laboratories have reported direct pituitary effects of IL-1 on ACTH secretion, whereas several others have not (see review, ref.

16). However, these *in vitro* studies are subject to the same kind of artifacts discussed above for adrenocortical tissue. Almost all of the positive studies used substantial periods of preincubation of the tissue. Several reports noted that the ACTH-secreting activity of IL-1 only appeared as the preincubation time was prolonged.[17,18] *In vivo* CRF appears to be required for the IL-1-induced secretion of ACTH. Sapolsky *et al.*[19] reported that IL-1 increased the concentrations of CRF in portal blood, and three groups found that pretreatment of rats with an antibody to CRF attenuated or prevented the ACTH or corticosterone response to IL-1.[19–21] We have now examined this in mice. In mice injected with CRF antibody one hour before injection with IL-1 or LPS, the ACTH and corticosterone responses were markedly attenuated (FIG. 5), but the MHPG response was not affected (data not shown). The residual response after CRF antibody pretreatment may have occurred because of incomplete neutralization of endogenous CRF, but it may also be because of peripheral release of catecholamines, which are known to stimulate ACTH release from the pituitary in rodents.[22]

Hypothalamus

Rivest and Rivier[23] initially showed that lesions of the PVN attenuated the HPA responses to IL-1. This suggests that this hypothalamic nucleus is necessary for the response to IL-1 and is consistent with the involvement of CRF. We have observed an almost perfect correlation between the increases in hypothalamic MHPG and those of plasma ACTH and corticosterone in a large number of studies. This led us to speculate that noradrenergic projections to the hypothalamus may be instrumental in the IL-1-induced stimulation of the HPA axis. To test this we used 6-hydroxydopamine (6-OHDA) to lesion the noradrenergic projections in the ventral noradrenergic ascending bundle (VNAB), known to be the main noradrenergic projection to the hypothalamus and the PVN in particular.[24] When these rats were challenged i.p. with IL-1, animals that exhibited depletions of PVN norepinephrine greater than 75% showed a markedly diminished increase in plasma corticosterone (FIG. 6). The same rats showed increases in plasma corticosterone to restraint that were indistinguishable from unlesioned rats. These results suggest that the noradrenergic innervation of the PVN is instrumental in the HPA response to i.p. IL-1 in the rat.

CYTOKINE MEDIATION OF CEREBRAL RESPONSES

Our next step was to study the involvement of cytokines and, specifically, IL-1 in the response to immune stimuli. We first chose to study LPS because it is known to be a robust stimulator of the HPA axis, and also stimulates cerebral catecholamine metabolism.[25] Furthermore, it is well known to stimulate the synthesis and secretion of IL-1,[26] and we have verified that LPS injection resulted in detectable concentrations of bioassayable IL-1. To test the involvement of IL-1 in the activation of the HPA axis and cerebral catecholamine metabolism by LPS, we used the IL-1-receptor antagonist protein (IRAP). FIGURE 7 shows the results of an experiment in which IRAP was injected 10 minutes before IL-1 or LPS.[27] IRAP markedly attenuated the increase in plasma corticosterone to IL-1β; however, the response to injection of LPS was not altered. The plasma ACTH and hypothalamic MHPG data paralleled the corticosterone results. These results suggest that IL-1 does not mediate the HPA and neurochemical responses to LPS. However, because we know that LPS induces IL-1 synthesis and secretion and that IL-1 will stimulate these responses, it is most likely that more than one pathway exists by which LPS can activate the HPA axis.

LPS has also been shown to stimulate the synthesis and secretion of tumor necrosis factor-α (TNF-α), and some evidence exists that TNF-α can activate the HPA axis, although it is considerably less potent in this respect than IL-1.[4,27,28] Therefore, we tested the ability of an antibody to murine TNF-α to alter the responses to LPS. FIGURE 8 shows that neither the TNF-α antibody nor the antibody in combination with IRAP was able to alter the HPA or neurochemical responses to LPS.[27] However, when pretreatment with IRAP was tested against NDV, IRAP was able to reverse the effects on plasma corticosterone in a majority of the mice (FIG. 9).

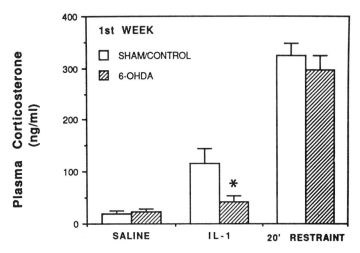

FIGURE 6. Effect of 6-hydroxydopamine (6-OHDA) lesions of the ventral noradrenergic ascending bundle (VNAB) on the plasma corticosterone response to IL-1. Rats were lesioned stereotaxically with a direct infusion of 6-OHDA into the VNAB. Five days later they were injected i.p. with saline, the next day with 0.5 μg recombinant human IL-1α, and the next day restrained for 20 minutes. Tail blood was collected for plasma corticosterone determination 2 hours after saline or IL-1, and directly after restraint. The response to IL-1 was significantly attenuated in VNAB-lesioned animals that showed depletions of PVN norepinephrine > 75%. Data from ref. 24.

BEHAVIORAL ACTIVITY OF IL-1

If cytokines can mediate the endocrine and neurochemical responses that occur during sickness, is it possible that they also mediate the behavioral effects? To test this, we examined the effects of IL-1 on two different behaviors that we had previously shown to be sensitive to restraint. Rats placed in a small enclosed chamber placed in an open field typically remain inside the chamber when they are unfamiliar with the behavioral apparatus, and reenter rapidly if they do emerge. After multiple exposures to the apparatus, the rats emerge rapidly and freely explore the open field. A brief period of restraint will cause them to behave like naive animals and to retreat into the chamber.[29] IL-1 injected intracerebroventricularly (i.c.v.) mimicked the effect of restraint (FIG. 10). In mice, investigation of novel objects in the multicompartment chamber is decreased by restraint or the i.c.v. injection of CRF.[30] There-

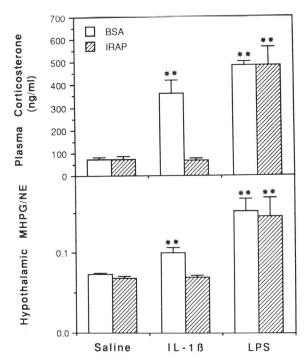

FIGURE 7. The effect of the IL-1-receptor antagonist protein (IRAP) on plasma corticosterone and hypothalamic MHPG/NE responses to IL-1β and LPS. Mice were injected i.p. with bovine serum albumin (BSA) or 10 μg IRAP immediately before 40 ng recombinant human IL-1β or 5 μg LPS. Plasma and brain samples were collected 2 hours later. Asterisks indicate statistically significant differences from saline ($p < 0.01$). Data from ref. 27.

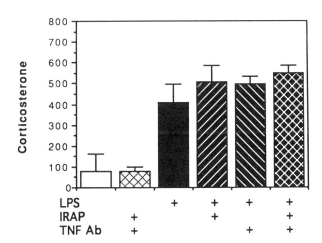

FIGURE 8. The effect of IRAP and TNF antibody on the plasma corticosterone response to LPS. Mice were pretreated i.p. with 0.05 mL antibody to murine TNF-α and 1 hour later injected with 10 μg of IRAP and/or 5 μg LPS. Plasma corticosterone was measured 2 hours later. Results from all LPS-treated groups were significantly higher than those in either control group. Data from ref. 27.

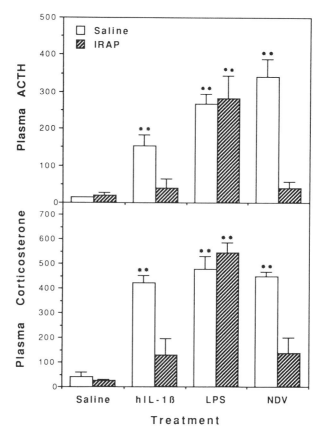

FIGURE 9. The effect of IRAP on the plasma ACTH and corticosterone responses to IL-1, LPS, and Newcastle disease virus (NDV). Mice were pretreated with 10 μg IRAP and then challenged with recombinant human IL-1β (100 ng), LPS (5 μg) or NDV (1000 hemagglutination units). Plasma ACTH and corticosterone were determined from blood samples collected 2 hours later. Asterisks indicate statistically significant differences from saline-treated mice ($p < 0.01$).

fore, we tested the ability of IL-1 to induce similar effects. Intraperitoneal doses of IL-1β as low as 1 ng were able to induce a reduction of investigatory behavior mimicking the effects of stress or CRF.[31] IL-1α or -β was also effective when administered i.c.v., in which case doses as low as 1 pg (about one-twentieth of a femtomole) were active.[32] To test whether the effect of IL-1 was mediated by CRF, we used the synthetic CRF antagonist, α-helical CRF[9–41]. This antagonist attenuated the effect of either i.c.v. IL-1[32] or i.p. IL-1.[31] These results suggest not only that IL-1 can elicit behaviors characteristic of stress, but that they may be mediated by cerebral CRF, just as we believe the responses to physical stressors are.[33,34] Thus our data complement those of other investigators indicating that IL-1 can elicit a number of behavioral responses characteristic of sickness, such as fever,[35] anorexia,[36] decreased locomotor activity,[37] and increased sleep.[38]

CONCLUSIONS

We have shown that, in common with physical and behavioral stressors, infections and other stimulators of the immune system can activate the HPA axis and cerebral catecholamine and indoleamine metabolism. These responses can be mimicked by administration of the cytokine, interleukin-1 (IL-1). The HPA response requires the pituitary and activation of hypothalamic CRF, probably via noradrenergic projections from the brain stem. IL-1 appears to mediate the neurochemical and endocrine responses to stimulation by Newcastle disease virus. It can also induce behavioral effects characteristic of sickness. All this suggests that IL-1 may be an

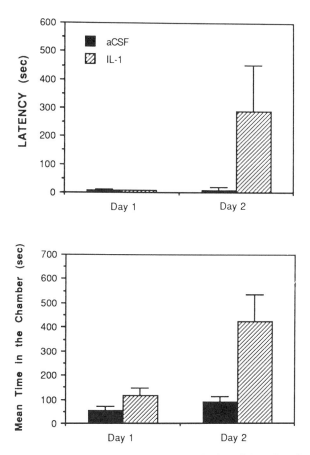

FIGURE 10. Defensive withdrawal of rats after i.c.v. injection of IL-1. Rats implanted with intracerebroventricular cannulae were thoroughly habituated to the behavioral apparatus and injected with saline (day 1), or saline or IL-1 (40 ng hIL-1α, day 2). Rats injected with IL-1 on day 2 showed a significantly elevated latency to exit from the enclosed chamber (*top*) and spent significantly more time in the chamber (i.e., a stress-like effect) than did saline-injected rats (*bottom*).

important mediator of endocrine, physiological, neurochemical, and behavioral responses during sickness. However, it is likely that other cytokines synthesized and secreted following immune stimulation (e.g., TNF-α, IL-6, and others not yet identified) may also participate in these responses.

ACKNOWLEDGEMENTS

We are grateful to Dr. P. Lomedico of Hoffmann-La Roche for the gift of recombinant human IL-1α; Dr. Y. Hirai of Otsuka Pharmaceutical Co. for recombinant human IL-1β; Dr. E. B. De Souza for recombinant murine IL-1β; Dr. D. Tracey of Upjohn for IRAP; and Dr. S. Kunkel of the University of Michigan for antibody to TNF.

REFERENCES

1. CHOWERS, I., H. T. HAMMEL, J. EISENMAN, R. M. ABRAMS & S. M. MCCANN. 1966. Comparison of effect of environmental and preoptic heating and pyrogen on plasma cortisol. Am. J. Physiol. **210:** 606–610.
2. BEISEL, W. R. & M. I. RAPOPORT. 1969. Inter-relations between adrenocortical functions and infectious illness. N. Engl. J. Med. **280:** 541–546.
3. BESEDOVSKY, H. O., A. E. DEL REY & E. SORKIN. 1985. Immune-neuroendocrine interactions. J. Immunol. **135:** 750–754s.
4. BESEDOVSKY, H. O., A. DEL REY, E. SORKIN & C. A. DINARELLO. 1986. Immunoregulatory feedback between interleukin-1 and glucocorticoid hormones. Science **233:** 652–654.
5. BESEDOVSKY, H., A. DEL REY, E. SORKIN, M. DA PRADA, R. BURRI & C. HONEGGER. 1983. The immune response evokes changes in brain noradrenergic neurons. Science **221:** 564–566.
6. DUNN, A. J., M. L. POWELL, C. MEITIN & P. A. SMALL. 1989. Virus infection as a stressor: Influenza virus elevates plasma concentrations of corticosterone, and brain concentrations of MHPG and tryptophan. Physiol. Behav. **45:** 591–594.
7. PLOTSKY, P., E. CUNNINGHAM & E. WIDMAIER. 1989. Catecholaminergic modulation of corticotropin-releasing factor and adrenocorticotropin secretion. Endocr. Rev. **10:** 437–458.
8. ROH, M. S., K. A. DRAZENOVICH, J. J. BARBOSE, C. A. DINARELLO & C. F. COBB. 1987. Direct stimulation of the adrenal cortex by interleukin-1. Surgery **102:** 140–146.
9. WINTER, J. S. D., K. W. GOW, Y. S. PERRY & A. H. GREENBERG. 1990. A stimulatory effect of interleukin-1 on adrenocortical cortisol secretion mediated by prostaglandins. Endocrinology **127:** 1904–1909.
10. ANDREIS, P. G., G. NERI, A. S. BELLONI, G. MAZZOCCHI, A. KASPRZAK & G. G. NUSSDORFER. 1991. Interleukin-1β enhances corticosterone secretion by acting directly on the rat adrenal gland. Endocrinology **129:** 53–57.
11. GWOSDOW, A. R., M. S. A. KUMAR & H. H. BODE. 1990. Interleukin 1 stimulation of the hypothalamic-pituitary-adrenal axis. Am. J. Physiol. **258:** E65–E70.
12. HARLIN, C. A. & C. R. PARKER. 1991. Investigation of the effect of interleukin-1β on steroidogenesis in the human fetal adrenal gland. Steroids **56:** 72–76.
13. CAMBRONERO, J. C., F. J. RIVAS, J. BORRELL & C. GUAZA. 1992. Is the adrenal cortex a putative site for the action of interleukin-1? Horm. Metab. Res. **24:** 48–49.
14. OLSEN, N. J., W. E. NICHOLSON, C. R. DEBOLD & D. N. ORTH. 1992. Lymphocyte-derived adrenocorticotropin is insufficient to stimulate adrenal steroidogenesis in hypophysectomized rats. Endocrinology **130:** 2113 2119.
15. BERNTON, E. W., J. E. BEACH, J. W. HOLADAY, R. C. SMALLRIDGE & H. G. FEIN. 1987. Release of multiple hormones by a direct action of interleukin-1 on pituitary cells. Science **238:** 519–521.

16. DUNN, A. J. 1990. Interleukin-1 as a stimulator of hormone secretion. Prog. NeuroEndo-crinImmunol. **3:** 26–34.
17. KEHRER, P., D. TURNHILL, J.-M. DAYER, A. F. MULLER & R. C. GAILLARD. 1988. Human recombinant interleukin-1 beta and -alpha, but not recombinant tumor necrosis factor stimulates ACTH release from rat anterior pituitary cells in vitro in a prostaglandin E2 and cAMP independent manner. Neuroendocrinology **48:** 160–166.
18. SUDA, T., F. TOZAWA, T. USHIYAMA, N. TOMORI, T. SUMITOMO, Y. NAKAGAMI, M. YAMADA, H. DEMURA & K. SHIZUME. 1989. Effects of protein kinase-C-related adrenocorticotropin secretagogues and interleukin-1 on proopiomelanocortin gene expression in rat anterior pituitary cells. Endocrinology **124:** 1444–1449.
19. SAPOLSKY, R., C. RIVIER, G. YAMAMOTO, P. PLOTSKY & W. VALE. 1987. Interleukin-1 stimulates the secretion of hypothalamic corticotropin-releasing factor. Science **238:** 522–524.
20. UEHARA, A., P. E. GOTTSCHALL, R. R. DAHL & A. ARIMURA. 1987. Interleukin-1 stimulates ACTH release by an indirect action which requires endogenous corticotro-pin releasing factor. Endocrinology **121:** 1580–1582.
21. BERKENBOSCH, F., J. VAN OERS, A. DEL REY, F. TILDERS & H. BESEDOVSKY. 1987. Corticotropin-releasing factor-producing neurons in the rat activated by interleukin-1. Science **238:** 524–526.
22. BRUHN, T., P. PLOTSKY & W. VALE. 1984. Effect of paraventricular lesions on corticotropin-releasing factor (CRF)-like immunoreactivity in the stalk-median eminence: Studies on the adrenocorticotropin response to ether stress and exogenous CRF. Endocrinology **114:** 57–62.
23. RIVEST, S. & C. RIVIER. 1991. Influence of the paraventricular nucleus of the hypothala-mus in the alteration of neuroendocrine functions induced by intermittent footshock or interleukin. Endocrinology **129:** 2049–2057.
24. CHULUYAN, H., D. SAPHIER, W. ROHN & A. J. DUNN. 1992. Noradrenergic innervation of the hypothalamus participates in the adrenocortical responses to interleukin-1. Neuro-endocrinology **56:** 106–111.
25. DUNN, A. J. 1992. Endotoxin-induced activation of cerebral catecholamine and serotonin metabolism—Comparison with interleukin-1. J. Pharmacol. Exp. Ther. **261:** 964–969.
26. ZUCKERMAN, S. H., J. SHELLHAAS & L. D. BUTLER. 1989. Differential regulation of lipopolysaccharide-induced interleukin-1 and tumor necrosis factor synthesis: Effects of endogenous and exogenous glucocorticoids and the role of the pituitary-adrenal axis. Eur. J. Immunol. **19:** 301–305.
27. DUNN, A. J. 1992. The role of interleukin-1 and tumor necrosis factor α in the neurochemi-cal and neuroendocrine responses to endotoxin. Brain Res. Bull. **29:** 807–812.
28. BESEDOVSKY, H. O., A. DEL REY, I. KLUSMAN, H. FURUKAWA, G. M. ARDITI & A. KABIERSCH. 1991. Cytokines as modulators of the hypothalamus-pituitary-adrenal axis. J. Steroid Biochem. Molec. Biol. **40:** 613–618.
29. YANG, X.-M., A. L. GORMAN & A. J. DUNN. 1990. The involvement of central noradrener-gic systems and corticotropin-releasing factor in defensive-withdrawal in rats. J. Phar-macol. Exp. Ther. **255:** 1064–1070.
30. BERRIDGE, C. W. & A. J. DUNN. 1986. Corticotropin-releasing factor elicits naloxone-sensitive stress-like alterations in exploratory behavior in mice. Regul. Pept. **16:** 83–93.
31. DUNN, A. J., M. ANTOON & Y. CHAPMAN. 1991. Reduction of exploratory behavior by intraperitoneal injection of interleukin-1 involves brain corticotropin-releasing factor. Brain Res. Bull. **26:** 539–542.
32. SPADARO, F. & A. J. DUNN. 1990. Intracerebroventricular administration of interleukin-1 to mice alters investigation of stimuli in a novel environment. Brain Behav. Immun. **4:** 308–322.
33. BERRIDGE, C. W. & A. J. DUNN. 1987. A corticotropin-releasing factor antagonist reverses the stress-induced changes of exploratory behavior in mice. Horm. Behav. **21:** 393–401.
34. DUNN, A. J. & C. W. BERRIDGE. 1990. Physiological and behavioral responses to corticotropin-releasing factor administration: Is CRF a mediator of anxiety or stress response? Brain Res. Rev. **15:** 71–100.
35. DINARELLO, C. A. 1984. Interleukin-1. Rev. Infect. Dis. **6:** 51–95.

36. McCarthy, D. O., M. J. Kluger & A. J. Vander. 1986. Effect of centrally administered interleukin-1 and endotoxin on food intake of fasted rats. Physiol. Behav. **36:** 745–749.
37. Otterness, I. G., P. A. Seymour, H. W. Golden, J. A. Reynolds & G. O. Daumy. 1988. The effects of continuous administration of murine interleukin-1α in the rat. Physiol. Behav. **43:** 797–804.
38. Opp, M. R., F. Obal & J. M. Krueger. 1991. Interleukin 1 alters rat sleep: Temporal and dose-related effects. Am. J. Physiol. **260:** R52–58.

Stress-Induced Immune Suppression

Role of the Autonomic Nervous System[a]

MICHAEL IRWIN

Department of Psychiatry
University of California
La Jolla, California 92093

San Diego VA Medical Center
San Diego, California 92161

The links between behavior, the central nervous system, and the immune system are being explored in an effort to understand the paths of communication between the brain and immune processes. This paper will discuss experimental evidence that describes the role of the central nervous system in coordinating neural and endocrine pathways important in the *in vivo* regulation of immune function. Studies that have shown alterations of immune function following severe life stress and depression in man or the administration of aversive stress in animals will be reviewed. Central corticotropin-releasing factor (CRF) is released after stress and is hypothesized to serve as an integrator of the behavioral, neuroendocrine, and autonomic responses to stress.[1,2] Our laboratory has expanded these data and evaluated the role of central CRF in the *in vivo* modulation of immune function.[3–5] Central CRF has been found to reduce cellular immune function and specific antibody responses via activation of the sympathetic nervous system,[3,6] a finding that may have implications for understanding the association between increased sympathetic outflow and reduction of immune function in aging as well as stress.[7,8]

STRESS—HEALTH RELEVANCE

Clinical Studies

Experimental and epidemiologic data have demonstrated that adverse life events, psychologic distress, and depressive symptoms are associated with the development and course of many human diseases.[9] For example, one of the most stressful life experiences, the death of a spouse, is associated with an elevated mortality rate in bereaved spouses, particularly during the early periods after the loss and among widowers between the ages of 55 and 75 years old.[10–12] In several but not all prospective studies,[13–18] depressed patients have been found to have an increase in the rate of cancer morbidity and mortality as compared to that in an age-matched general population. In addition, as compared with controls, a higher incidence and higher titers of herpes simplex virus antibodies have been demonstrated in depressed patients,[19–21] and other studies have revealed correlations between increased herpes simplex virus titers and examination stress,[22] increased herpes simplex virus recur-

[a]This work was supported by grants from the Veterans Affairs Merit Review (MI); the National Institute of Mental Health (NIMH) grants MH 44275-04, MH 46867-01A2, and MH 42840-03; NIMH Mental Health Clinical Research Center grant MH30914; and General Clinical Research Center grant M01 RR00827.

rence rate and depressive affect,[23,24] and chronic fatigue syndrome (chronic Epstein-Barr virus infection) and major depression.[25] Finally, Cohen and colleagues[26] have demonstrated a dose-response relationship between psychologic stress and increased risk of acute infectious respiratory illness. In subjects who were given nasal drops containing one of five respiratory viruses, rates of both respiratory infection and clinical colds increased with increases in the degree of psychologic stress independent of the contribution of age, sex, education, allergic status, or virus-specific antibody status at baseline before challenge.[26]

Preclinical Studies

Stress associated with physical and psychologic stimuli has also been associated with increased susceptibility of animals to a number of immune-related disorders such as infectious and neoplastic disease.[27] For example, psychosocial stimulation of animals involving either avoidance conditioning, physical restraint, or auditory stimulation can produce decreased resistance to herpes simplex, coxsackie B, poliomyelitis, or vesicular stomatitis virus.[28] High-population density affects the susceptibility of mice to the malarial parasite *Plasmodium berghei*,[29] and isolation housing is associated with increased risk of encephalomyocarditis virus infections.[30] It appears that both the virulence of the organism as well as the psychophysiologic state of the animal affects disease risk. If the infectious agent produces a chronic or insidious infection and the animals are stressed at the time of exposure, then symptoms of disease are more likely.[27,31,32]

Findings from studies of the role of stress in susceptibility to neoplastic disease are diverse, depending upon the age and species of the animal, the type of tumor (viral or chemically induced), the timing of the stressor in relation to tumor inoculation, and the quality of the stressor (inescapable or escapable).[27,33–35] However, in general, it appears that exposure of rats or mice to inescapable shock at the time the stressor is experienced facilitates tumor growth, whereas administration of the stressor before implantation inhibits its growth.[36] Exposure to escapable shock has no impact on tumor development.[36]

STRESS AND IMMUNITY

Clinical Studies

Clinical research has begun to evaluate the association between depression, life stress, and reduced cell-mediated immunity,[37–39] hypothesizing that decrements of immune function might contribute to changes of health status during stress. In persons undergoing bereavement or other severe, threatening life adversity, *in vitro* correlates of cellular immune function such as natural killer (NK) cell activity or lymphocyte responses to mitogen stimulation are reduced as compared to values in nonstressed comparison subjects.[40–42] Likewise, the stress associated with other life difficulties, such as caregiving for a family member with Alzheimer's disease,[43] or even modest changes such as academic examinations,[22,44–46] is associated with a reduction in the function or response of a number of immune responses *in vitro*.

Inasmuch as severity of depressive symptoms is negatively correlated with values of immune function such as NK lytic activity in persons undergoing such life stress,[41,47] the association between depression and immune function has also been examined, demonstrating immunologic changes similar to those found in stress. For example, depressed patients show a reduction in natural cytotoxicity as compared to age-matched controls,[48–50] and additional clinical studies have described a suppressed ability of lymphocytes to respond to mitogenic stimulation in depressed patients.[51,52] Importantly, subgroups of depressed patients who show increased severity of depressive symptoms, who are older, or who have past histories of alcohol abuse appear to be at the greatest risk to show changes in the function of the immune system.[50,53]

Preclinical Studies

Behavioral responsiveness to inescapable aversive stimulation has served as an animal model of clinical depression,[54] and such aversive stress has been found to produce alterations in a number of immune responses. With respect to *in vitro* measures of cellular immune responses, the administration of aversive stressors such as sound exposure,[55,56] rotation,[33,57] intermittent shock[54,58,59] or forced immobilization[60] affects lymphocyte responses to mitogen stimulation and/or NK activity in a manner that depends on their dose- and time-response profiles. For example, using an audiogenic stressor repeated at daily intervals, Irwin *et al.*[56] have replicated the findings of Monjan and Collector[55] who found that the initial stress-induced immune suppression is followed by an increase or enhancement of natural cytotoxicity. With respect to the effects of dose of the stressor, studies by Keller *et al.*[54] have demonstrated a relationship between the intensity of an acute stressor and the degree of suppression of T cell function. As compared to home cage controls, lymphocyte proliferation is reduced in a dose-dependent manner by apparatus stress, low-level tail shock, and high-level electric tail shock.[58]

Cellular *in vivo* immune and antibody responses are also altered by aversive stressors. Delayed hypersensitivity reactions are decreased in mice exposed to heat stress,[61] and the graft-versus-host response is suppressed in animals subjected to limited feeding,[62] an effect that is independent of adrenocortical levels.[62] Reduced antibody responses are found in monkeys exposed to a number of aversive stimuli,[63,64] in mice housed in high- versus low-density grouping,[65] and in mice subjected to changes in housing condition (either from individual to group housing or from a group to the return to an individual cage).[66] Similar to the effects of stressor timing on susceptibility to infectious or neoplastic disease, restraint produces a significant reduction in antibody response to sheep red blood cells only if the stress is applied before the time of immunization; no change in antibody production occurs when the stress is applied after antigen injection.[67]

CENTRAL NERVOUS SYSTEM EFFECTS ON IMMUNITY

The influence of the brain on immune function was first evaluated by performing experiments involving electrolytic or other destructive lesions in the central nervous system (CNS).[68,69] Associated alterations in lymphoid tissue architecture were demonstrated such as impairment or enhancement of lymphoid cell activation,[69–71] impairment of delayed type hypersensitivity,[72,73] and suppression of NK cell activity.[69] In addition to these studies, the administration of pharmacologic agents or neuropeptides into the CNS has been found to alter immune function. For example, depletion of CNS catecholamines by central injection of the neurotoxin, 6-hydroxydopamine, into the cisterna magna impairs the primary antibody immune response[74] by inducing T-suppressor cell activity.[75] Similarly, administration of a small dose of morphine given into the cerebral ventricle or intracerebral infusion of morphine into the periaqueductal grey, but not other brain regions, produces a suppression of splenic NK activity.[76,77]

CENTRAL CRF MODULATION OF STRESS-INDUCED SUPPRESSION OF IMMUNITY

CRF is one neuropeptide that has been hypothesized to have a role in mediating stress-induced changes of immune functions. CRF initiates biologic responses within the brain that are observed in response to stress, including effects on behavior,[78,79] and activation of both the hypothalamic-pituitary-adrenal axis[80] and the autonomic nervous system.[81–83] To expand these earlier observations involving the effects of CRF on behavior and visceral function, our laboratory examined the role of central CRF on immune function.

In the first series of studies,[5] we tested the hypothesis that the increased release of CRF after exposure to a stressor has a *physiologic* role in mediating suppression of splenic NK cytotoxicity. Using an intermittent footshock paradigm (1.5 mA, 1 s duration 60 Hz sine wave, delivered randomly twice per min for 30 min, repeated twice daily over a 48-h period consistent with previously described protocols)[59] we found a reduction of splenic NK activity in stressed animals as compared to home cage controls. The stressor was not associated with statistically significant alterations in splenic weights, number of total lymphocytes, or percentage of T-helper, T-suppressor, or NK cells.

The role of central release of CRF in mediating footshock-induced suppression of NK activity was assessed using polyclonal antibodies to CRF (anti-CRF serum). By administering anti-CRF serum either centrally or peripherally prior to each stress session, these experiments evaluated the action of central-versus-peripheral mechanisms in altering immune responses after stress. The results showed that intracerebroventricular (i.c.v.) injection of anti-CRF serum completely antagonized the immunosuppressive action of footshock stress, yielding values of NK activity comparable to that obtained after injection with i.c.v. anti-CRF alone. Furthermore, when the polyclonal anti-CRF serum had been affinity-purified against CRF, similar results were obtained. These findings, together with the work of Jain et al,[84] demonstrate that central immunoneutralization of CRF completely antagonizes stress-induced suppression of cellular immune function.

In contrast to the action of central anti-CRF serum in antagonizing stress-induced suppression of immunity, intraperitoneal (i.p.) injection of anti-CRF serum failed to alter the stress-induced reduction of splenic NK activity. Animals that received peripheral doses of anti-CRF serum before each stress session had values of NK activity that were significantly lower than in control rats treated with i.p. anti-CRF serum alone.

The acute immunosuppressive effect of footshock stress appears to be dissociated from stress-induced activation of the pituitary adrenal axis. Measurement of plasma levels of ACTH and corticosterone demonstrated that footshock stress produced about a 10-fold increase in the circulating concentrations of these hormones. Whereas peripheral administration of the anti-CRF serum antagonized stress-induced release of ACTH and corticosterone, peripheral anti-CRF serum did not alter the immunosuppressive effects of footshock stress. Conversely, central anti-CRF serum abrogated stress-associated changes of immunity but failed to antagonize stress-related activation of the pituitary adrenal axis. Together, these observations are consistent with the hypothesis that activation of the pituitary-adrenal axis is dissociated from stress-induced reduction of cellular immunity such as splenic NK activity, suggesting that other efferent pathways such as the autonomic nervous system may play a role in stress-induced immune suppression.[85]

CRF IN THE BRAIN SUPPRESSES IMMUNE FUNCTION

The demonstration that central nervous system release of CRF plays a role in modulating NK activity following stress also implies that CRF in the brain may be involved in the *in vivo* regulation of this distinct functional population of lymphocytes. To further examine this hypothesis, studies have been conducted involving the exogenous intracerebral injection of CRF (1.0 μg) and measurement of immune function.[3,4,6,86] Central infusion of CRF produces a dose-dependent reduction of several cellular immune measures such as splenic and peripheral blood NK activity and lymphocyte responses to mitogenic stimulation.[86] Additional observations also indicate that central doses of CRF slow the kinetics and reduce the magnitude of the IgG response to a specific T-cell-dependent antigen.[87] The effects of central CRF on cellular and humoral immune responses *in vivo* are likely mediated by CRF in the brain because central coadministration of the CRF antagonist, α-helical ovine CRF$_{9-41}$ blocks CRF-induced suppression of NK cytotoxicity.[4] In contrast, peripheral administration of the CRF antagonist has no effect on CRF modulation of immunity, even at doses capable of inhibiting CRF-induced ACTH release.[4,87]

CRF AND AUTONOMIC NERVOUS SYSTEM MODULATION OF IMMUNITY

The autonomic nervous system is one pathway for communication between the brain and cells of the immune system. Anatomic studies have revealed an extensive presence of autonomic fibers in primary and secondary lymphoid organs,[88-92] innervating the vasculature and the parenchyma of the tissues. In a pattern of classic anatomic connection, preganglionic cell bodies are located in the intermediolateral cell column of the spinal cord synapse with the ganglion cells that are found either in the sympathetic chain or in collateral ganglia.[91] They enter the lymphoid organs such as the spleen along with the vasculature; immunohistochemical studies have demonstrated that nerve fibers branch into the parenchyma[90] and areas in which lymphocytes (primarily T cells) reside.[90,93] These noradrenergic fibers are not only adjacent to T cells but, at the electron microscopic level, end in synaptic-like contacts with lymphocytes in the spleen.[94] Together these observations establish an anatomic link between the brain and the immune system.

In the adult animal, norepinephrine appears to act as a neurotransmitter in the spleen. Norepinephrine is released within the spleen; early studies by von Euler[95] found that splenic nerve stimulation yields a release of norepinephrine. Furthermore, *in vivo* dialysis techniques have preliminarily documented a 1-μM concentration of norepinephrine in the rat spleen,[96] a concentration that is more than 100-fold higher than that in blood, suggesting local release of norepinephrine within the spleen.

Lymphocytes have been found to receive signals from the sympathetic neurons by adrenoreceptor binding of norepinephrine, epinephrine, and dopamine.[97-102] These beta receptors are linked to adenylate cyclase[103-105] and appear to have a functional role in the modulation of cellular immunity. *In vitro* incubation of lymphocytes with varying concentrations of norepinephrine or epinephrine decreases NK activity[106] and mitogenic responses.[107] Because preincubation with a beta antagonist reverses the inhibitory effects of norepinephrine *in vitro*,[106] the concept has emerged that beta adrenoreceptor binding mediates an inhibition of cellular immunity.[108]

In vivo studies have shown that either surgical denervation of the spleen or chemical sympathectomy using the neurotoxin, 6-hydroxydopamine, produces an augmented antibody response to thymus-dependent antigens such as sheep red blood cells,[109] an enhanced plaque-forming cell response to thymus-independent antigens,[110] and altered T and B cell responsiveness to mitogen stimulation.[108,111] Others have found in humans that infusion of adrenergic agonists results in a down-regulation of beta adrenergic receptors in circulating mononuclear cells[97,112] and acute changes in NK cell function and mitogen responses.[108,113]

CRF is anatomically localized at brain sites important in the control of autonomic outflow,[82] and central administration of CRF induces an activation of the sympathetic nervous system as measured by elevations of plasma levels of epinephrine and norepinephrine.[83] To further examine the functional significance of noradrenergic innervation of lymphoid tissue in the link between the brain and immune cells, CRF has been used as a neuropeptide probe to alter autonomic outflow, testing the role of autonomic activation in mediating suppression of immune function after the administration of CRF.

In these studies, central administration of CRF produces a significant elevation in circulating levels of norepinephrine, which is completely abolished by the preadministration of the ganglionic blocker, chlorisondamine.[6] Measurement of NK activity again demonstrated that an acute central dose of CRF reduced splenic NK activity to values 50% of those in vehicle-infused controls.[6] When the ganglionic blocker chlorisondamine was preadministered, CRF-induced suppression of NK activity was antagonized. Chlorisondamine had no intrinsic effect on NK activity. These data showed that treatment with ganglionic blockade abolishes CRF-induced elevations in norepinephrine levels and completely antagonizes CRF suppression of NK activity, demonstrating that autonomic nervous system mechanisms have a role in mediating CRF-induced suppression of NK activity.

To extend these studies regarding the role of the autonomic nervous system in immune modulation *in vivo,* the involvement of the sympathetic nervous system in CRF-induced suppression of immunity has been examined using chemical sympathectomy or β-receptor antagonists.[3] Animals were administered CRF intracerebroventricularly, and measurement of splenic NK activity demonstrated a reduction of cytotoxicity as compared to values in the saline-infused control group. Intraperitoneal pretreatment with the neurotoxin 6-hydroxydopamine prevents CRF-induced activation of the sympathetic nervous system as shown by the complete blockade of the elevations of plasma concentrations of epinephrine and norepinephrine. Similar to the observations using ganglionic blockade, 6-hydroxydopamine pretreatment also antagonized the immunosuppressive action of CRF. Injection with 6-hydroxydopamine alone had no intrinsic effect on NK activity as compared with vehicle-injected controls. To further establish the role of sympathetic activation in mediating CRF-induced suppression of NK cytotoxicity, β-adrenergic receptor antagonists were also administered.[3] Intraperitoneal injection of either the nonselective β_2-antagonist propranolol or the selective β_2-antagonist butoxamine antagonized the immunosuppressive action of CRF. Although propranolol alone significantly reduced NK activity as compared to vehicle-injected controls, butoxamine had no intrinsic effect on NK activity. These findings using either chemical sympathectomy or β-receptor antagonism suggest that acute activation of the sympathetic nervous system and β_2-adrenergic receptors are involved in mediating intraventricular CRF suppression of NK cytotoxicity.

In an effort to extend previous observations on sympathetic regulation of immunity, immune changes have also been examined in humans after administration of a stressor known to produce an activation of the sympathetic nervous system.[114] In these studies, the effects of exercise stress on immune changes were examined. In addition, β-receptor antagonists were used to evaluate the mediating role of sympathetic mechanisms on exercise-induced alterations in the distribution and function of immune cells. Because lymphocytes express β_2-adrenergic receptors,[115] nonelective β_{1-2}-adrenergic receptor blockade, but not β_1-receptor antagonism, was anticipated to alter exercise stress-induced changes of immunity.

Consistent with previous observations, exercise stress was found to produce marked increases in circulating levels of plasma catecholamines, to alter the distribution of T cell subpopulations, and to reduce lymphocyte responses to mitogen stimulation.[114] Pretreatment with the nonselective β_{1-2}-receptor antagonist propranolol altered exercise-induced changes in T cell traffic and antagonized the reduction of lymphocyte responses following acute exercise stress. In contrast, exercise-induced suppression of lymphocyte responses was not altered by pretreatment with the β_1-selective receptor antagonist metoprolol. These observations together with preclinical findings demonstrate that acute activation of the sympathetic nervous system has a role in mediating a suppression of cellular immune function, likely via β_2-adrenergic receptor mechanisms.

AGE, SYMPATHETIC ACTIVATION, AND SUPPRESSION OF IMMUNITY

The finding that activation of the sympathetic nervous system has a role in the suppression of cellular immunity after stress may also have relevant implications for understanding the reduction of cellular immune function found in other conditions such as aging. Aged humans and animals show chronic and sustained increase in sympathetic nervous system outflow,[7,116–118] in which circulating concentrations of catecholamines are elevated because of an increased appearance rate of plasma norepinephrine.[119] Furthermore, microneurographic techniques have found that the resting burst rate of sympathetic nerves innervating the muscle increases with advancing age.[117]

Aging is also characterized by a decline of immune responses to exogenous stimuli (mainly involving T-cell-dependent functions), dysregulation, and a loss of self-tolerance.[120–122] For example, in animal models of aging, there is general agreement that NK activity diminishes with age, despite no change or even an increase in the numbers of circulating NK cells.[123–126] In addition, an age-related decline of *in vivo* immune function occurs mainly in responses mediated by T lymphocytes, that is, delayed type hypersensitivity (DTH) or primary antibody responses that require T cells as controlling elements.[127,128] Finally, the decline of *in vivo* function of T cells in primary antibody responses is mirrored by *in vitro* findings.[122] T cells isolated from peripheral blood or lymphoid organs such as the spleen show altered *in vitro* responses including impaired proliferation to antigens, mitogenic antibodies (i.e., anti-CD3 and WT31) and lectins.[122,129–133] Despite the decline of *in vitro* T cell function, no change in T cell numbers or shift in the ratio of helper to suppressor T cells occurs with age to account for the decrement in functional responses.[134]

In view of the role of CRF in regulating sympathetic outflow and immune function, an age-related change in the secretion of CRF has been hypothesized to contribute to the dysregulation of the autonomic nervous system and, possibly, immune decrements with age.[7,8] Indeed, hypersecretion of hypothalamic CRF has been proposed to occur in aging. For example, studies have found an increased *in vitro* release of CRF from hypothalamic fragments at rest and after acetylcholine stimulation in aged rats,[135] dampened anterior pituitary response to CRF *in vivo* in aged animals,[136] and a decrease in hypothalamic and anterior pituitary CRF receptors in aged rats.[137]

To evaluate possible age-related changes in central CRF systems, our laboratory recently studied the effects of aging on CRF-induced elevations in sympathetic activity as measured by the release of catecholamines.[8] Furthermore, because of the association between resting levels of sympathetic activity and NK cytotoxicity independent of pituitary adrenal activation, values of splenic NK activity and circulating concentrations of corticosterone were also measured. Briefly, Fisher 344 rats, ages 3 months or 23 months, were compared after central infusion of either saline or CRF by the measurement of plasma levels of epinephrine, norepinephrine, neuropeptide Y, and NK activity.

Basal levels of epinephrine were similar in the aged and young animals, and CRF induced a significant increase in plasma levels of epinephrine in both groups of rats. However, CRF-induced elevations of epinephrine in the aged rats occurred more rapidly, reached higher peak values, and were more likely to remain elevated throughout the blood sampling period as compared to the CRF-induced epinephrine responses of the young rats. Moreover, measurement of norepinephrine demonstrated that basal levels were significantly higher in the aged rats than in the young animals. Similar to the exaggerated CRF-induced response of epinephrine in the aged rats, norepinephrine responses to CRF infusion in the aged animals occurred more rapidly and remained elevated throughout the experiment. CRF-treated young rats showed only a modest increase in norepinephrine 15 minutes after intracerebroventricular infusion, and levels of norepinephrine returned to baseline by 60 minutes. Age-related differences in neuropeptide Y were similar to findings with norepinephrine levels. Basal plasma levels of neuropeptide Y were elevated in the aged animals as compared to the young rats. CRF induced a transient increase in circulating concentrations of neuropeptide Y in the aged animals, but not in the young rats. Neither basal levels nor responses of corticosterone to CRF infusion differed between the aged and young rats. CRF induced a similar increase in plasma corticosterone which was sustained in both age groups of animals throughout the testing interval.

As for assessment of immune function, the aged animals showed a reduction of NK activity at baseline as compared to values in the young animals. In addition, CRF produced a further decrease in splenic NK cytotoxicity in the aged animals, whereas NK activity in the young Fisher 334 animals did not change following CRF.

These findings demonstrated that sympathetic activity is increased with aged rats, consistent with the observations of McCarty.[138] Resting plasma concentrations of norepinephrine and neuropeptide Y are significantly elevated in aged rats as compared to young animals. In addition, the responsivity of the sympathetic nervous system to acute challenge is altered in the aged animals. Administration of a central dose of CRF produces a greater elevation of plasma levels of epinephrine, norepinephrine, and neuropeptide Y in the aged rat, and the CRF-induced increase in catecholamines persists for up to 3 hours after central infusion of CRF in the aged rat. In young animals, levels of epinephrine and norepinephrine return to resting concentrations after 1 hour and 15 minutes, respectively. The present study extends previous observations that sympathetic measures of catecholamines are increased at rest and suggests that regulation of the sympathetic nervous system after central activation of autonomic outflow is impaired in the aged rat.

Of additional interest is the association between activation of the sympathetic nervous system and reduction of immune function. The present study has extended our clinical findings reporting a negative correlation between levels of circulating catecholamines and neuropeptide Y[7] and values of natural cytotoxicity in elderly persons; aged rats also show an increase in circulating levels of norepinephrine and neuropeptide Y and a reduction in basal levels of NK activity. Although an association between sympathetic measures and cytotoxicity does not demonstrate a causative link, administration of central CRF further produced an activation of the sympathetic nervous system, release of norepinephrine, and reduction of NK activity in the aged rats but not in the young animals. In contrast, CRF induced a similar elevation of plasma corticosterone levels in both the aged and young animals. These data further suggest that changes of NK activity in aging might be at the level of altered release of catecholamines, rather than a defect in the NK cell per se.

The mechanisms that mediate the differential effects of age on CRF-induced elevations in catecholamines and NK activity remain to be elucidated, including an age-associated increase in the release of CRF *in vivo* and/or augmentation of an ultrashort positive feedback loop of CRF on its own release, as hypothesized by Ono *et al.*[139] In addition, the persistent elevation of plasma catecholamines after central CRF in the aged rat suggests a decreased sensitivity with age to the inhibitory feedback signal of increased sympathetic activity. Nevertheless, because CRF acts within the brain to stimulate the activity of the sympathetic nervous system and to reduce splenic NK activity,[3] increased responsivity to CRF with age implicates the CNS as an important influence in the abnormal regulation of the sympathetic nervous system and natural cytotoxicity with aging.

The pathophysiologic consequences of the abnormal regulation of autonomic outflow and immune function in the aged rats has not been investigated in the present study. However, some evidence exists that stress-induced tumor growth after inoculation with virally transformed cells is accelerated in aged rats.[140] In addition, NK cells have a demonstrated ability to lyse target cells that have undergone malignant transformation.[141] Finally, in experiments in animals, NK cells have been shown to play an important part in immune surveillance against the establishment of primary tumors as well as in controlling the spread of distant metastases.[141]

CRF acts within the brain to stimulate the activity of the sympathetic nervous system and to reduce splenic NK activity. These findings show an age-related increase of autonomic outflow after the administration of CRF. Furthermore, these data are consistent with the hypothesis that age-related changes in central nervous system regulation of sympathetic activity may influence *in vivo* modulation and suppression of natural cytotoxicity in aging.

SUMMARY

Experimental data together with clinical studies have generated information about the association between sympathetic nervous system activity and immunity as measured by *in vitro* correlates of cellular immune function. In addition, studies on the *in vivo* role of central CRF in coordinating sympathetic outflow and modulating immune function have provided an opportunity to examine central mechanisms important in the link between brain, behavior, and immune function. Finally, use of CRF as a neuropeptide probe will likely continue to give information about the central mechanisms relevant to the abnormal regulation of sympathetic nervous activity and immune function in stress and possibly in aging.

REFERENCES

1. DUNN, A. J. & C. W. BERRIDGE. 1990. Physiological and behavioral responses to corticotropin-releasing factor administration: Is CRH a mediator of anxiety or stress responses? Brain Res. Rev. **15:** 71–100.
2. OWENS, M. J. & C. B. NEMEROFF. 1991. Physiology and pharmacology of corticotropin-releasing factor. Pharmacol. Rev. **91:** 425–473.
3. IRWIN, M., R. L. HAUGER, L. JONES, M. PROVENCIO & K. T. BRITTON. 1990. Sympathetic nervous system mediates central corticotropin-releasing factor induced suppression of natural killer cytotoxicity. J. Pharmacol. Exp. Ther. **255:** 101–107.
4. IRWIN, M. R., W. VALE & K. T. BRITTON. 1987. Central corticotropin-releasing factor suppresses natural killer cytotoxicity. Brain Behav. Immun. **1:** 81–87.
5. IRWIN, M., W. VALE & C. RIVIER. 1990. Central corticotropin-releasing factor mediates the suppressive effect of stress on natural killer cytotoxicity. Endocrinology **126:** 2837–2844.
6. IRWIN, M., R. L. HAUGER, M. BROWN & K. T. BRITTON. 1988. CRH activates autonomic nervous system and reduces natural killer cytotoxicity. Am. J. Physiol. **255:** R744–747.
7. IRWIN, M., M. BROWN, T. PATTERSON, R. HAUGER, A. MASCOVICH & I. GRANT. 1991. Neuropeptide Y and natural killer cell activity: Findings in depression and Alzheimer caregiver stress. FASEB J. **5:** 3100–3107.
8. IRWIN, M., R. HAUGER & M. BROWN. 1992. Central corticotropin releasing hormone activates the sympathetic nervous system and reduces immune function: Increased responsivity of the aged rat. Endocrinology **131(3):** 1047–1053.
9. WEINER, H. 1991. The behavioral biology of stress and psychosomatic medicine. *In* Stress: Neurobiology and Neuroendocrinology. M. R. Brown, G. F. Koob & C. Rivier, Eds.: 22–51. Dekker. New York, NY.
10. JACOBS, S. & A. OSTFELD. 1977. An epidemiological review of the mortality of bereavement. Psychosom. Med. **39:** 344–357.
11. OSTERWEIS, M., F. SOLOMON & F. GREEN. 1984. Bereavement reactions, consequences, and care. National Academy Press. Washington, D.C.
12. HELSING, K. J., M. SZKLO & E. W. COMSTOCK. 1981. Mortality after bereavement. Am. J. Public Health **71:** 802–809.
13. WHITLOCK, F. A. & M. SISKING. 1979. Depression and cancer: A follow-up study. Psychol. Med. **9:** 747–752.
14. NIEMI, T. & T. TASSKELAINEN. 1978. Cancer morbidity in depressed persons. J. Psychosom. Res. **22:** 117–120.
15. PERSKY, V. W., J. KEMPTHORNE-RAWSON & R. B. SHEKELLE. 1987. Personality and risk of cancer: 20-year follow-up of the Western Electric Study. Psychosom. Med. **49:** 435–449.
16. VARSAMIS, J., T. ZUCHOWSKI & K. K. MAIN. 1972. Survival rate and causes of death of geriatric psychotic patients. Can. Psychiatr. Assoc. J. **17:** 17–21.
17. ZONDERMAN, A. B., P. T. COSTA, JR. & R. R. MCCRAE. 1989. Depression as a risk for cancer morbidity and mortality in a nationally representative sample. JAMA **262:** 1191–1195.
18. FOX, B. H. 1989. Depressive symptoms and risk of cancer. JAMA **262:** 1231.
19. CAPPELL, R., F. GREGOIRE, L. THIRY & S. SPRECHER. 1978. Antibody and cell-mediated immunity to herpes simplex virus in psychotic depression. J. Clin. Psychiatry **39:** 266–268.
20. RIMON, R., P. HALONEN, E. ANTTINEN & E. EVOLA. 1971. Complement fixing antibody to herpes simplex virus in patients with psychotic depression. Dis. Nerv. Syst. **32:** 822–824.
21. CLEOBURY, J. F., G. R. B. SKINNER, M. E. THOULESS & P. WIDLY. 1971. Association

between psychopathic disorders and serum antibody to herpes simplex virus (type 1). Br. Med. J. **1:** 438–439.

22. GLASER, R., J. K. KIECOLT-GLASER, C. E. SPEICHER & J. E. HOLLIDAY. 1985. Stress, loneliness and changes in herpes virus latency. J. Behav. Med. **8:** 249–260.

23. KEMENY, M. E., L. ZEGANS & F. COHEN. 1987. Stress, mood, immunity and recurrence of genital herpes. Ann. N.Y. Acad. Sci. **496:** 735–736.

24. LEVENSON, J. L., R. M. HAMER, T. MYERS, R. P. HART & L. G. KAPLOWITZ. 1987. Psychological factors predict symptoms of severe recurrent genital herpes infection. J. Psychosom. Res. **31:** 153–159.

25. KRUESI, M. J. P., J. DALE & S. E. STRAUS. 1989. Psychiatric diagnoses in patients who have chronic fatigue syndrome. J. Clin. Psychiatry **50:** 53–56.

26. COHEN, S., D. A. TYRRELL & A. P. SMITH. 1991. Psychological stress and susceptibility to the common cold. N. Engl. J. Med. **325(9):** 606–656.

27. GRIFFIN, J. F. T. 1989. Stress and immunity: A unifying concept. Vet. Immunol. Immunopathol. **20:** 263–312.

28. FRIEDMAN, S. B. & L. A. GLASGOW. 1966. Psychologic factors and resistance to infectious disease. Pediatr. Clin. North Am. **13:** 315–355.

29. PLAUT, S. M., R. ADER, S. B. FRIEDMAN & A. L. RITTERSON. 1969. Social factors and resistance to malaria in the mouse: Effects of group vs. individual housing on resistance to *Plasmodium berghei* infection. Psychosom. Med. **31:** 536–552.

30. FRIEDMAN, S. B., L. A. GLASGOW & R. ADER. 1969. Psychosocial factors modifying host resistance to experimental infections. Ann. N.Y. Acad. Sci. **164:** 381–392.

31. FRIEDMAN, S. B., R. ADER & L. A. GLASGOW. 1965. Effects of psychological stress in adult mice inoculated with Coxsackie B viruses. Psychosom. Med. **27:** 361–368.

32. ADER, R. 1983. Developmental psychoneuroimmunology. Dev. Psychobiol. **16:** 251–267.

33. RILEY, V. 1981. Psychoneuroendocrine influences on immunocompetence and neoplasia. Science **212:** 1100–1109.

34. SKLAR, L. S. & H. ANISMAN. 1981. Stress and cancer. Psychol. Bull. **89:** 369–406.

35. JUSTICE, A. 1985. Review of the effects of stress on cancer in laboratory animals: Importance of time of stress application and type of tumour. Psychol. Bull. **98:** 108–138.

36. SHAVIT, Y., G. W. TERMAN, F. C. MARTIN, J. W. LEWIS, J. C. LIEBSKIND & R. P. GALE. 1985. Stress, opioid peptides, the immune system, and cancer. J. Immunol. **135:** 834s–837s.

37. R. ADER, D. L. FELTEN & N. COHEN, EDS. 1991. Psychoneuroimmunology, 2nd edit. Academic Press. San Diego, CA.

38. IRWIN, M. & H. STRAUSBAUGH. 1991. Stress and immune changes in humans: A biopsychosocial model. *In* Psychoimmunology Update. J. M. Gorman & R. M. Kertzner, Eds.: 55–79. American Psychiatric Press, Washington, D.C.

39. KIECOLT-GLASER, J. K. & R. GLASER. 1991. Stress and immune function in humans. *In* Psychoneuroimmunology, 2nd edit. R. Ader, D. L. Felten & N. Cohen, Eds.: 849–868. Academic Press. San Diego, CA.

40. BARTROP, R. W., L. LAZARUS, E. LUCKHURST, L. G. KILOH & R. PENNY. 1977. Depressed lymphocyte function after bereavement. Lancet **1:** 834–836.

41. IRWIN, M., M. DANIELS, T. L. SMITH, E. BLOOM & H. WEINER. 1987. Life events, depressive symptoms, and immune function. Am. J. Psychiatry **144:** 437–441.

42. SCHLEIFER, S. J., S. E. KELLER, M. CAMERINO & J. C. THORNTON. 1983. Suppression of lymphocyte stimulation following bereavement. JAMA **250(3):** 374–377.

43. KIECOLT-GLASER, J. K., R. GLASER, C. S. DYER, E. C. SHUTTLEWORTH, P. OGROCKI & C. E. SPEICHER. 1991. Chronic stress and immunity in family caregivers of Alzheimer's disease victims. Psychosom. Med. **49(5):** 523–535.

44. GLASER, R., S. KENNEDY, W. P. LAFUSE, R. H. BONNEAU, C. SPEICHER, J. HILLHOUSE & J. K. KIECOLT-GLASER. 1990. Psychological stress-induced modulation of interleukin-2 receptor gene expression and interleukin-2 production in peripheral blood leukocytes. Arch. Gen. Psychiatry **47:** 707–712.

45. KIECOLT-GLASER, J. K., W. GARNER, C. SPEICHER, G. M. PENN, J. HOLLIDAY & R.

GLASER. 1984. Psychosocial modifiers of immunocompetence in medical students. Psychosom. Med. **46:** 7–14.

46. GLASER, R., J. RICE, C. E. SPEICHER, J. C. STOUT & J. K. KIECOLT-GLASER. 1986. Stress depresses interferon production by leukocytes concomitant with a decrease in natural killer cell activity. Behav. Neurosci. **100:** 625–678.

47. IRWIN, M., M. DANIELS, T. L. SMITH, E. BLOOM & H. WEINER. 1987. Impaired natural killer cell activity during bereavement. Brain Behav. Immun. **1:** 98–104.

48. IRWIN, M., T. L. SMITH & J. C. GILLIN. 1987. Low natural killer cytotoxicity in major depression. Life Sci. **41:** 2127–2133.

49. IRWIN, M. R., T. L. PATTERSON, T. L. SMITH, C. CALDWELL, S. A. BROWN, J. C. GILLIN & I. GRANT. 1990. Reduction of immune function in life stress and depression. Biol. Psychiatry **27:** 22–30.

50. IRWIN, M., C. CALDWELL, T. L. SMITH, S. BROWN, M. A. SCHUCKIT & J. C. GILLIN. 1990. Major depressive disorder, alcoholism, and reduced natural killer cell cytotoxicity: Role of severity of depressive symptoms and alcohol consumption. Arch. Gen. Psychiatry **47:** 713–719.

51. KRONFOL, Z., J. SILVA, J. GREDEN, S. DEMBINSKI, R. GARDNER & B. CARROLL. 1983. Impaired lymphocyte function in depressive illness. Life Sci. **33:** 241–247.

52. SCHLEIFER, S. J., S. E. KELLER, A. T. MEYERSON, M. J. RASKIN, K. L. DAVIS & M. STEIN. 1984. Lymphocyte function in major depressive disorder. Arch. Gen. Psychiatry **41:** 484–486.

53. SCHLEIFER, S. J., S. E. KELLER, R. N. BOND, J. COHEN & M. STEIN. 1989. Major depressive disorder and immunity: Role of age, sex, severity, and hospitalization. Arch. Gen. Psychiatry **46:** 81–87.

54. KELLER, S. E., J. M. WEISS, S. J. SCHLEIFER, N. E. MILLER & M. STEIN. 1981. Suppression of immunity by stress: Effect of a graded series of stressors on lymphocyte stimulation in the rat. Science **213:** 1397–1400.

55. MONJAN, A. A. & M. I. COLLECTOR. 1977. Stress-induced modulation of the immune response. Science **196:** 307–308.

56. IRWIN, M. R., D. S. SEGAL, R. L. HAUGER & T. L. SMITH. 1989. Individual behavioral and neuroendocrine differences in responsiveness to audiogenic stress. Pharmacol. Biochem. Behav. **32:** 913–917.

57. KANDIL, O. & M. BORYSENKO. 1987. Decline of natural killer cell target binding and lytic activity in mice exposed to rotation stress. Health Psychol. **6(2):** 89–99.

58. KELLER, S. E., J. M. WEISS, S. J. SCHLEIFER, N. E. MILLER & M. STEIN. 1983. Stress-induced suppression of immunity in adrenalectomized rats. Science **221:** 1301–1304.

59. SHAVIT, Y., J. W. LEWIS, G. W. TERMAN, R. P. GALE & J. C. LIEBESKIND. 1984. Opioid peptides mediate the suppressive effect of stress on natural killer cell cytotoxicity. Science **223:** 188–190.

60. IRWIN, M. R. & R. L. HAUGER. 1988. Adaptation to chronic stress: Temporal pattern of immune and neuroendocrine correlates. Neuropsychopharmacology **1:** 239–242.

61. PITKIN, D. H. 1965. Effect of psychological stress on the delayed hypersensitivity reaction. Proc. Soc. Exp. Biol. Med. **120:** 350–351.

62. AMKRAUT, A. A., G. F. SOLOMON, P. KASPER & A. PURDUE. 1973. Stress and hormonal intervention in the graft-versus-host response. *In* Microenvironmental Aspects of Immunity. B. D. Jankovic & K. Isakovic, Eds.: 667–674. Plenum Publishing Corp. New York, NY.

63. FELSENFELD, O., C. W. HILL & W. E. GREER. 1966. Response of Cercepitheaus aethiops to Cholera vibrio lipopolysaccharide and psychological stress. Trans. R. Soc. Trop. Med. Hyg. **60:** 514–518.

64. HILL, C. W., W. E. GREER & O. FELSENFELD. 1967. Psychological stress, early response to foreign protein, and blood cortisol in vervets. Psychosom. Med. **29:** 279–283.

65. SOLOMON, G. F. 1969. Stress and antibody response in rats. Int. Arch. Allergy **35:** 97–104.

66. EDWARDS, E. A., R. H. RAHE, P. M. STEPHENS & J. P. HENRY. 1980. Antibody response to bovine serum albumin in mice: The effects of psychosocial environmental change. Proc. Soc. Exp. Biol. Med. **164:** 478–481.

67. OKIMURA, T., M. OGAWA & T. YAMAUCHI. 1986. Stress and immune responses. III. Effect of restraint stress on delayed type hypersensitivity (DTH) response, natural killer (NK) activity and pyagocytosis in mice. Jpn. J. Pharmacol. **41:** 229–235.

68. ISAKOVIC, K. & B. D. JANKOVIC. 1973. Neuroendocrine correlates of immune response. II. Changes in the lymphatic organs of brain lesioned rats. Int. Arch. Allergy **45:** 373–384.

69. CROSS, R. J., W. R. MARKESBERY, W. H. BROOKS & T. L. ROSZMAN. 1984. Hypothalamic immune interactions: Neuromodulation of natural killer activity by lesioning of the anterior hypothalamus. Immunology **51:** 399–405.

70. KELLER, S. E., M. STEIN, M. S. CAMERINO, S. J. SCHLEIFER & J. SHERMAN. 1980. Suppression of lymphocyte stimulation by anterior hypothalamic lesions in the guinea pig. Cell. Immunol. **52:** 334–340.

71. BROOKS, W. H., R. J. CROSS, T. L. ROSZMAN & W. R. MARKESBERY. 1980. Neuroimmunomodulation: Neural anatomical basis for impairment and facilitation. Ann. Neurol. **12:** 56–61.

72. MACRIS, N. T., R. C. SCHIAVI & M. CAMERINO. 1970. Effect of hypothalamic lesions on immune processes in the guinea pig. Am. J. Physiol. **219:** 1205–1209.

73. STEIN, M., R. C. SCHIAVI & M. CAMERINO. 1976. Influence of brain and behavior on the immune system. Science **191:** 435–440.

74. CROSS, R. J., J. C. JACKSON, W. H. BROOKS, D. L. SPARKS, W. R. MARKESBERY & T. L. ROSZMAN. 1986. Neuroimmunomodulation: Impairment of humoral immune responsiveness by 6-hydroxydopamine treatment. Immunology **57:** 145–152.

75. CROSS, R. J. & T. L. ROSZMAN. 1988. Central catecholamine depletion impairs *in vivo* immunity but not *in vitro* lymphocyte activation. J. Neuroimmunol. **19:** 33–45.

76. SHAVIT, Y., A. DEPAULIS, F. C. MARTIN, G. W. TERMAN, R. N. PECHNICK, C. J. ZANE, R. P. GALE & J. C. LIEBSKIND. 1986. Involvement of brain opiate receptors in the immune suppressive affect of morphine. Proc. Natl. Acad. Sci. USA **83:** 7114–7117.

77. WEBER, R. J. & A. PERT. 1989. The periaqueductal gray matter mediates opiate-induced immunosuppression. Science **245:** 188–190.

78. SUTTON, R. E., G. F. KOOB, M. LEMOAL, J. RIVIER & W. VALE. 1982. Corticotropin releasing factor produces behavioral activation in rats. Nature **297:** 331–333.

79. BRITTON, K. T., G. F. KOOB & J. RIVIER. 1982. ICV—CRH enhanced behavioral effects of novelty. Life Sci. **31:** 363–367.

80. RIVIER, J., C. RIVIER & W. VALE. 1984. Synthetic competitive antagonists of corticotropin-releasing factor: Effect on ACTH secretion in the rat. Science **224:** 889–891.

81. BROWN, M. R., L. A. FISHER, J. SPIESS, C. RIVIER, J. RIVIER & W. VALE. 1982. Corticotropin releasing factor: Actions on the sympathetic nervous system and metabolism. Endocrinology **111:** 928–931.

82. BROWN, M. R. 1986. Corticotropin releasing factor: Central nervous system sites of action. Brain Res. **399:** 10–14.

83. FISHER, L. A., J. RIVIER, C. RIVIER, J. SPIESS, W. W. VALE & M. R. BROWN. 1982. CRH: Central effects on mean arterial pressure and heart rate in rats. Endocrinology **110:** 2222–2224.

84. JAIN, R., D. ZWICKLER, C. S. HOLLANDER, H. BRAND, A. SAPERSTEIN, B. HUTCHINSON, C. BROWN & T. AUDHYA. 1991. Corticotropin-releasing factor modulates the immune response to stress in the rat. Endocrinology **128:** 1329–1336.

85. CUNNICK, J. E., D. T. LYSLE, B. J. KUCINSKI & B. S. RABIN. 1990. Evidence that shock-induced immune suppression is mediated by adrenal hormones and peripheral β-adrenergic receptors. Pharmacol. Biochem. Behav. **36:** 645–651.

86. STRAUSBAUGH, H. & M. IRWIN. 1992. Central corticotropin releasing hormone reduces cellular immunity. Brain Behav. Immun. **6:** 11–17.

87. IRWIN, M. R. 1993. Brain corticotropin releasing hormone and interleukin-1β induced suppression of specific antibody production. Endocrinology. In press.

88. FELTEN, D. L., J. M. OVERHAGE, S. Y. FELTEN & J. F. SCHMEDTJE. 1984. Noradrenergic and peptidergic innervation of lymphoid tissue. Brain Res. Bull. **13:** 693–699.

89. FELTEN, D. L., S. LIVNAT, S. Y. FELTEN, S. L. CARLSON, D. L. BELLINGER & P. YEH. 1984. Sympathetic innervation of lymph nodes in mice. Brain Res. Bull. **13:** 693–699.

90. FELTEN, D. L., S. Y. FELTEN, S. L. CARLSON, J. A. OLSCHOWKA & S. LIVNAT. 1985. Noradrenergic and peptidergic innervation of lymphoid tissue. J. Immunol. **135:** 755s–765s.

91. FELTEN, D. L., K. D. ACKERMAN, S. J. WIEGAND & S. Y. FELTEN. 1987. Noradrenergic sympathetic innervation of the spleen. I. Nerve fibers associate with lymphocytes and macrophages in specific compartments of the splenic white pulp. J. Neurosci. Res. **18:** 28–36.

92. BULLOCH, K. & W. POMERANTZ. 1984. Autonomic nervous system innervation of thymic-related lymphoid tissue in wild-type and nude mice. J. Comp. Neurol. **228:** 57–68.

93. ACKERMAN, K. D., S. Y. FELTEN, D. L. BELLINGER & D. L. FELTEN. 1987. Noradrenergic sympathetic innervation of the spleen. III. Development of innervation in the rat spleen. J. Neurosci. Res. **18:** 49–54.

94. FELTEN, S. Y. & J. OLSCHOWKA. 1987. Noradrenergic sympathetic innervation of the spleen. II. Tyrosine hydroxylase (TH)-positive nerve terminals form synaptic-like contacts on lymphocytes in the splenic white pulp. J. Neurosci. Res. **18:** 37–48.

95. VON EULER, U. S. 1946. The presence of a substance with sympathin E properties in spleen extracts. Acta Physiol. Scand. **11:** 168.

96. FELTEN, S. Y., J. HOUSEL & D. L. FELTEN. 1986. Use of in vivo dialysis for evaluation of splenic norepinephrine and serotonin. Soc. Neurosci. Abstr. **12:** 1065.

97. AARONS, R. D. & P. B. MOLINOFF. 1982. Changes in the density of beta adrenergic receptors in rat lymphocytes, heart, and lung after chronic treatment with propranolol. J. Pharmacol. Exp. Ther. **221:** 439–443.

98. BIDART, J. M., P. H. MOTTE, M. ASSICOT, C. BOHOUN & D. BELETT. 1983. Catechol-o-methyltransferase activity and aminergic binding site distribution in human peripheral blood lymphocyte subpopulations. Clin. Immunol. Immunopathol. **26:** 1.

99. BRODDE, O. E., G. ENGEL, D. HOVER, K. D. BOCK & F. WEBER. 1981. The beta-adrenergic receptor in human lymphocytes. Life Sci. **29:** 2189–2198.

100. MILES, K., S. ATWEH, G. OTTEN, B. G. ARNASON & E. CHELMICKA-SCHOOR. 1984. Beta-adrenergic receptors on splenic lymphocytes from axotomized mice. Int. J. Immunopharmacol. **6:** 171.

101. MOTULSKY, H. J. & P. A. INSEL. 1982. Adrenergic receptors in man: Direct identification, physiologic regulation, and clinical alterations. N. Engl. J. Med. **307(1):** 18–29.

102. WILLIAMS, L. T., R. SNYDERMAN & R. J. LEFKOWITZ. 1976. Identification of β-adrenergic receptors in human lymphocytes by (−)[3H]alprenolol binding. J. Clin. Invest. **57:** 149–155.

103. KATZ, P., A. M. ZAYTOUN & A. S. FAUCI. 1982. Mechanisms of human cell-mediated cytotoxicity. I. Modulation of natural killer cell activity by cyclic nucleotides. J. Immunol. **129:** 287–296.

104. WATSON, J. J. 1975. The influence of intracellular levels of cyclic nucleotides on cell proliferation and the induction of antibody synthesis. Exp. Med. **141:** 97–111.

105. STROM, T. D., A. P. LUNDIN & C. B. CARPENTER. 1977. Role of cyclic nucleotides in lymphocytes activation and function. Prog. Clin. Immunol. **3:** 115–153.

106. HELLSTRAND, K., S. HERMODSSON & Ö. STRANNEGÅRD. 1985. Evidence for a β-adrenoceptor-mediated regulation of human natural killer cells. J. Immunol. **134:** 4095–4099.

107. HADDEN, J. W., E. M. HADDEN & E. MIDDLETON. 1970. Lymphocyte blast transformation. I. Demonstration of adrenergic receptors in human peripheral lymphocytes. Cell. Immunol. **1:** 583–595.

108. LIVNAT, S., S. Y. FELTEN, S. L. CARLSON, D. L. BELLINGER & D. L. FELTEN. 1985. Involvement of peripheral and central catecholamine systems in neural-immune interactions. J. Neuroimmunol. **10:** 5–30.

109. DEL REY, A., H. O. BESEDOVSKY, E. SORKIN, M. DA PRADA & S. ARRENBRECHT. 1981. Immunoregulation mediated by the sympathetic nervous system, II. Cell. Immunol. **63:** 329–334.

110. MILES, K., J. QUINTANS, E. CHELMICKS-SCHOOR & B. G. W. ARNASON. 1981. The sympathetic nervous system modulates antibody response to thymus independent antigens. J. Neuroimmunol. **1:** 101–105.

111. HALL, N. R. & A. L. GOLDSTEIN. 1981. Neurotransmitters and the immune system. *In* Psychoneuroimmunology. R. Ader, D. L. Felten & N. Cohen, Eds.: 521–544. Academic Press. San Diego, CA.

112. KRALL, J. F., M. CONNELLY & M. L. TUCK. 1980. Acute regulation of beta adrenergic catecholamine sensitivity in human lymphocytes. J. Pharmacol. Exp. Ther. **214:** 554–560.

113. TONNESEN, E., J. TONNESEN & N. J. CHRISTENSEN. 1984. Augmentation of cytotoxicity by natural killer cells after adrenaline administration in man. Acta Pathol. Microbiol. Immunol. Scand. C **92:** 81–83.

114. MURRAY, D. R., M. IRWIN, C. A. REARDEN, M. ZIEGLER, H. MOTULSKY & A. S. MAISEL. 1992. Sympathetic and immune interactions during dynamic exercise: Mediation via a β2-adrenergic dependent mechanism. Circulation **86:** 203–213.

115. ACKERMAN, K. D., D. L. BELLINGER, S. Y. FELTEN & D. L. FELTEN. 1991. Ontogeny and senescence of noradrenergic innervation of the rodent thymus and spleen. *In* Psychoneuroimmunology, Second edit. R. Ader, D. L. Felten & N. Cohen, Eds.: 72–115. Academic Press. San Diego, CA.

116. PFEIFER, M. A., C. R. WEINBERG, D. COOK, J. D. BEST, A. REENAN & J. B. HALTER. 1983. Differential changes of autonomic nervous system function with age in man. Am. J. Med. **75:** 249–258.

117. IWASE, S., T. MANO, T. WATANABE, M. SAITO & F. KOBAYASHI. 1991. Age-related changes of sympathetic outflow to muscles in humans. J. Gerontol. **46(1):** M1–M5.

118. ZIEGLER, M. G., C. R. LAKE & J. J. KOPIN. 1976. Plasma noradrenaline increases with age. Nature **261:** 333–335.

119. VEITH, R. C., J. A. FEATHERSTONE, O. A. LINARES & J. B. HALTER. 1986. Age differences in plasma norepinephrine kinetics in humans. J. Gerontol. **41(3):** 319–324.

120. HALLGREN, H. M., C. E. BUCKLEY, V. A. GILBERTSON & E. J. YUNIS. 1973. Lymphocyte phytohemagglutinin responsiveness, immunoglobulins and autoantibodies in aging humans. J. Immunol. **111:** 1101–1107.

121. O'LEARY, J. J. & H. M. HALLGREN. 1991. Aging and lymphocyte function: A model for testing gerontologic hypotheses of aging in man. Arch. Gerontol. Geriatr. **12:** 199–218.

122. MAKINODAN, T. & M. M. KAY. 1980. Age influence on the immune system. Adv. Immunol. **29:** 287–330.

123. SHIGEMOTO, S., S. KISHIMOTO & Y. YAMAMURA. 1975. Change of cell-mediated cytotoxicity with aging. J. Immunol. **115:** 307–309.

124. WEINDRUCH, R., B. H. DEVENS, H. V. RAFF & R. L. WALFORD. 1983. Influence of dietary restriction and aging on natural killer cell activity in mice. J. Immunol. **130:** 993–996.

125. BLAIR, P. B., M. O. STASKAWICZ & J. S. SAM. 1987. Suppression of natural killer cell activity in young and old mice. Mech. Ageing Dev. **40:** 57–70.

126. BASH, J. A. & D. VOGEL. 1984. Cellular immunosenescence in F344 rats: Decreased natural killer (NK) cell activity involves changes in regulatory interactions between NK cells, interferon, prostaglandin and macrophages. Mech. Ageing Dev. **24:** 49–65.

127. BOVBJERG, D. H., Y. T. KIM, R. SCHWAB, K. SCHMITT, T. DEBLASIO & M. E. WEKSLER. 1991. Cross-wiring of the immune response in old mice: Increased autoantibody response despite reduced antibody response to nominal antigen. Cell. Immunol. **135:** 519–525.

128. THOMAN, M. L. & W. O. WIEGLE. 1989. The cellular and subcellular basis of immunosenescence. Adv. Immunol. **46:** 221–261.

129. ADLER, W. H. & J. E. NAGEL. 1977. Studies of immune function in a human population. *In* Immunological Aspects of Aging. D. Segre & L. Smith, Eds.: 295–310. Dekker. New York, NY.

130. HALLGREN, H. M., N. BERGH, K. J. RODYSILL & J. J. O'LEARY. 1988. Lymphocyte proliferative response to PHA and anti-CD3/Ti monoclonal antibodies, T cell surface marker expression, and serum IL-2 receptor levels as biomarkers of age and health. Mech. Ageing Dev. **43:** 175–185.

131. HALLGREN, H. M. & E. J. YUNIS. 1977. Immune function, immune regulation, and survival in an aging human population. *In* Immunological Aspects of Aging. D. Segre & L. Smith, Eds.: 281–293. Dekker. New York, NY.

132. ROBERTS-THOMSON, I. C., S. WHITTINGHAM, U. YOUNGCHAIYUD & I. R. MACKAY. 1974. Ageing, immune response and mortality. Lancet **2:** 368–370.
133. MURASKO, D. M., P. WEINER & D. KAYE. 1988. Association of lack of mitogen-induced lymphocyte proliferation with increased mortality in the elderly. *In* Aging: Immunology and Infectious Disease.: 1–5. Mary Ann Liebert, Inc. New York, NY.
134. JENSEN, T. L., H. M. HALLGREN, W. G. YASMINEH & J. J. O'LEARY. 1986. Do immature T cells accumulate in advanced age? Mech. Ageing Dev. **33:** 237–245.
135. SCACCIANOCE, S., A. DESCIULLO & L. ANGELUCCI. 1990. Age-related changes in hypothalamo-pituitary-adrenocortical axis activity in the rat. Neuroendocrinology **52:** 150–155.
136. HYLKA, V., W. SONNTAG & J. MEITES. 1984. Reduced ability of old male rats to release ACTH and corticosterone in response to CRH administration. Proc. Soc. Exp. Biol. Med. **175:** 1.
137. HEROUX, J. A., D. E. GRIGORIADIS & E. B. DE SOUZA. 1991. Age-related decreases in corticotropin-releasing factor (CRF) receptors in rat brain and anterior pituitary gland. Brain Res. **542:** 155–158.
138. MCCARTY, R. 1985. Sympathetic-adrenal medullary and cardiovascular responses to acute cold stress in adult and aged rats. J. Auton. Nerv. Syst. **12:** 15–22.
139. ONO, N., J. C. B. DE CASTRO & S. M. MCCANN. 1985. Ultrashort-loop positive feedback of corticotropin (ACTH)-releasing factor to enhance ACTH in stress. Proc. Natl. Acad. Sci. USA **82:** 3528–3531.
140. SAPOLSKY, R., C. RIVIER, G. YAMAMOTO, P. PLOTSKY & W. VALE. 1987. Interleukin-1 stimulates the secretion of hypothalamic corticotropin-releasing factor. Science **238:** 522–524.
141. RITZ, J. 1989. The role of natural killer cells in immune surveillance. N. Engl. J. Med. **320:** 1748–1749.

CRF and Related Peptides
as Anti-Inflammatory Agonists[a]

H. A. THOMAS,[b,c] N. LING,[d] AND E. T. WEI[b]

[b]School of Public Health
University of California
316 Warren Hall
Berkeley, California 94720

[d]Department of Molecular Endocrinology
Whittier Institute
La Jolla, California 92037

Modulation of the responses of living tissues to injury by pituitary and adrenal hormones was demonstrated by Selye over 50 years ago.[1] Today, as more biomolecules are discovered, it appears that certain peptides share with adrenocorticotropin (ACTH) the ability to stimulate biological processes that suppress the immediate manifestations of inflammation. These agents, of which the 41-residue peptide corticotropin-releasing factor (CRF) is the prototype, may be called anti-inflammatory peptide agonists.[2,3] In this brief review, we describe the ability of CRF to inhibit inflammation in various short-term models of tissue injury, and present data on a new class of anti-inflammatory peptides, called mystixins.

ANTI-INFLAMMATORY PROPERTIES OF CRF

Leakage of plasma contents from small blood vessels into the interstitial spaces is a characteristic response of tissues to local injury.[4] In this immediate phase of inflammation, increased vascular permeability can be measured as changes in tissue volume, as increases in tissue water and protein content, or as alterations in morphology. Peptides of the CRF superfamily potently reduce vascular leakage in experimental animals.[5] For example, human/rat (h/r) CRF (used in our studies, unless specified otherwise), at systemic doses of 10 to 60 µg/kg, decreased vascular leakage induced in the paws of anesthetized rats by exposure to heat or to extreme cold, in tracheal mucosa by exposure to formaldehyde, in lung alveoli by an intravenous injection of epinephrine, in skeletal muscle by a knife cut, and in brain cortex by freezing (TABLE 1).[6]

The ability of CRF to suppress vascular leakage was independent of steroid release or hypotensive effects[6–9] (TABLE 2). For example, CRF inhibited heat-induced swelling in the paws of anesthetized adrenalectomized or hypophysectomized rats, and its effect was not mimicked by injection of dexamethasone, a potent synthetic glucocorticoid. TABLE 2 shows three models of tissue injury[5–9] in which CRF has anti-inflammatory activity; the rank order of CRF's ability to suppress

[a]These studies were supported in part by National Institute on Drug Abuse Research Grant DA-00091, the Northern California Occupational Health Center, the Chevron Risk Assessment Research Program, and the University of California Toxic Substances Teaching and Research Program.

[c]Corresponding author.

TABLE 1. Situations In Which CRF Attenuates Vascular Leakage

Tissue	Conditions or Agents Producing Leakage	Method for Quantifying Vascular Leakage
Skin Abdomen, paw	Immersion in warm (48 to 58 °C) or cold (−20 °C) solutions Exposure to concentrated inorganic acids Antidromic stimulation of saphenous nerve Intradermal injection of inflammatory mediators	Fluid displacement method Evans blue dye leakage Water content
Trachea Mucous membranes	Formaldehyde vapors Antidromic stimulation of vagus Subcutaneous injection of substance P	Evans blue dye and Monastral blue pigment leakage
Esophagus Mucous membranes	Subcutaneous injection of substance P	Monastral blue pigment leakage
Skeletal muscle	Surgical incision Local injection of substance P	Monastral blue pigment leakage
Brain cortex and meninges	Cold probe (−50 °C) applied to skull	Monastral blue pigment leakage; water content
Lung alveoli	Intratracheal instillation of formalin Intravenous epinephrine injection	Water content

leakage in these models, based on dose estimates, is: pulmonary edema > skin, mucous membrane = muscle edema. In all three models, CRF's actions were fully antagonized by α-helical-CRF$_{9-41}$, a putative antagonist of CRF at its receptor.[10]

Pain, like increased vascular permeability, is a sign of inflammation, and it is interesting to note that CRF shows positive activity in tests of antinociception. CRF inhibits the abdominal constrictor response to intraperitoneal injection of phenylbenzoquinone in mice,[11] the paw withdrawal response of anesthetized rats to 48 °C water,[7] and the paw-lick response of rats in the hot-plate test.[12] Neurophysiological

TABLE 2. Summary of Conditions Under Which Anti-Inflammatory Actions of CRF Were Expressed

	CRF Actions					
	Present after	Present after	Not Mimicked by	Independent of Changes in	Antagonized by	
Model	Adx	Hypx	Dex	MAP	αCRF$_{9-41}$	Ref. No.
Skin/heat	Yes	Yes	Yes	Yes	Yes	5, 8
Muscle/cut	Yes	NT	Yes	Yes	Yes	6
Lung/epi	NT	NT	Yes	Yes	Yes	9

Abbreviations: Adx, adrenalectomy; Hypx, hypophysectomy; Dex, pretreatment with dexamethasone; MAP, mean arterial pressure; αCRF$_{9-41}$, pretreatment with α-helical CRF$_{9-41}$; Epi, intravenous injection of epinephrine bitartrate; NT, not tested.

studies suggest that CRF interacts with peripheral sensory nerves to decrease afferent transmission of nociceptive signals. The rate of firing of wide dynamic range trigeminal neurons in anesthetized rats, increased by noxious heat applied to the whisker pad, is reduced by intravenously administered CRF.[13] Low doses of CRF inhibit vascular leakage induced by antidromic stimulation of sensory nerves, a process called neurogenic inflammation.[11,14] Anti-inflammatory actions of CRF, however, appear to be unrelated to its actions on peripheral sensory nerves because drugs which interfere with neurogenic inflammation, such as morphine, ethylketocyclazocine, and CP-96,345 (a potent nonpeptide substance P antagonist) are relatively ineffective in reducing heat-induced ($\geq 58\ °C$) swelling in the paw of the rat.[3,7]

Localized suffusion of CRF onto the hamster cheek pouch preparation (a standard model for examining vascular permeability) prevented histamine-induced leaks from postcapillary venules of the mucosa.[15] Displaceable binding sites for iodinated-Tyr°-CRF were found on the rabbit aorta,[16] and binding was reduced after removal of the endothelium. Clusters of CRF-binding sites have been demonstrated on blood vessels and on epithelial cells of the rat esophagus, in close proximity to sites of vascular leakage labeled by Monastral blue pigment.[17] These results suggest that CRF acts at peripheral sites in inhibiting vascular leakage.

MYSTIXINS—CRF-RELATED ANTI-INFLAMMATORY PEPTIDES

To search for sequences in CRF that might retain anti-inflammatory activity without ACTH-releasing properties, we synthesized and tested various peptides in animal models of heat-induced swelling and pulmonary edema. Because the amino terminus of CRF is thought to be required for ACTH release,[10] we focused initially on the carboxyl termini of ovine (o) and h/rCRF. Through a search of the Protein Identification Resource database (National Biomedical Foundation, Georgetown University, Washington, D.C.), we noted that sequences within a group of intermediate filament proteins were similar to the carboxyl terminus of oCRF and h/rCRF. Within the coil region of these proteins—keratin, desmin, vimentin, neurofilament, and other intermediate filament proteins—the highly conserved sequence (indicated by the single-letter amino acid code) -RKLLE- is found[18,19] (TABLE 3). This sequence is similar to h/rCRF$_{35-39}$, -RKLME-, and to oCRF$_{35-39}$, -RKLLD-. Because intermediate filaments may be important for the maintenance of cell morphology and regulation of vascular permeability,[20–23] we also tested short peptides containing these sequences.

Ovine CRF Fragments

oCRF has approximately the same activity as h/rCRF in inhibiting thermogenic edema in the paw of the anesthetized rat.[5,7] However, the synthetic fragments oCRF$_{21-41}$NH$_2$, oCRF$_{26-41}$NH$_2$, oCRF$_{30-41}$NH$_2$, and the free carboxylic acid fragment oCRF$_{21-41}$OH did not inhibit edema when tested at 5 mg/kg intravenously (i.v.) (FIG. 1).

Peptide Mixtures with Bioactivity

Peptides were synthesized by solid phase methodology[24] with sequences based on the carboxyl terminus of h/rCRF$_{31-41}$ and on an 11-residue segment of human type II

TABLE 3. Examples of Sequences Similar to h/rCRF$_{35-39}$ (-RKLME-) and oCRF$_{35-39}$ (-RKLLD-) in Various Proteins[a]

I.D. Code in Database	Residue No.	Primary Structure			
KRHUEA	259	LALDVEIATY	RKLLE	GEECRLNGEG	
KRHUEB	464	LALDVEIATY	RKLLE	GEECRLNGEG	**Keratins**
KRBO2B	31	LALDVEIATY	RKLLE	GEECRMSGEC	
DMHU	405	MALDVEIATY	RKLLE	GEESRINLPI	
DMPG	74	MALDVEIATY	RKLLE	GEESRINLPI	
DMHY	234	MALDVEIATY	RKLLE	GEESRINLPI	**Desmins**
DMCH	397	MALDVEIATY	RKLLE	GEENRISIPM	
VEHY	399	MALDIEIATY	RKLLE	GEESRISLPL	
VEMSGF	337	LALDIEIATY	RKLLE	GEENRITIPV	
VEHULA	377	LALDMEIHAY	RKLLE	GEEERLRLSP	**Vimentins**
VEHULC	377	LALDMEIHAY	RKLLE	GEEERLRLSP	
QFHUH	403	MALDIEIAAY	RKLLE	GEECRIGFGP	
QFPGL	389	MALDIEIAAY	RKLLE	GEETRLSFTS	
QFMSL	150	MALDIEIAAY	RKLLE	GEETRLSFTS	**Neurofilaments**
QFPGM	402	MALDIEIAAY	RKLLE	GEETRFSTFA	
DDBY18	371	MKSNGKSSSY	RKLLE	NFKNDKFNRK	
GNFF42	1157	YRLEVAYARA	RKLLE	AHKEKNKENY	
VCFFGY	97	LSESFPHSHM	RKLLE	VDTDHLRTLL	**Miscellaneous**
VHXPLJ	468	VITCQGSDDI	RKLLE	SQGRKDIKLI	
NUBSSA	159	TEPAIAFRIF	RKLLE	EKYGKEEARK	

[a]A scan for -RKLLE- was conducted on the Protein Information Resource database, National Biomedical Foundation, Georgetown University, Washington, D.C. The residue number is the position in the protein where the beginning of the sequence -RKLLE- is found.

keratin(255–265)[18] (I.D. code KRHUEA in TABLE 3) that corresponds to the region similar to h/rCRF$_{35-39}$, namely, the region containing the sequence -RKLLE-. D-Amino acid substitutions (denoted by the lower case of the single-letter code) were made as a possible means of enhancing potency. Because of cost considerations, we first tested the unpurified synthetic products. We found that the crude preparations from the synthesis of aHSnRKL(L/M)EIl-NH$_2$ and lATyRKLLEIl-HN$_2$ inhibited

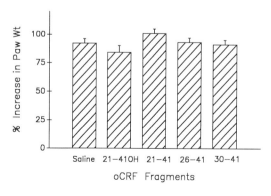

FIGURE 1. oCRF fragments do not inhibit heat-induced edema. Saline (1 mL/kg i.v.) or oCRF fragments (5 mg/kg i.v.) were injected (via a branch of the femoral vein) into pentobarbital-anesthetized rats 10 minutes before immersion of a hind paw into 58 °C water for 1 minute. Edema was measured 30 minutes later as percent increase in paw weight of the heated versus the contralateral unheated paw.

thermogenic edema at doses of 1 to 2 mg/kg i.v. High-performance liquid chromato-
graphic (HPLC) analysis of the synthetic peptide lATyRKLLEIl-NH$_2$ indicated that
the sample was at least 95% pure, with the mass spectrum showing a molecular ion
peak corresponding to the molecular mass of the expected peptide (1332 Da).
However, we found that a minor fraction obtained from HPLC of larger samples was
active at doses of less than 0.1 mg/kg i.v. in the heat-induced edema assay. The mass
spectrum of the more active fraction showed a molecular ion peak at a molecular
mass of 1422 Da, 90 Da higher than that of the major peptide.

Characterization of Anisolylated Glutamyl Peptides

Amino acid composition data and sequence analysis of the more active fraction
showed that the glutamic acid residue (E) of the expected peptide, lATyRKLLEIl-
NH$_2$, had been modified. The glutamyl residue was not detected in amino acid
analysis, and Edman degradation did not yield any more sequence information when
the cycle for this residue was reached. We attributed the 90-Da increase in mass to
anisolylation of the glutamyl residue to form a γ-methoxybenzoyl-α-aminobutyric
acid residue (*) and assigned a tentative structure (FIG. 2). Anisolylation of the

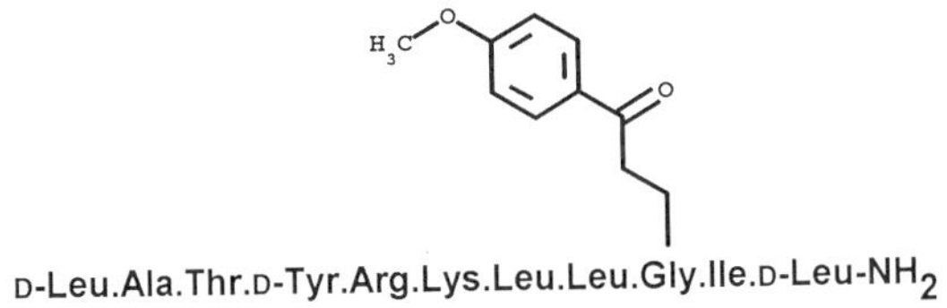

D-Leu.Ala.Thr.D-Tyr.Arg.Lys.Leu.Leu.Gly.Ile.D-Leu-NH$_2$

FIGURE 2. Assigned structure of bioactive constituent. The increase in molecular mass and
modification of the glutamyl residue are attributed to anisolylation, resulting in the formation
of a para- (major product) or ortho- (minor product) γ-methoxybenzoyl-α-aminobutyric acid
derivative, shown in the figure as a modified Gly residue.

side-chain carboxyl function of glutamic acid is known to occur from the temperature-
dependent Friedel-Crafts acylation reaction that takes place during hydrogen fluoride cleavage of glutamyl-containing peptides in the presence of anisole (methoxybenzene)[25,26] (FIG. 3). In the standard procedure for peptide synthesis, it is recommended
that the cleavage reaction be carried out at 0 °C for about 30 minutes to minimize
anisolylation.[25]

Synthesis of Anisolylated Glutamyl Peptides

Our attempt to synthesize lATyRKLL*Il-NH$_2$ by direct introduction of the
N$^\alpha$-Boc (butyloxycarbonyl) protected γ-para-methoxybenzoyl-α-aminobutyric acid
residue to the peptide chain was not successful because of rapid internal cyclization
of the deprotected amino group to the benzoyl ketone moiety after treatment with
trifluoroacetic acid in methylene chloride, which in turn terminated the synthesis of
the desired peptide (FIG. 4).

To obtain lATyRKLL*Il-NH$_2$ by an indirect method, we cleaved resin containing
the protected lATyRKLLEIl peptide at room temperature for 3 hours in excess
anisole and purified the product by gel and ion-exchange chromatography. The

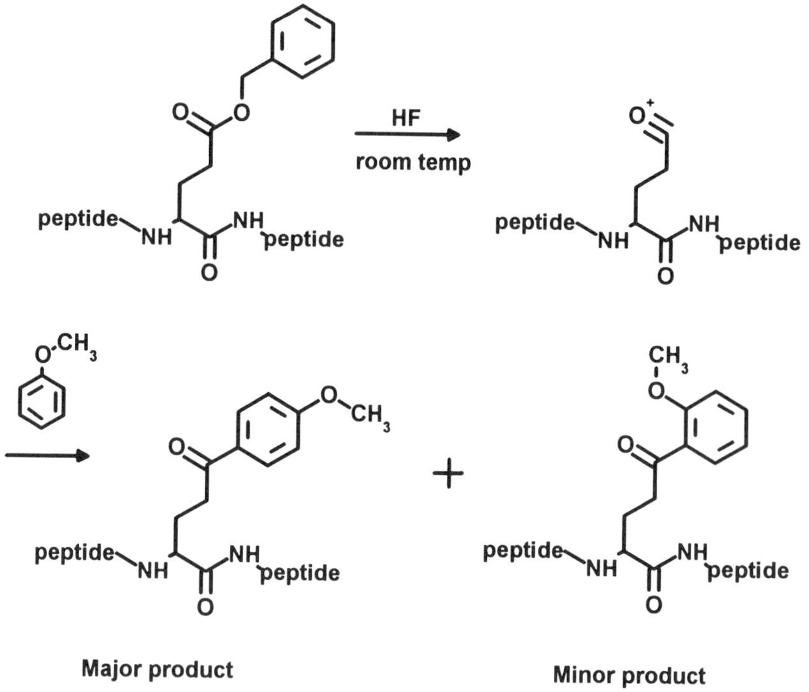

FIGURE 3. Anisolylation of glutamic acid in a Friedel-Crafts acylation reaction. During hydrogen fluoride cleavage of glutamyl-containing peptides, a reactive carbonyl is produced. In the presence of anisole, acylation of the scavenger results in the formation of para-methoxy and ortho-methoxy products.

purity and identity of the purified product were determined by HPLC, mass spectrometry, and amino acid analysis. Using a similar procedure, we synthesized and evaluated a group of undecapeptides with sequences based on the carboxyl terminus of h/rCRF (TABLE 4).

Acylation of anisole by glutamyl-containing peptides can occur on the para- or ortho- positions of anisole, as shown in FIGURE 2. The relative proportion of these two isomers has not been measured directly, although a larger proportion of

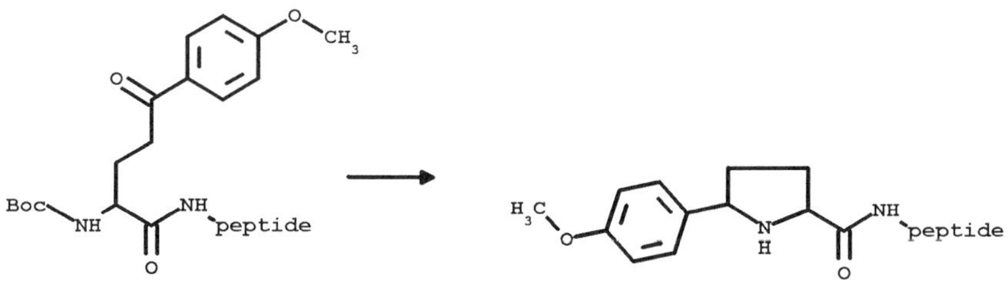

FIGURE 4. Internal cyclization reaction prevents synthesis of the desired peptide.

para-isomers would be predicted based on steric hindrance by the ortho-methoxy group. To address this question, we synthesized, cleaved, and purified a heptapeptide, RKLM*Il-NH$_2$, using the modified conditions described above, that is, hydrogen fluoride cleavage in excess anisole at room temperature for 3 hours. Proton nuclear magnetic resonance spectrum of the purified RKLM*Il-NH$_2$ was compared with the spectra of para- and ortho- Boc-anisolylated glutamic acid standards synthesized by Professor H. Rapoport of the College of Chemistry at Berkeley. Analysis of the heptapeptide spectrum indicated that over 95% of the synthetic product was the para-isomer, though there were minor peaks in the spectrum matching those of the ortho-isomer. In the heat-induced edema model (see below), the heptapeptide had a median effective dose[27] (ED$_{50}$) of 1.6 (95% CL, 0.7–3.6) mg/kg i.v. Development of methods for the direct synthesis of both para- and ortho-isomers, perhaps by coupling with a Boc-dipeptide containing the desired isomer, will help to establish the relative contributions of these two isomers to bioactivity.

TABLE 4. Anti-Inflammatory Potencies of Mystixins[a]

Synthetic Peptide	ED$_{50}$ (95% C.L.) mg/kg i.v.	
	Heat-Edema	Pulmonary Edema
aHSnRKLLEIl-NH$_2$	2.2 (1.4–3.6)	NT
lATyRKLLEIl-NH$_2$	1.9 (1.1–3.8)	NT
AHSNRKLM*Il-NH$_2$	0.88 (0.52–1.49)	NT
aHSnRKLM*Il-NH$_2$	0.24 (0.09–0.60)	NT
aHSnRKLL*Il-NH$_2$	0.11 (0.04–0.29)	0.04 (0.03–0.07)
lATyRKLL*Il-NH$_2$	0.05 (0.02–0.12)	0.04 (0.02–0.07)

[a]The ED$_{50}$ (dose inhibiting edema by 50%) and 95% C.L. (confidence limits) were according to Litchfield & Wilcoxon.[25] Heat-edema was induced in the pentobarbital-anesthetized rat by immersion of the paw in 58 °C water for 1 min. The weights of the heated and contralateral unheated paws were measured 30 minutes later. Pulmonary edema was produced by i.v. injection of epinephrine bitartrate (30 μg/kg), and the weights of the lungs determined 30 minutes later. Comparisons were to values in saline-injected animals. Lower case denotes D-amino acid; NT, not tested; *, is an anisolylated glutamic acid derivative—methoxybenzene (anisole) reacts with the free carboxyl group of glutamic acid to yield a γ-methoxybenzoyl-α-aminobutyric acid residue in place of Glu(E).

Bioactivity of Anisolylated Glutamyl Peptides

Intravenous injection of the peptides listed in TABLE 4 into the pentobarbital-anesthetized rat caused, like i.v. CRF,[28] a rapid fall in blood pressure. The duration of this hypotension was dose-dependent, pressure being lowered for up to 40 min after a 0.4 mg/kg i.v. dose of lATyRKLL*Il-NH$_2$ before returning to pre-injection levels. The skin of animals injected with these peptides did not show the flushed appearance that is characteristic of the vasodilatory action of CRF.[29]

The anti-inflammatory activities of the peptides listed in TABLE 4 were assayed in the heat-induced edema model wherein the paw of the anesthetized rat was immersed in 58 °C water for 1 minute, and the increase in paw weight measured 30 minutes later was taken as an index of increased vascular permeability.[2] Saline or peptides were injected 1 hour before exposure to heat to reduce the possibility of hypotension contributing to the observed effects. Replacement of the glutamyl residue by the anisolylated derivative enhanced potency 20–47-fold. The D-amino acid-containing peptide aHSnRKLM*Il-NH$_2$ was about three times more potent than the similar sequence (AHSNRKLM*Il-NH$_2$) containing only L-amino acids. Replacement of Met with Leu in position 8 yielded an undecapeptide with increased potency. The two most potent peptides, aHSnRKLL*Il-NH$_2$ and IATyRKLL*Il-NH$_2$, were also tested in the epinephrine-induced pulmonary edema model where they had ED$_{50}$ values of 40 μg/kg i.v. These results suggested that the undecapeptides, like CRF, may be effective in reducing edema caused by increased hydrostatic pressure in the lower respiratory tract.[9]

As shown in FIGURE 5, the putative CRF receptor antagonist α-helical CRF$_{9-41}$, which is effective against the central and peripheral vascular actions of CRF but less so against its ACTH-releasing properties,[10,30] blocked the inhibitory effects of CRF on thermogenic edema. This antagonist, at an agonist:antagonist molar ratio of approximately 3:1, did not prevent the antiedema effects of the undecapeptide aHSnRKLL*Il-HN$_2$.

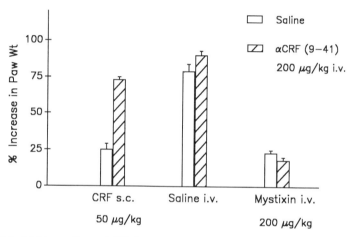

FIGURE 5. Inhibitory effects of aHSnRKLL*Il-NH$_2$ on heat-induced edema were not blocked by α-helical-CRF$_{9-41}$. h/rCRF injected s.c. 30 minutes before heat exposure inhibited edema, an effect antagonized by α-helical-CRF$_{9-41}$ injected 5 minutes before heat. α-Helical-CRF$_{9-41}$ injected 5 minutes before aHSnRKLL*Il-NH$_2$ and 15 minutes before heat exposure did not prevent the anti-inflammatory effects of aHSnRKLL*Il-NH$_2$.

We have called these short anti-inflammatory peptides containing the sequence -RKL(M/L)*Il-NH$_2$, with an N-terminal protecting group, mystixins because their powerful mode of action is unknown, mysterious, and intriguing.

SUMMARY

The permeability of endothelial surfaces increases in response to injury. We have shown that vascular leakage in experimental models of tissue injury can be inhibited by CRF and by a novel class of peptides that we call mystixins. Binding sites for iodinated-Tyr^o-CRF have been revealed in mucous membranes, and immunoreactive CRF-like materials have been found in inflamed tissues.[31,32] Perhaps the breakdown of cytoskeletal intermediate filaments after insult generates or exposes peptide domains similar to mystixins. Endogenous CRF-like or mystixin-like peptides, if activated or released locally in injured tissues, may function as agonists to counteract the immediate inflammatory response. If this is so, the peripheral actions of these peptides add a new dimension to the idea that CRF and related substances organize and regulate an organism's response to stress.

REFERENCES

1. SELYE, H. 1950. The Physiology and Pathology of Exposure to Stress: A Treatise on the Concepts of the General-Adaptation-Syndrome and the Diseases of Adaptation. Acta, Inc. Medical Publishers. Montreal.
2. WEI, E. T. & H. A. THOMAS. 1993. Anti-inflammatory peptide agonists. Annu. Rev. Pharmacol. Toxicol. **33:** 91–108.
3. WEI, E. T., G. C. GAO & H. A. THOMAS. 1993. Peripheral anti-inflammatory actions of CRF. *In* Corticotropin-Releasing Factor. D. J. Chadwick, J. Marsh & K. Ackrill, Eds. Ciba Found. Symp. **172:** 258–268. Wiley. Chichester.
4. COTRAN, R. S., V. KUMAR & S. L. ROBBINS. 1989. Inflammation and repair. *In* Pathologic Basis of Disease. 4th edit. S. L. Robbins, Ed. **2:** 39–86. W. B. Saunders. Philadelphia, PA.
5. WEI, E. T. & J. G. KIANG. 1989. Peptides of the corticoliberin superfamily inhibit thermal and neurogenic inflammation. Eur. J. Pharmacol. **168:** 81–86.
6. WEI, E. T. & G. C. GAO. 1991. Corticotropin-releasing factor: An inhibitor of vascular leakage in rat skeletal muscle and brain cortex after injury. Regul. Pept. **33:** 93–104.
7. KIANG, J. G. & E. T. WEI. 1987. Corticotropin-releasing factor inhibits thermal injury. J. Pharmacol. Exp. Ther. **243:** 517–520.
8. WEI, E. T., J. C. WONG & J. G. KIANG. 1990. Decreased inflammatory responsiveness of hypophysectomized rats to heat is reversed by a corticotropin-releasing factor (CRF) antagonist. Regul. Pept. **27:** 317–323.
9. SERDA, S. M. & E. T. WEI. 1992. Epinephrine-induced pulmonary edema in rats is inhibited by corticotropin-releasing factor. Pharmacol. Res. **26:** 85–91.
10. RIVIER, J., C. RIVIER & W. VALE. 1984. Synthetic competitive antagonists of corticotropin-releasing factor: Effect on ACTH secretion in the rat. Science **224:** 889–891.
11. WEI, E. T., J. G. KIANG, P. BUCHAN & T. W. SMITH. 1986. Corticotropin-releasing factor inhibits neurogenic plasma extravasation in the rat paw. J. Pharmacol. Exp. Ther. **238:** 783–787.
12. HARGREAVES, K. M., G. P. MUELLER, R. DUBNER, D. GOLDSTEIN & R. A. DIONNE. 1987. Corticotropin-releasing factor (CRF) produces analgesia in humans and rats. Brain Res. **422:** 154–157.
13. POREE, L., A. H. DICKENSON & E. T. WEI. 1989. Corticotropin-releasing factor inhibits the response of trigeminal neurons to noxious heat. Brain Res. **502:** 349–355.
14. LEMBECK, F. & P. HOLZER. 1979. Substance P as a neurogenic mediator of antidromic vasodilitation and neurogenic plasma extravasation. Arch. Pharmacol. **310:** 175–183.
15. JOYNER, W. L. & E. T. WEI. 1989. Mechanism for the anti-inflammatory effect of corticotropin-releasing factor (CRF). FASEB J. **3:** 272.
16. DASHWOOD, M. R., H. E. ANDREWS & E. T. WEI. 1987. Binding of [^{125}I]Tyr-corticotropin-releasing factor to rabbit aorta is reduced by removal of the endothelium. Eur. J. Pharmacol. **135:** 111–112.
17. GAO, G. C., M. R. DASHWOOD & E. T. WEI. 1991. Corticotropin-releasing factor inhibition of substance P-induced vascular leakage in rats: Possible sites of action. Peptides **12:** 639–644.
18. HANUKOGLU, I. & E. FUCHS. 1983. The cDNA sequence of a type II cytoskeletal keratin reveals constant and variable structural domains among keratins. Cell **33:** 915–924.
19. QUAX, W., W. V. EGBERTS, W. HENDRIKS, Y. QUAX-JEUKEN & H. BLOEMENDAL. 1983. The structure of the vimentin gene. Cell **35:** 215–223.
20. NAGLE, R. B. 1988. Intermediate filaments: A review of the basic biology. Am. J. Surg. Pathol. **12** (Suppl. 1): 4–16.

21. GOLDMAN, G., R. WELBOURN, S. ALEXANDER, J. M. KLAUSNER & M. WILES. 1991. Modulation of pulmonary permeability in vivo with agents that effect the cytoskeleton. Surgery **109**: 533–538.
22. ALEXANDER, J. S., W. F. PATTON, M. U. YOON & D. SHEPRO. 1991. Cytokeratin filament modulation in pulmonary microvascular endothelial cells by vasoactive agents and culture confluency. Tissue & Cell **23**: 141–150.
23. LETAI, A., P. A. COULOMBE & E. FUCHS. 1992. Do the ends justify the mean? Proline mutations at the ends of the keratin coiled-coil rod segment are more disruptive than internal mutations. J. Cell Biol. **116**: 1181–1195.
24. MERRIFIELD, R. B. 1963. Solid phase peptide synthesis. I. The synthesis of a tetrapeptide. J. Am. Chem. Soc. **85**: 2149–2154.
25. STEWART, J. M. & J. D. YOUNG. 1984. Solid Phase Peptide Synthesis: 43. Pierce Chemical Co. Rockford, IL.
26. CHIBBER, B. A. K., S. URANO & F. J. CASTELLINO. 1990. Synthesis, purification, and properties of a peptide that enhances the activation of human [Glu^1]plasminogen by tissue plasminogen activator and retards fibrin polymerization. Int. J. Pept. Protein Res. **35**: 73–80.
27. LITCHFIELD, J. T. & F. WILCOXON. 1949. A simplified method of evaluating dose-effect experiments. J. Pharmacol. Exp. Ther. **96**: 99–113.
28. VALE, W., J. SPEISS & J. RIVIER. 1981. Characterization of a 41-residue ovine hypothalamic peptide that stimulates secretion of corticotropin and β-endorphin. Science **213**: 1394–1397.
29. OWENS, M. J. & C. B. NEMEROFF. 1991. Physiology and pharmacology of corticotropin-releasing factor. Pharmacol. Rev. **43**: 425–473.
30. FISHER, L., C. RIVIER, J. RIVIER & M. BROWN. 1991. Differential antagonist activity of alpha-helical corticotropin-releasing factor 9–41 in three bioassay systems. Endocrinology **129**: 1312–1316.
31. HARGREAVES, K. M., A. H. COSTELLO & J. L. JORIS. 1989. Release from inflamed tissue of a substance with properties similar to corticotropin-releasing factor. Neuroendocrinology **49**: 476–482.
32. KARALIS, K., H. SANO, J. REDWINE, S. LISTWAK & R. L. WILDER. 1991. Autocrine or paracrine inflammatory actions of corticotropin-releasing hormone in vivo. Science **254**: 421–423.

"Restraint Ulcer" as a Model
of Stress-Induced Gastric Lesion

A Historical Note

SERGE BONFILS

INSERM U.10, Hôpital Bichat
F-75877 Paris Cedex 18, France

In 1936, Hans Selye presented a short note in *Nature* entitled "A syndrome produced by diverse nocuous agents."[1] In a few lines, Selye introduced revolutionary concepts that remain, nearly 60 years later, the background of countless scientific works. "... if the organism is severely damaged by acute non-specific noxious agents such as exposure to cold, surgical injury, production of spinal shock ... a syndrome develops in three stages: during the first stage ... are observed ... formation of acute erosions in the digestive tract, particularly in the stomach...."[1] This was the modest announcement of the birth of the stress ulcer.

Since that time the topic has widely developed, with each year leading to a variety of new research aims but sharing the same concept of the nonspecificity of the triggering process and the same damage response of erosions (or ulcers) to the glandular stomach of the rat.

In the world of animal experiments, stress ulcers are used in two fundamental ways. First, they are used in considering the pathophysiological model of stress itself and the cascade of events following its introduction; gastric lesions appear to be the easiest obtainable evidence that a "stress" mechanism is involved or conversely that animals are protected from stress (whatever the protective mechanism involved) when the stomach remains intact. Second, stress ulcers are used by gastroenterologists and people interested in ulcer pathophysiology, particularly in relation to the psychosomatic aspects of ulcer disease in man.

In both animals and humans the pathogenesis of gastric lesions is a complex process. Psychological variables that are experiential in nature and behavioral characteristics may play a significant role in ulcerogenesis, as stated by Ader on the basis of a large compilation of data in 1971.[2] Among the multiple techniques used, it is difficult to be certain that no physical aggression was involved even if the handling of the rat was very limited. TABLE 1 gives a sample of methods published since 1956: none of them is safe from bodily intervention and it is likely that the interaction between the physical disturbance and the psychological factor(s) is responsible for ulcer occurrence. Conversely, one can hypothesize that for any experimental method of ulcer production, the pathogenesis of the digestive disturbance must take cognizance of the role of psychological influences. The fact that psychological stress-induced lesions are constantly observed in the glandular part of the stomach, and that they are macroscopically and histologically indistinguishable regardless of the specific stimulus conditions used to induce the lesion, makes all these models, to some extent, comparable and useful for several purposes; for example, in studies on stress pathophysiology, pharmacological testing, and analysis of biological predisposition (perhaps genetically determined).

One major problem in the comparative assessment of the various techniques, as well as the adequate use of them, is stress quantitation. A 100% positive result (i.e.,

TABLE 1. Stress Ulcer in the Rat—Psychological Aggressions[a]

Standard restraint		
Immobilization	1936	Selye
	1956	Rossi, Bonfils
	1959	Sines
	1960	Brodie
Variant restraints		
Restriction curve test (variable volumes)	1960	Bonfils
Electric grid	1960	Desmarez
Fasting	1962	Brodie
Shortening	1962	Brodie
Fasting and cold (hemorrhage)	1963	Brodie
Cold	1966	Buchel
Cold and electro-stress	1967	Rosenberg
Approach-avoidance	1956	Sawrey
Prolonged modification of environment	1959	Levrat, Lambert
Activity-Stress	1964	Paré

[a]From R. Ader.[2]

ulcer frequency) is generally considered as an adequate baseline. We are very skeptical concerning this a priori viewpoint, the validity of which is highly disputable. If precise pathophysiological processes are obtained by a given technique, a dose-dependent response should be observed; only variations of stress intensity with precise quantitation are able to give such a result. Reaching lesion production of 100% means that no further increase in response frequency might be obtained, but the stronger the stimulus the less specific the response. In other words, it is likely that with an ulcer frequency of 100%, in some circumstances various nonspecific mechanisms would intervene as additional pathogenetic factors. Thus the analysis of protective actions or conditioning factors would be rendered difficult or incorrect. Our work on the restraint-induced stress ulcer was largely focused on this kind of problem.

The fact that immobilization is a stressful situation for the rat was suggested in another paper of Selye *et al.* dated 1936[3] and further mentioned in the classic 1950 issue of his book[4] *The Physiology and Pathology of Exposure to Stress.* "This possibility has not yet been adequately studied, but observations on the rat suggest that forced restraint can produce GAS [general adaptation syndrome] changes."

When starting our work, Selye's name was world renowned but gastroenterologists were not keenly interested in the GAS concept. We were mainly working on gastric secretion. Our initial observations of ventricular ulcers in experimental animals were obtained by chance, in gastric fistula rats undergoing several hours of immobilization for easy juice collection. Following various types of control, we finally concluded that immobilization and/or restraint was the pathogenic factor for these lesions. In accordance with our first publication on this subject in 1956,[5] we kept working on immobilized rats without performing a gastric fistula. In 1960, we experienced one of the major rewards of our research: we met and became friends with David Brodie, whose article[6] (with H. Hanson) was fundamental to a wide diffusion of the model, either directly (320 citations in the literature until 1986) or by referring others to our work[5] (140 citations for our paper of 1956).

The originality of our work, as emphasized by David Brodie, was that we were the first to use restraint stress on rats with the specific aim of producing experimental ulcers rather than as general stressors. This was 20 years after Selye's work. Presented first as a simple pathophysiological model, then as a pharmacological tool, the restraint-induced ulcer was extended to a psychosomatic model. It was explored along these lines by our group as well as by numerous colleagues, with special contribution from D. Brodie,[7,8] R. Ader,[2] J. O. Sines,[9] and W. Paré[10] (TABLE 1).

For over 10 years, our group published a variety of results concerning histological lesions, healing, duration of restraint, volume of restraint, acid secretion variations, body motility patterns, the influence of vagotomy, adrenalectomy, hypophysectomy (TABLE 2), and more general pharmacological tests. Among these 23 papers, the main interest of our group (particularly of M. Dubrasquet[11]) was related to a quantitation of the psychological stimulus by modifying the volume of restraint (using a restriction curve test). Thus the percentage of animals presenting gastric ulcers may vary from 25% (760-mL restriction volume) to 83% (180-mL restriction volume). According to the chosen volume one could find evidence for either the protection or aggravation of the pathophysiological process. Another interest of restriction volume variations resulted in the pathophysiological analysis of the model. If the importance of the pituitary-adrenal axis, as suggested by Selye, was not to be reduced, other factors may have played an important role, either quantitatively or as "gate controls." This was evidenced by Bonfils and Lambling using the restriction curve test.[12]

TABLE 2. Pathophysiology of Restraint-Induced Ulcers

Main stimulus: Volumetric restriction	
Additional stimuli: Starvation, cold, sensory stimulation	
Transmission Pathways	
Endocrine (adrenal cortex, pituitary): Specific, nutritional	
Nervous, vagal: Secretory, nutritional	
Autonomic nervous action on the gastric capillary bed	
Target Organ	
Gastric secretion maintained	
Indetermined Factors	
Genetic	Strain
Dietetic	Circadian rhythms
Breeding (weaning)	Gastric hypersecretion
CNS excitability	Adaptation to reiteration

In conclusion, although described more than 30 years ago as a tool for both pharmacological and pathophysiological studies, restraint-induced stress ulcer still appears to be a useful model. Very simple and reproducible, it allows the study of drugs not only for their protective or aggravating effect, but also for assessing the rapidity of healing. For scientists devoted to the study of stress it is largely accepted as a valid model, but often without absolute control of the gastric lesions induced. We strongly believe that even by carrying out a technique repeatedly, with utmost care and precision, we are limited in our control in targeting the pathophysiological process. Gastric lesions are *the* correct evidence for an adequate performance of the model; however, it cannot be accepted as ultimately defining the involvement of a unique biological mechanism.

REFERENCES

1. SELYE, H. 1936. A syndrome produced by diverse nocuous agents. Nature **138:** 32.
2. ADER, R. 1971. Experimentally induced gastric lesions. Results and implications of studies in animals. Adv. Psychosom. Med. **6:** 1–39.
3. SELYE, H., R. I. STEHLE & J. P. COLLIP. 1936. Recent advances in experimental production of gastric ulcer. Can. Med. Assoc. J. **347:** 339.
4. SELYE, H. 1950. The physiology and pathology of exposure to stress. Acta Inc. Montreal.
5. ROSSI, G., S. BONFILS, F. LIEFOOGHE & A. LAMBLING. 1956. Une technique nouvelle pour produire des ulcérations gastriques chez le rat blanc: l'ulcère de contrainte. C. R. Soc. Biol. (Paris) **150:** 2124–2126.
6. BRODIE, D. A. & H. M. HANSON. 1960. A study of the factors involved in the production of gastric ulcers by the restraint technique. Gastroenterology **38:** 353–360.
7. BRODIE, D. 1962. Ulceration of the stomach produced by restraint in rats. Gastroenterology **43:** 107–109.
8. BRODIE, D. A., R. W. MARSHALL & O. M. MORENO. 1962. Effect of restraint on gastric acidity in the rat. Am. J. Physiol. **202(4):** 812–814.
9. SINES, J. O. 1962. Strain differences in activity, emotionality, body weight and susceptibility to stress induced stomach lesions. J. Genet. Psychol. **101:** 209–217.
10. PARÉ, W. P. 1980. Psychological studies of stress ulcer in the rat. Brain Res. Bull. **5(Suppl. 1):** 73–79.
11. BONFILS, S., G. LIEFOOGHE, X. GELLE, M. DUBRASQUET & A. LAMBLING. 1960. Experimental restraint "ulcer" of the white rat. III. Demonstration and analysis of the role of certain psychological factors. Rev. Fr. Etud. Clin. Biol. **5:** 571–581.
12. BONFILS, S. & A. LAMBLING. 1963. Psychological factors and psychopharmacological actions in the restraint-induced gastric ulcer. In Pathophysiology of Peptic Ulcer. S. C. Skoryna, Ed.: 153–171. McGill University Press. Montreal.

Role of CRF in Stress-Related Alterations of Gastric and Colonic Motor Function[a]

YVETTE TACHÉ,[b,c] HUBERT MÖNNIKES,[b]
BRUNO BONAZ,[b] AND JEAN RIVIER[d]

[b]CURE/Digestive Disease Center
V.A. Wadsworth Medical Center, and
Department of Medicine and Brain Research Institute
University of California at Los Angeles
Los Angeles, California 90073

[d]The Clayton Foundation Laboratories for Peptide Biology
The Salk Institute
La Jolla, California 92037

The impact of emotion on digestive function was recognized nearly 200 years ago. In 1802, the French physiologist, Pierre Jean Georges Cabanis, reported: "Should a man receive bad news, or should sad and baneful passions suddenly arise in his soul, his stomach and intestines will immediately cease to act on the foods contained in them ... digestion ceases entirely."[1] In 1833, Beaumont noticed in his fistulous subject that "fear, anger, or whatever depresses or disturbs his nervous system suppresses gastric secretion and delays gastric digestion and emptying of the stomach."[2] A century later, experimental evidence provided by Cannon[3] established that the fight or flight response is associated with a reduction in gastric acid secretion and motor activity. In 1934, Hall proposed using defecation scores as a measure for individual differences in fearfulness in rodents exposed to unfamiliar surroundings or arousing situations.[4] Selye[5] developed in 1936 the unifying concept of stress and drew attention to the omnipresent sign of alterations in the stomach as part of the bodily response to stress. Since then, the influence and mechanisms of action of stress on gastrointestinal secretory and motor function have been the object of intense investigation in experimental animals and in humans.[6–8]

Over the past decade, the characterization of the hypothalamic corticotropin-releasing factor, CRF, by Vale et al.,[9] followed by the development of a specific CRF antagonist by Rivier et al.,[10] has paved the way to the study of the central mechanisms underlying stress-related alterations of gastrointestinal function. This paper reviews compelling experimental evidence that supports a role of CRF in mediating the stress-related inhibition of gastric motor function and the acceleration of colonic motor activity. The relevance of these findings to the underlying mechanisms of postoperative gastric ileus and irritable bowel syndrome (IBS) is also addressed.

[a]This work was supported by the National Institutes of Health grants MH 00663 (Y.T.), DK-33061 (Y.T.), and DK-26741 (J.R.).
[c]Address correspondence to Y. Taché, Ph.D., V.A. Wadsworth Medical Center, Building 115, Room 115, Wilshire and Sawtelle Blvd., Los Angeles, California 90073.

ROLE OF CRF IN STRESS-RELATED INHIBITION
OF GASTRIC MOTOR FUNCTION

Inhibition of Gastric Motor Function by Central CRF

CRF and the amphibian related peptide, sauvagine, injected into the cisterna magna or the lateral ventricle are well documented as inhibiting gastric emptying of a liquid noncaloric or a solid caloric meal in various experimental animals including rats, mice, and dogs.[11-17] The delay in gastric emptying is associated with an inhibition of gastric contractility in fasted rats and dogs and in fed sheep.[18-21] Although the central injection of CRF has consistently been reported to have an inhibitory effect on gastric emptying in rodents, one group of investigators has presented evidence that CRF injected intracerebroventricularly (i.c.v.) in mice has a stimulatory effect on the gastric emptying of a milk solution.[22-24]

CRF antibody or the CRF antagonist, α-helical CRF$_{9-41}$, injected peripherally at doses that blocked the gastric stasis induced by peripheral injection of CRF, did not alter the inhibition of gastric emptying induced by CRF injected into the cerebrospinal fluid (CSF) in rats and mice.[12,16] These data demonstrated that CRF injected into the CSF acts in the brain to delay gastric emptying and not after peptide leakage into the periphery. Further studies have established that responsive brain sites for CRF to influence gastric motor function are located in the paraventricular nucleus of the hypothalamus (PVN) and the dorsal vagal complex (DVC) in rats.[25,26] By contrast, the lateral hypothalamus, central amygdala, and locus coeruleus did not influence gastric emptying when microinjected with CRF.[25,27] In addition, intrathecal injection of CRF inhibits gastric emptying of a noncaloric solution in mice, suggesting a possible spinal site of action.[16] The CRF antagonist, α-helical CRF$_{9-41}$, injected into the CSF with CRF at 10–100:1 fold ratio blocked CRF-induced inhibition of gastric emptying in rats and mice.[13,16,28,29] These data show that the central action of CRF is mediated through a specific interaction with CRF receptors.

From results obtained in dogs injected intravenously with ACTH or cortisol or in hypophysectomized rodents, it was inferred that central CRF-induced inhibition of gastric motor function occurs independently of the stimulation of the pituitary-adrenal axis.[15,16,18] Several sets of evidence suggest that the pathways through which intracisternal CRF delays gastric emptying is vagal dependent. First, CRF injected into the cisterna magna or the dorsal vagal complex inhibited gastric contractions that had been stimulated by central vagal activation using thyrotropin releasing hormone or 2-deoxy-glucose in fasted rats.[21,26] By contrast, intracisternal CRF had no effect on carbachol-stimulated gastric motility.[21] Second, intracisternal injection of CRF decreased efferent activity recorded from the gastric branch of the vagus in urethane-anesthetized rats.[30] Third, vagotomy prevented intracisternal CRF-induced inhibition of gastric emptying in rats whereas adrenalectomy had no effect.[12] However, when the peptide was injected into the lateral ventricle, vagotomy had no effect and when microinjected into the PVN, it reduced the inhibition of gastric emptying by 50%. In addition, sympathetic blockade or adrenalectomy prevented or attenuated i.c.v. CRF-induced delay in gastric emptying in rats and mice.[15,16,25] These data suggest that different autonomic pathways may be involved in inhibiting gastric emptying, depending upon whether CRF acts on medullary or forebrain sites. Peripheral mechanisms mediating the inhibition of gastric motor function are still to be investigated. Naloxone-sensitive opioid mechanisms have been ruled out in rats and mice.[12,16] In dogs there is evidence that the inhibition of cyclic release of motilin may play a role.[19]

Inhibition of Gastric Motor Function by Peripheral CRF

CRF and the related peptide, sauvagine, are equal or less potent in their ability to inhibit gastric emptying and contractility when injected peripherally (intravenously, intraperitoneally, subcutaneously) than when injected centrally in rats, mice, and dogs.[11-13,15,16,28,31-34] Such an effect is transduced by peripheral CRF receptors because it can be completely prevented by peripheral but not CSF injection of the CRF antagonist in rats and mice.[13,16,28] The action of CRF is independent of opioid mechanisms and sympathetic nervous system pathways in mice, rats, and dogs.[16,31,32,34] The integrity of vagal pathways is required for the full expression of peripherally injected CRF and sauvagine-induced inhibition of gastric emptying and contractility in rats and mice.[34,35] *In vitro* studies using rat antral longitudinal muscles further demonstrated that CRF inhibits spontaneous contractions.[34] CRF action is not directly exerted on smooth muscle cells, but involves neural transmission within the enteric nervous system.[34]

Reversal by CRF Antagonists of Stress-Induced Inhibition of Gastric Motor Function: Implications for the Understanding of Postoperative Gastric Ileus

In humans, various stressors including fear, labyrinthine stimulation, painful stimuli on the hand, preoperative anxiety, viewing of stressful films, playing video-games, or high-intensity exercises delay gastric emptying and postprandial antral motility.[6,36-39] Likewise, in experimental animals, different stressors such as radiation, acoustic stress, passive avoidance, hemorrhage, electric footshocks, brain surgery, and restraint inhibit gastric emptying of a caloric or noncaloric liquid meal.[37] However, variations in the response exist depending upon the intensity and the nature of the stressors.[6,37,40]

The activation of CRF synthesis and release in the brain by various stressors[41-44] and the inhibition of gastric motor function by central CRF suggest a role of endogenous CRF in the gastric response to stress. Further evidence of such a role came from the demonstration that α-helical CRF_{9-41} injected intracisternally or into the lateral ventricle prevented the alteration of gastric emptying induced by all stressors investigated so far, namely, restraint, ether anesthesia, cold exposure, noise, trephination, and footshock in rats and mice.[22,24,25,28,29] Two sets of evidence indicate that the PVN is a site of action where endogenous CRF triggers the delay in gastric emptying in response to restraint. First, restraint-induced delay in gastric emptying is prevented by bilateral microinjections of the CRF antagonist into the PVN.[25] Second, restraint activates CRF-containing neurons and increases CRF expression in the PVN as shown by the induction of c-fos mRNA and CRF mRNA by *in situ* hybridization.[44-46]

Another interesting observation in rats was the demonstration that intracisternal injection of α-helical CRF_{9-41} or another recently developed CRF antagonist, $[DPhe^{12},Nle^{21,38},C^{\alpha}\text{-}MeLeu^{37}]rCRF_{12-41}$, dose-dependently inhibited gastric stasis induced by surgical stress (laparotomy and cecal manipulation).[29,47] The new CRF analog proved to be fivefold more potent than α-helical CRF_{9-41} in antagonizing central CRF-induced delay in gastric emptying.[47] By contrast, the CRF receptor antagonists do not influence resting gastric motor function.[22,24,25,28,29] Recent neuro-anatomical studies have provided further support for the role of brain CRF in postoperative gastric ileus. Abdominal surgery activates CRF as well as arginine vasopressin (AVP), and oxytocin neurons in the PVN. This has been shown by the high number of neurons in the parvocellular part of the PVN that express c-fos immunoreactivity after abdominal surgery and double immunostaining of c-fos positive cells with the peptide antibody.[48] Activation of peptidergic PVN neurons including CRF may be conveyed by A1, A2, and A6 catecholaminergic systems, which are also activated by abdominal surgery and are well established as having an excitatory synaptic input on CRF neurons in the PVN.[48–51] The inhibition of gastric emptying of caloric solution induced by intraperitoneal injection of 0.6% acetic acid was also dose-dependently reversed by the intracisternal injection of α-helical $CRF_{9–41}$ in rats.[52] In addition, we recently demonstrated that the inhibition of gastric emptying induced by intracisternal injection of interleukin-1β is partly reversed by prior intracisternal injection of α-helical $CRF_{9–41}$.[53] These results reveal a role of brain CRF in mediating gastric stasis after abdominal surgery, peritonitis, and situations that activate the production of inflammatory mediators.

The role of peripheral CRF has been the object of fewer investigations. However, peripheral injection of the CRF antagonist can reverse, in part, abdominal surgery-induced delay in gastric emptying in rats.[54] The site of action of endogenous CRF is independent of capsaicin-sensitive afferents.[54]

ROLE OF CRF IN STRESS-RELATED STIMULATION OF COLONIC MOTOR FUNCTION

Stimulation of Colonic Motor Function by Central CRF

Marked stimulation of colonic transit and fecal output have been consistently observed after injection of CRF into the lateral brain ventricle in rats.[13,15,28,55] The PVN and the locus coeruleus are the two responsive sites which have so far been identified. Following microinjection of CRF into the PVN or the locus coeruleus at a maximal effective dose, colonic transit time is reduced by fivefold, and fecal output is increased up to 20 times in fed or fasted rats.[25,27,56] By contrast, microinjection of CRF into the lateral hypothalamus or central amygdala had no effect.[25,56] In addition, one-third of the animals developed watery diarrhea within 15–20 minutes of CRF injection into the CSF or PVN at the maximal effective dose.[25] CRF action is mediated through interactions with central CRF receptors. This was shown by the complete reversal of the stimulatory effect of i.c.v. CRF on colonic motor function by α-helical $CRF_{9–41}$ injected into the CSF, but not intravenously.[13,15,28] The stimulation of colonic transit and fecal output induced by CRF injected into the lateral ventricle or PVN is well correlated with the increase in intraluminal pressure and phasic contractility or frequency of spike burst recorded in the cecum and proximal colon of conscious fasted or fed rats.[57–59]

There is evidence that the central action of CRF to stimulate colonic contractility involves brain AVP receptors. AVP antagonist injected i.c.v. blocked the increase in spike burst in the proximal colon induced by i.c.v. CRF.[60] In addition, AVP injected into the CSF stimulates the occurrence of colonic spike bursts.[60] Pharmacological studies revealed that several transmitters can modulate i.c.v. CRF-induced stimulation of colonic motility[61] (see also Junien and Gué, this volume). The central action of CRF and mental stress (fear conditioning) to increase cecal motility are blocked by i.c.v. injection of neuropeptide Y (NPY), sigma ligands, *d*-NANM (+ N-allyl-normetazocine) and JO 1784,[62] and cholecystokinin (CCK) and peripheral injection of the 5HT$_{1A}$ agonist.[57,63–65] The NPY antagonistic effect appears to be conveyed by an interaction with sigma and CCK$_A$ receptors.[63,64]

The peripheral mechanisms whereby central CRF stimulates colonic transit and the frequency of spike burst are not related to endocrine changes. A similar colonic motor response is observed in sham-operated and hypophysectomized, adrenalecto-mized or naloxone-treated rats.[15,59] Moreover, peripheral injection of ACTH or β-endorphin does not reproduce the effects of central CRF.[15,59] Pharmacological studies indicate that the stimulation of colonic motor function induced by CRF injected i.c.v. or into the PVN is transduced mainly by the parasympathetic component of the autonomic nervous system and muscarinic mechanisms. Chlor-isondamine, vagotomy, and atropine blocked CRF action whereas a sympathetic blockade did not modify the CRF effects in rats and dogs.[15,25,56,58] Direct projections from the locus coeruleus to the sacral spinal cord have been established,[66] although the pathways conveying CRF action at that site are still unknown.

Reversal by Central CRF Antagonist of Stress-Induced Stimulation of Colonic Motor Function

Various acute stressors such as immersion of the hand in ice water, psychologi-cally stressful tests or fear reportedly increased colonic contractility in healthy sub-jects.[67–71] Recently, several non-ulcerogenic models of psychological stress stimulat-ing colonic motor function (transit, fecal excretion, and frequency of spike burst) have been developed in fasted or fed rats. These stressors include partial or complete re-straint at room temperature or in cold, voluntary confinement by standing on a small platform to avoid a surrounding aversive stimulus (water) and conditioned fear triggered by placing rats in an environment where they previously experienced inescapable footshocks.[13,25,28,56,59,72–74] The autonomic nervous system is involved in mediating stress-related stimulation of colonic motor function, independently of the release of pituitary-adrenal derived factors as demonstrated for the central action of CRF.[59,72,73]

α-Helical CRF$_{9–41}$ injected i.c.v. blocks the increases in colonic transit and fecal output induced by partial restraint or water avoidance stress while having no effect on resting colonic motor function in rats.[13,28,75] Likewise, the increase in the fre-quency of colonic spike burst induced by conditioned fear in fed or fasted rats is blocked by an i.c.v. injection of the CRF antagonist.[59] A recent study also indicates that i.c.v. injection of the CRF antagonist prevents i.c.v. interleukin-1β induced stimulation of cecocolonic contractions.[76]

Further neuropharmacological and neuroanatomical studies established that the PVN is an important site of action for endogenous CRF to mediate stress-induced stimulation of colonic transit. CRF neurons in the PVN are activated by various stressors including restraint and water avoidance stress as shown by the localization of c-fos expression in this nucleus.[45,46,75,77] In addition, i.c.v. injection of α-helical CRF$_{9–41}$ mainly decreases the water avoidance stress-induced stimulation of c-fos expression in the PVN and the locus coeruleus and colonic transit.[75] In addition, α-helical CRF$_{9–41}$ microinjected into the PVN prevents restraint and water avoidance stress-induced increase in colonic transit and fecal output.[25,56]

The role of peripheral CRF has not been fully explored although evidence from one study shows that intravenous injection of CRF enhanced colonic transit and that the CRF antagonist prevented wrap restraint-induced stimulation of colonic transit and fecal output.[13] However, further studies are required to address the site and mechanisms of action of peripheral CRF in the colonic response to stress.

Central CRF Activation during Stress: Relevance to the Irritable Bowel Syndrome

The irritable bowel syndrome is a prevalent functional bowel disorder characterized by abnormality of motor function resulting in either diarrhea or constipation or an alternation of both and acute or chronic abdominal pain.[78,79] However, the underlying pathogenesis still defies explanation because the disorder of motor function of the gut cannot be linked with defined structural or biochemical disturbances. On the one hand, IBS is recognized as ". . . an illness of distressed persons, not of the colon"[80] and, on the other hand, as an "organic disorder of gut function." The question, IBS: an irritable mind or an irritable bowel?[79] is still an intriguing one. In support of the former view, clinical surveys indicate that 50–100% of outpatients with IBS fulfill diagnostic criteria of psychiatric illnesses involving mood disturbances, anxiety, depression, somatization disorders or psychological distress.[78,80] In addition, the improvement of emotional status with psychological treatment led to an amelioration in bowel symptomatology, particularly in the subset of patients suffering from diarrhea and intermittent abdominal pain exacerbated by stress and diagnosed with anxiety/depression.[81]

In experimental animals including monkeys, central CRF has been involved in mediating stress-related behavioral changes including increased emotionality, anxiety, and fear[82] (see also Menzaghi *et al.*, this volume). In a previous study, we observed that CRF microinjected into the PVN increases grooming, locomotor activity and, at the highest dose, induces freezing behavior reflecting fear[83] while a marked stimulation of colonic fecal output and watery diarrhea is present.[25,84] Similar behavioral and colonic alterations were reported when CRF was microinjected into the locus coeruleus.[27,82,85,86] By contrast, CRF microinjected into the lateral hypothalamus and sites nearby, but outside the boundaries of the PVN or locus coeruleus, did not alter colonic transit and behavior.[25,27,56,84] These data suggest a possible interaction between CRF-induced behavioral anxiogenic response and the alterations in colonic motor function, particularly because i.c.v. CRF no longer stimulated colonic transit in anesthetized rats.[55]

In this respect, microinjection of CRF into the PVN or the locus coeruleus may provide a relevant experimental model to further elucidate the central and peripheral mechanisms of functional alterations of colonic motor activity and the relationship between the anxiogenic behavioral and colonic responses. The study of the role of CRF in the PVN and locus coeruleus may be clinically relevant for a subset of patients showing a relationship between stress and the initiation and exacerbation of IBS or for those with demonstrated psychiatric illness.[81] This is further supported by evidence that patients with depression have hypercortisolemia associated with elevated CSF levels of CRF.[82]

Recent evidence indicates that colonic hypersensitivity manifested by a lowered threshold for colonic distention is observed in 57% of IBS patients with diarrhea-predominant symptoms.[87] These findings are particularly interesting in light of experimental evidence that distention of the distal colon increases the firing rate of locus coeruleus neurons in a manner that is correlated with the increase in colonic pressure.[88] In addition, visceral stimuli reached CRF-containing neurons in the PVN through aminergic neuronal afferents.[88–91] It is tempting to speculate that the altered threshold of activation of sensory mechanoreceptors in the hypersensitive colon and rectum may cause a more pronounced, sustained and/or frequent activation of CRF neurons in the locus coeruleus and the PVN. CRF action in these nuclei will trigger both the anxiogenic reactions[85,90,92] and activation of colonic motor activity and watery diarrhea.[25,27,56] Such a functional loop may explain the association of colon hypersensitivity, psychopathological disturbance, and diarrhea in a subset of IBS patients.

SUMMARY AND CONCLUSIONS

Major advances have been made in the understanding of the pathophysiology of stress-related alteration of gut function. A wealth of information indicates that CRF is involved in the central mechanisms by which stress inhibits gastric emptying while stimulating colonic motor function. CRF acts in the PVN to trigger both the inhibition of gastric emptying and the stimulation of colonic motor function in response to stress, in addition to previously established endocrine and behavioral responses. Preliminary evidence exists that CRF acts in the locus coeruleus to induce a selective stimulation of colonic transit without influencing gastric emptying. The central actions of CRF to alter gastric and colonic motor function are conveyed by autonomic pathways and are unrelated to the associated stimulation of pituitary hormone secretion. The demonstration that central CRF plays a role in mediating gastric stasis resulting from surgery, peritonitis or high levels of central interleukin-1 provides new insight into the mechanisms involved in gastric ileus induced postoperatively or by infectious disease. Likewise, the demonstration that CRF in the PVN and locus coeruleus induce the anxiogenic and colonic motor responses to stress and that colonic distention activates neurons in the locus coeruleus opens new avenues for the understanding of the pathogenesis of a subset of IBS patients with colonic hypersensitivity associated with psychopathological disturbance and diarrhea-predominant symptoms.

ACKNOWLEDGMENTS

Paul Kirshbaum is acknowledged for helping in the preparation of the manuscript.

REFERENCES

1. CABANIS, P. J. G. 1981. Introduction. *In* On the Relation Between the Physical and Moral Aspects of Man. G. Mora, Ed. John Hopkins University Press. Baltimore, MD.
2. BEAUMONT, W. 1833. *In* Experiments and Observations on the Gastric Juice and the Physiology of Digestion. W. Osler, Ed.: 1–280. Dover Publications Inc., New York, NY.
3. CANNON, W. B. 1929. Bodily Changes in Pain, Hunger, Fear and Rage. Appleton. New York, NY.
4. HALL, C. S. 1934. Emotional behavior in the rat. 1. Defecation and urination as measures of individual differences in emotionality. J. Comp. Psychol. **18:** 385–403.
5. SELYE, H. 1936. Syndrome produced by diverse nocuous agents. Nature **138:** 32.
6. BUÉNO, L., S. COLLINS & J. L. JUNIEN. 1989. Stress and Digestive Motility.: 3–258. John Libbey Eurotext. Montrouge.
7. TACHÉ, Y. 1991. Effect of stress on gastric ulcer formation. *In* Stress: Neurobiology and Neuroendocrinology. M. R. Brown, G. F. Koob & C. Rivier, Eds.: 549–564. Marcel Dekker Inc., New York, NY.
8. BURKS, T. F. 1991. Role of stress in the development of disorders of gastrointestinal

motility. *In* Stress: Neurobiology and Neuroendocrinology. M. R. Brown, G. F. Koob & C. Rivier, Eds.: 565–583. Marcel Dekker Inc. New York, NY.

9. VALE, W., J. SPIESS, C. RIVIER & J. RIVIER. 1981. Characterization of a 41-residue ovine hypothalamic peptide that stimulates secretion of corticotropin and β-endorphin. Science **213:** 1394–1397.

10. RIVIER, J., C. RIVIER & W. VALE. 1984. Synthetic competitive antagonists of corticotropin-releasing factor: Effect on ACTH secretion in the rat. Science **224:** 889–891.

11. BROCCARDO, M., G. IMPROTA & P. MELCHIORRI. 1982. Effect of sauvagine on gastric emptying in conscious rats. Eur. J. Pharmacol. **85:** 111–114.

12. TACHÉ, Y., M. MAEDA-HAGIWARA & C. M. TURKELSON. 1987. Central nervous system action of corticotropin-releasing factor to inhibit gastric emptying in rats. Am. J. Physiol. **253:** G241–G245.

13. WILLIAMS, C. L., J. M. PETERSON, R. G. VILLAR & T. F. BURKS. 1987. Corticotropin-releasing factor directly mediates colonic responses to stress. Am. J. Physiol. **253:** G582–G586.

14. LENZ, H. J. 1987. Brain regulation of gastric secretion, emptying and blood flow by neuropeptides in conscious dogs. Gastroenterology **92:** 1500.

15. LENZ, H. J., M. BURLAGE, A. RAEDLER & H. GRETEN. 1988. Central nervous system effects of corticotropin-releasing factor on gastrointestinal transit in the rat. Gastroenterology **94:** 598–602.

16. SHELDON, R. J., J. A. QI, F. PORRECA & L. A. FISHER. 1990. Gastrointestinal motor effects of corticotropin-releasing factor in mice. Regul. Pept. **28:** 137–151.

17. BARQUIST, E., T. GARRICK, M. PRINCE, H. MÖNNIKES, M. J. ZINNER & Y. TACHÉ. 1992. Central action of CRF inhibits gastric emptying of solid meal in conscious rats. Dig. Dis. Sci. **37:** 982.

18. BUÉNO, L. & J. FIORAMONTI. 1986. Effects of corticotropin-releasing factor, corticotropin and cortisol on gastrointestinal motility in dogs. Peptides **7:** 73–77.

19. BUÉNO, L., M. J. FARGEAS, M. GUÉ, T. L. PEETERS, V. BORMANS & J. FIORAMONTI. 1986. Effects of corticotropin-releasing factor on plasma motilin and somatostatin levels and gastrointestinal motility in dogs. Gastroenterology **91:** 884–889.

20. RUCKEBUSCH, Y. & C. H. MALBERT. 1986. Stimulation and inhibition of food intake in sheep by centrally-administered hypothalamic releasing factors. Life Sci. **38:** 929–934.

21. GARRICK, T., A. VEISEH, A. SIERRA, H. WEINER & Y. TACHÉ. 1988. Corticotropin-releasing factor acts centrally to suppress stimulated gastric contractility in the rat. Regul. Pept. **21:** 173–181.

22. GUÉ, M., J. FIORAMONTI & L. BUÉNO. 1987. Comparative influences of acoustic and cold stress on gastrointestinal transit in mice. Am. J. Physiol. **253:** G124–G128.

23. GUÉ, M. & L. BUÉNO. 1988. Involvement of CNS corticotropin-releasing factor in the genesis of stress-induced gastric motor alterations. *In* Nerves and the Gastrointestinal Tract. M. V. Singer & H. Goebell, Eds.: 417–425. Kluwer Academic. Dordrecht.

24. BUÉNO, L. & M. GUÉ. 1988. Evidence for the involvement of corticotropin-releasing factor in the gastrointestinal disturbances induced by acoustic and cold stress in mice. Brain Res. **441:** 1–4.

25. MÖNNIKES, H., B. G. SCHMIDT, H. E. RAYBOULD & Y. TACHÉ. 1992. CRF in the paraventricular nucleus mediates gastric and colonic motor response to restraint stress. Am. J. Physiol. **262:** G137–G143.

26. HEYMANN-MÖNNIKES, I., Y. TACHÉ, M. TRAUNER, H. WEINER & T. GARRICK. 1991. CRF microinjected into the dorsal vagal complex inhibits TRH analog- and kianic acid-stimulated gastric contractility in rats. Brain Res. **554:** 139–144.

27. MÖNNIKES, H., B. G. SCHMIDT & T. TACHÉ. 1992. Corticotropin releasing factor (CRF) microinfused into the locus ceruleus complex (LCC) stimulates colonic transit in the conscious rats. Gastroenterology **102:** A488.

28. LENZ, H. J., A. RAEDLER, H. GRETEN, W. W. VALE & J. E. RIVIER. 1988. Stress-induced gastrointestinal secretory and motor responses in rats are mediated by endogenous corticotropin-releasing factor. Gastroenterology **95:** 1510–1517.

29. TACHÉ, Y., E. BARQUIST, R. L. STEPHENS & J. RIVIER. 1991. Abdominal surgery- and

trephination-induced delay in gastric emptying is prevented by intracisternal injection of CRF antagonist in the rat. J. Gastrointest. Motil. **3:** 19–25.

30. WEI, J. Y. & Y. TACHÉ. 1990. Alterations of efferent discharges of the gastric branch of the vagus nerve by intracisternal injection of peptides influencing gastric function in rats. Gastroenterology **98:** A531.

31. PAPPAS, T., H. DEBAS & Y. TACHÉ. 1985. Corticotropin-releasing factor inhibits gastric emptying in dogs. Regul. Pept. **11:** 193–199.

32. PAPPAS, T. N., M. WELTON, Y. TACHÉ & J. RIVIER. 1988. Corticotropin-releasing factor inhibits gastric emptying in dogs: Studies on its mechanism of action. Peptides **8:** 1011–1014.

33. KONTUREK, S. J., J. BILSKI, W. PAWLIK, P. THOR, K. CZARNOBILSKI, B. SZOKE & A. V. SCHALLY. 1985. Gastrointestinal secretory, motor and circulatory effects of corticotropin releasing factor (CRF). Life Sci. **37:** 1231–1240.

34. RAYBOULD, H. E., C. B. KOELBEL, E. A. MAYER & Y. TACHÉ. 1990. Inhibition of gastric motor function by circulating corticotropin-releasing factor in anesthetized rats. J. Gastrointest. Motil. **2:** 265–272.

35. IMPROTA, G. 1991. Evolutionary aspects of peripheral peptidergic signals: CRF-like peptides and modulation of G.I. functions. In Sensory Nerves and Neuropeptides in Gastroenterology. M. Costa, Ed.: 75–83. Plenum Press, New York, NY.

36. FONE, D. R., M. HOROWITZ, A. MADDOX, L. M. AKKERMANS, N. W. READ & J. DENT. 1990. Gastroduodenal motility during the delayed gastric emptying induced by cold stress. Gastroenterology **98:** 1155–1161.

37. TACHÉ, Y. 1989. Stress-induced alterations of gastric emptying. In Stress and Digestive Motility. L. Buéno, S. Collins & J. L. Junien, Eds.: 123–132. John Libbey Eurotext. Montrouge.

38. NEUFER, P. D., A. J. YOUNG & M. N. SAWKA. 1989. Gastric emptying during exercise: Effects of heat stress and hypohydration. Eur. J. Appl. Physiol. **58:** 433–439.

39. HAUSKEN, T., S. SVEBAK, I. WILHELMSEN, Y. T. HAUG, K. OLAFSEN, E. PETTERSSON, K. HVEEM & A. BERSTAD. 1993. Low vagal tone and antral dysmotility in patients with functional dyspepsia. Psychosom. Med. **55:** 12–22.

40. NEUFER, P. D., A. J. YOUNG & M. N. SAWKA. 1989. Gastric emptying during walking and running: Effects of varied exercise intensity. Eur. J. Appl. Physiol. **58:** 440–445.

41. HAAS, D. A. & S. R. GEORGE. 1988. Single or repeated mild stress increases synthesis and release of hypothalamic corticotropin-releasing factor. Brain Res. **461:** 230–237.

42. CHAPPELL, P. B., M. A. SMITH, C. D. KILTS, G. BISSETTE, J. RITCHIE, C. ANDERSON & C. B. NEMEROFF. 1986. Alterations in corticotropin-releasing factor-like immunoreactivity in discrete rat brain regions after acute and chronic stress. J. Neurosci. **6:** 2908–2914.

43. HARBUZ, M. S. & S. L. LIGHTMAN. 1989. Responses of hypothalamic and pituitary mRNA to physical and psychological stress in the rat. J. Endocrinol. **122:** 705–711.

44. MAMLAKI, E., R. KVETNANSKY, L. S. BRADY, P. W. GOLD & M. HERKENHAM. 1993. Repeated immobilization stress alters tyrosine hydroxylase, corticotropin-releasing hormone and corticosteroid receptor messenger ribonucleic acid levels in rat brain. J. Neuroendocrinol. **4:** 689–699.

45. IMAKI, T., T. SHIBASAKI, M. HOTTA & H. DEMURA. 1992. Early induction of c-fos precedes increased expression of corticotropin-releasing factor messenger ribonucleic acid in the paraventricular nucleus after immobilization stress. Endocrinology **131:** 240–246.

46. CECCATELLI, S., M. J. VILLAR, M. GOLSTEIN & T. HOKFELT. 1989. Expression of c-fos immunoreactivity in transmitter-characterized neurons after stress. Proc. Natl. Acad. Sci. USA **86:** 9569–9573.

47. HERNANDEZ, J. F., W. KORNREICH, C. RIVIER, A. MIRANDA, G. YAMAMOTO, J. ANDREWS, Y. TACHÉ, W. VALE & J. RIVIER. 1993. Synthesis and relative potency of new constrained CRF antagonists. J. Med. Chem. In press.

48. BONAZ, B., V. PLOURDE & Y. TACHÉ. 1993. Abdominal surgery induces c-fos expression in the hypothalamus and nucleus tractus solitarius. Gastroenterology **104:** A815.

49. CUNNINGHAM, E. T., JR. & P. E. SAWCHENKO. 1988. Anatomical specificity noradrenergic inputs to the paraventricular and supraoptic nuclei of the rat hypothalamus. J. Comp. Neurol. **274:** 60–76.

50. PLOTSKY, P., E. T. J. CUNNINGHAM & E. P. WIDMAIER. 1989. Catecholaminergic modulation of corticotropin-releasing factor and adrenocorticotropin secretion. Endocr. Rev. **10**: 437–458.

51. WHITNALL, M. H. 1993. Regulation of hypothalamic corticotropin-releasing hormone neurosecretory system. Prog. Neurobiol. **40**: 573–629.

52. RIVIERE, P. J. M., X. PASCAUD, E. CHEVALIER & J. L. JUNIEN. 1993. Fedotozine acts on the afferent side of the extrinsic inhibitory nervous pathways activated during peritonitis in rats. Gastroenterology **104**: A571.

53. SÜTÓ, G., Á. KIRÁLY, D. NOVIN & Y. TACHÉ. 1993. Potent inhibition of gastric emptying by intracisternal (ic) injection of interleukin-1β (IL-1β). Soc. Neurosci. **19**: 226.

54. BARQUIST, E., M. ZINNER, J. RIVIER & Y. TACHÉ. 1992. Abdominal surgery-induced delayed gastric emptying in rats: Role of CRF and sensory neurons. Am. J. Physiol. **262**: G616–G620.

55. TACHÉ, Y. & H. MÖNNIKES. 1993. CRF in the central nervous system mediates stress-induced stimulation of colonic motor function: Relevance to pathophysiology of the IBD. *In* Basic and Clinical Aspect of Chronic Abdominal Pain. E. A. Mayer & H. Raybould, Eds.: 141–151. Elsevier Science Publishers. Amsterdam.

56. MÖNNIKES, H., B. G. SCHMIDT & Y. TACHÉ. 1993. Psychological stress-induced accelerated colonic transit in rats involves hypothalamic corticotropin-releasing factor. Gastroenterology **104**: 716–723.

57. JIMÉNEZ, M. & L. BUÉNO. 1990. Inhibitory effects of neuropeptide Y (NPY) on CRF and stress-induced cecal motor response in rats. Life Sci. **47**: 205–211.

58. MÖNNIKES, H., H. E. RAYBOULD, B. SCHMIDT & Y. TACHÉ. 1993. CRF in the paraventricular nucleus of the hypothalamus stimulates colonic motor activity in fasted rats. Peptides **14**: 743–747.

59. GUÉ, M., J. L. JUNIEN & L. BUÉNO. 1991. Conditioned emotional response in rats enhances colonic motility through the central release of corticotropin-releasing factor. Gastroenterology **100**: 964–970.

60. BUÉNO, L., M. GUÉ & C. DEL RIO. 1992. CNS vasopressin mediates emotional stress and CRH-induced colonic motor alterations in rats. Am. J. Physiol. **262**: G427–G431.

61. GUÉ, M. 1993. Neuromodulation of corticotropin-releasing factor-induced gastrointestinal motility alterations. *In* Innervation of the Gut: Pathophysiological Implications. Y. Taché, D. L. Wingate & T. F. Burks, Eds.: 13–37. CRC Press. Boca Raton, FL.

62. WALKER, J. M., W. D. BOWEN, F. O. WALKER, R. R. MATSUMOTO, B. DE COSTA & K. C. RICE. 1990. Sigma receptors: Biology and function. Pharmacol. Rev. **42**: 355–402.

63. JUNIEN, J. L., M. GUÉ & L. BUÉNO. 1991. Neuropeptide Y and sigma ligand (JO 1784) act through a Gi protein to block the psychological stress and corticotropin-releasing factor-induced colonic motor activation in rats. Neuropharmacology **30**: 1119–1124.

64. GUÉ, M., J. L. JUNIEN, C. DEL RIO & L. BUÉNO. 1992. Neuropeptide Y and sigma ligand (JO 1784) suppress stress-induced colonic motor disturbances in rats through sigma and cholecystokinin receptors. J. Pharmacol. Exp. Ther. **261**: 850–855.

65. MARTINEZ, J. A. & L. BUÉNO. 1991. Busbirone inhibits corticotropin-releasing factor and stress-induced cecal motor response in rats by acting through 5-HT1A receptors. Eur. J. Pharmacol. **202**: 379–383.

66. CLARK, F. M. & H. K. PROUDFIT. 1991. The projection of locus coeruleus neurons to the spinal cord in the rat determined by anterograde tracing combined with immunohistochemistry. Brain Res. **538**: 231–245.

67. NARDUCCI, F., W. J. SNAPE, W. M. BATTLE, JR., R. L. LONDON & S. COHEN. 1985. Increased colonic motility during exposure to a stressful situation. Dig. Dis. Sci. **30**: 40–44.

68. WELGAN, P., H. MESHKINPOUR & F. HOEHLER. 1985. The effect of stress on colon motor and electrical activity in irritable bowel syndrome. Psychosom. Med. **47**: 139–149.

69. FUKUDO, S. & J. SUZUKI. 1987. Colonic motility, autonomic function, and gastrointestinal hormones under psychological stress and irritable bowel syndrome. Tohoku J. Exp. Med. **151**: 373–385.

70. ALMY, T. P., L. E. HINKLE, B. BERLE & F. KERN, JR. 1949. Alterations in colonic function

in man under stress. III. Experimental production of sigmoid spasm in patients with spastic constipation. Gastroenterology **12:** 437–449.

71. ALMY, T. P., F. KERN, JR. & M. TULIN. 1949. Alterations in colonic function in man under stress. II. Experimental production of sigmoid spasm in healthy persons. Gastroenterology **12:** 425–436.

72. BARONE, F. C., J. F. DEEGAN, W. J. PRICE, P. J. FOWLER, J. D. FONDACARO & H. S. ORMSBEE III. 1990. Cold-restraint stress increases rat fecal pellet output and colonic transit. Am. J. Physiol. **258:** G329–G337.

73. WILLIAMS, C. L., R. G. VILLAR, J. M. PETERSON & T. F. BURKS. 1988. Stress-induced changes in intestinal transit in the rat: A model for irritable bowel syndrome. Gastroenterology **94:** 611–621.

74. ENCK, P., V. MERLIN, J. F. ERCKENBRECHT & M. WIENBECK. 1989. Stress effects on gastrointestinal transit in the rat. Gut **30:** 455–459.

75. BONAZ, B. & Y. TACHÉ. 1993. Psychological stress-induced c-fos expression in the rat brain and stimulation of fecal output. Gastroenterology **104:** A479.

76. FARGEAS, M.-J., J. FIORAMONTI, L. PONS & L. BUÉNO. 1993. Central action of interleukin-1β on intestinal motility in rats: Mediation by two mechanisms. Gastroenterology **104:** 377–383.

77. KONONEN, J., J. HONKANIEMI, H. ALHO, J. KIOSTINAHO, M. IADAROLA & M. PELTO-HUIKKO. 1992. Fos-like immunoreactivity in the rat hypothalamic pituitary axis after immobilization stress. Endocrinology **130:** 3041–3047.

78. DROSSMAN, D. A., D. W. POWEL & J. T. SESSIONS. 1977. The irritable bowel syndrome. Gastroenterology **73:** 811–822.

79. ZIGHELBOIM, J. & N. J. TALLEY. 1993. What are functional bowel disorders? Gastroenterology **104:** 1196–1201.

80. WEINER, H. 1992. Perturbing the Organisms: The Biology of Stressful Experience. University of Chicago Press. Chicago, IL.

81. GUTHRIE, E., F. CREED, D. DAWSON & B. TOMENSON. 1991. A controlled trial of psychological treatment for the irritable bowel syndrome. Gastroenterology **100:** 450–457.

82. OWENS, M. J. & C. B. NEMEROFF. 1991. Physiology and pharmacology of corticotropin-releasing factor. Pharmacol. Rev. **43:** 425–473.

83. BINDRA, D. & W. R. THOMPSON. 1953. An evaluation of defecation and urination as measure of fearfulness. J. Comp. Physiol. Psychol. **46:** 43–45.

84. MÖNNIKES, H., I. HEYMANN-MÖNNIKES & Y. TACHÉ. 1992. CRF in the paraventricular nucleus of the hypothalamus induces dose-related behavioral profile in rats. Brain Res. **574:** 70–76.

85. VALENTINO, R. J. 1988. CRH effects on central noradrenergic neurons: Relationship to stress. *In* Mechanisms of Physical and Emotional Stress. G. P. Chrousos, D. L. Loriaux & P. W. Gold, Eds.: 47–64. Plenum Press, New York, NY.

86. VALENTINO, R. J., M. PAGE, E. VAN BOCKSTAELE & G. ASTON-JONES. 1992. Corticotropin-releasing factor innervation of the locus coeruleus region: Distribution of fibers and sources of input. Neuroscience **48:** 689–705.

87. MAYER, E. A. & H. E. RAYBOULD. 1990. Role of visceral afferent mechanisms in functional bowel disorders. Gastroenterology **99:** 1688–1704.

88. ELAM, M., P. THOREN & T. H. SVENSSON. 1986. Locus ceruleus neurons and sympathetic nerves: Activation by visceral afferents. Brain Res. **375:** 117–125.

89. SWANSON, L. W., P. E. SAWCHENKO & R. W. LIND. 1986. Regulation of multiple peptides in CRF parvocellular neurosecretory neurons: Implications for the stress response. Prog. Brain Res. **68:** 169–190.

90. REDMOND, D. E. & Y. H. HUANG. 1979. II. New evidence for a locus coeruleus-norepinephrine connection with anxiety. Life Sci. **25:** 2149–2162.

91. PALKOVITS, M. 1987. Organization of the stress response at the anatomical level. Prog. Brain Res. **72:** 47–55.

92. BUTLER, P. D., J. M. WEISS, J. C. STOUT & C. B. NEMEROFF. 1990. Corticotropin-releasing factor produces fear-enhancing and behavioral activating effects following infusion into the locus coeruleus. J. Neurosci. **10:** 176–183.

Interaction between Neuropeptide Y and Sigma Ligands in the Modulation of CRF and Stress-Induced Alteration of Gastrointestinal Function

J. L. JUNIEN AND M. GUÉ

Institut de Recherche Jouveinal
P.O. Box 100
94265 Fresnes, France

Martin *et al.*[1] were the first to use the term opioid/sigma receptors to characterize the psychopharmacological action of a series of benzomorphans, compounds with opiate activity. It was later shown[2] that the (+)-enantiomeric form bound preferentially to two sites, one termed the PCP (phencyclidine) site associated with the NMDA (N-methyl-D-aspartate) receptor to which the psychopharmacological effects of these compounds are attributed, and the other termed the sigma site whose nature and role remain less well understood.

This paper will first introduce general background information on sigma receptors and then will focus on the interaction of sigma ligand and neuropeptide Y (NPY) peptides with stress and/or corticotropin-releasing factor (CRF) gastrointestinal (GI)-induced effects.

CHARACTERIZATION OF SIGMA SITES

Localization and Subtypes

Sigma sites are widely distributed in the organism. They have been characterized in the central nervous system, in particular, in the sensorimotor area of the limbic region where the dopaminergic fibers are also located.[3,4] Sigma sites have also been demonstrated in the digestive tract,[5] liver,[6] the endocrine organs, and lymphocytes.[7] Further characterization of these sites was hampered by the lack of specific ligands. In addition to the benzomorphans such as (+)-SKF 10047 and (+)-pentazocine, these sites also have a high affinity for haloperidol and (+)-3PPP (but none for naloxone and the nonbenzomorphan opiates). However, (+)-SKF 10047 [(+)-N-allyl-normetazocine] has the drawback of binding to both sigma and PCP sites, and haloperidol binds as well to dopaminergic and serotoninergic receptors. Fortunately, new compounds that are highly selective for sigma sites have been developed in the last few years (FIG. 1).

In fact at least two sigma sites exist[8,9] because the relative affinities of the different compounds for this receptor vary with the tritiated ligand used, and the binding of such ligands is affected differently by physical treatments (UV irradiation) or by the addition of derivatives of GTP.[10] These two sites have been differentiated as sigma 1 and 2. Whereas (+)-pentazocine, (+)-SKF 10047, and dextromethorphan have high affinity for site 1, they bind only moderately to site 2. In addition, there is a high selectivity, (+) ≫ (−), for site 1, and an inverse selectivity for site 2. Phenytoin modulates allosterically site 1 but not site 2. Only sigma 1 is sensitive to chronic treatment with haloperidol.[11] Roman et al.[5] characterized sigma sites in a guinea pig myenteric plexus membrane preparation using [³H](+)-SKF 10047. These authors demonstrated the presence of two sites of high and low affinity (K_d = 46 and 342 nM, respectively). The high-affinity site was not sensitive to naloxone or morphine or other dopaminergic compounds but had a high affinity for haloperidol (IC_{50} = 14 nM) and a low affinity for PCP as do cerebral sigma sites.[3]

In order to investigate the distribution of sigma and any PCP sites in guinea pig digestive tract, the same authors[12] used autohistoradiographical methods. Sections of tissue from the esophagus, stomach, intestine, and colon were incubated for 45 minutes in the presence of tritiated ligands, [³H](+)-SKF 10047 or [³H]PCP, and treated with hematoxylin-eosin for histological characterization. Nonspecific binding

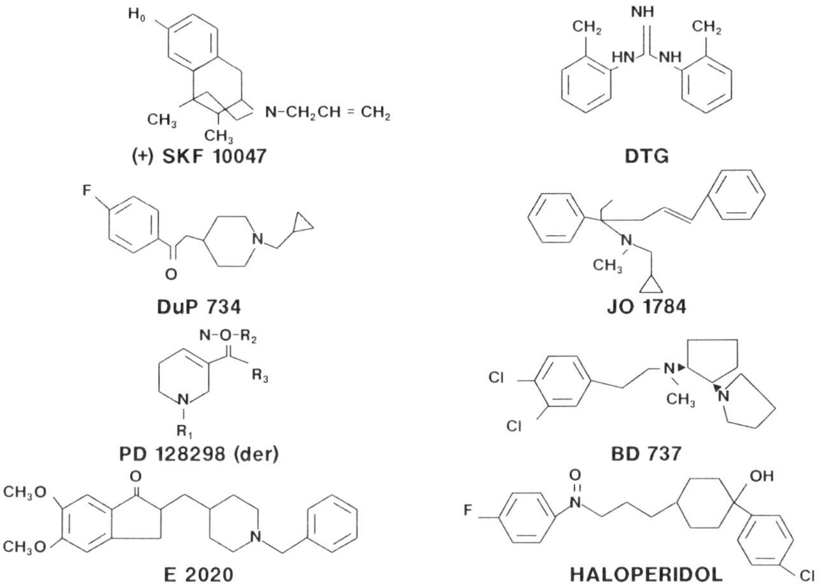

FIGURE 1. Chemical structures of various sigma ligands.

was evaluated in the presence of 1 µM haloperidol or 100 µM PCP. With [³H](+)-SKF 10047, all tissues examined showed an identical profile, that is, an intense preferential localization in the mucosal regions and the submucosal plexuses. The highest concentration was found in the submucosal plexuses of the duodenum. At the mucosal level, the fundus and the duodenum showed the highest concentration. Muscular regions were poorly labeled by [³H](+)-SKF 10047, with the exception of the colon. These results correspond to the low density of high-affinity sites reported by Roman et al.[5] using a myenteric plexus membrane preparation (about 10-fold lower compared to cerebral tissues). No PCP site was characterized in this study. Roman et al.[13] confirmed the presence of sigma sites in human digestive tract. As in the guinea pig, a high density of sites labeled with [³H](+)-SKF 10047 was found in the mucosal and submucosal regions of the duodenum, ileum, cecum, and colon. In the colon, a relatively high concentration of grains was demonstrated in the circular muscular layer.

Endogenous Ligands

Various endogenous peptide ligands whose exact sequences are not known have been proposed by different groups.[14–17] Roman et al., [18] using [³H](+)-SKF 10047, reported in vitro an interaction between the peptides of the NPY family and the sigma sites using rodent brain membrane preparation, whereas Tam and Mitchell[19] did not find such an interaction. Bouchard et al.[20] and Roman et al.[21] demonstrated in vivo in mouse hippocampus a partial displacement (30 to 45%) of [³H](+)-SKF 10047 from its binding site by peptides of the NPY family. This result seems to indicate that only a portion of the sites labeled by this ligand recognize the peptide, whereas 100% displacement is obtained with reference sigma ligands.[22] Although at the present time the existence and thus the nature of this sigma/NPY interaction is not clearly established, it has been shown that NPY mimics in a certain number of experimental models the functional activity of sigma ligands in the brain[21,23,24] and in the gastrointestinal tract.[25,26]

Second Messengers and Ion Channels

It seems likely that at least one of the sigma sites is associated with a G protein.[10,27,28] On the other hand, no second messenger directly related to the activation of these sites has been identified. Some studies, however, have reported an interaction with the formation of inositol phosphates and cGMP. Bowen et al.[29] demonstrated that sigma ligands inhibited the increase in the rate of formation of inositol phosphates produced by carbachol and norepinephrine in rat brain synaptosome preparations. This effect is well correlated with the affinity of substances for the site labeled with [³H](+)3-PPP in guinea pig brain. All the ligands studied, including haloperidol, DTG, and (+)3-PPP behave as inhibitors, and the concentrations necessary are of the order of 10^{-5} M. (+)-Benzomorphan and (+)-morphinan are as active as DTG and haloperidol.

Rao et al.[30] studied the effects of sigma ligands on the formation of cGMP in mouse cerebellum. They showed that most ligands, including (+)-SKF 10047, (+)-pentazocine, BMY 14802, dextromethorphan, and opipramol modulate the formation of cGMP negatively. This effect is mediated by indirect inhibition of the NMDA receptor.

Electrophysiological studies have demonstrated a relationship between sigma sites and potassium current. Bell et al.[31] used the patch-clamp technique on NCB20 cells. They showed that tonic potassium outward current is blocked by sigma ligands. The rank order of activity of the different ligands is well correlated with their affinity for a low-affinity site found in these cells and which differs from the sigma 2 site. With the exception of haloperidol, the effects occur at micromolar concentrations.

In binding studies with [³H]DTG using a guinea pig brain membrane preparation, Rothman et al.[32] described the presence of two high-affinity sites (K_d, 12 and 37 nM). The first has a high affinity for (+)-benzomorphans and the other sigma ligands. The relative affinity of the different compounds corresponds to that of sigma 1 site, whereas the second site is not very sensitive to (+)-benzomorphans and more resembles sigma 2 site. The two sites are, however, sensitive to the presence of inorganic cations that block calcium channels and to verapamil. These results suggest an association between sigma sites and the calcium channels.

SIGMA SITES AND THE GASTROINTESTINAL TRACT

Numerous functional effects have been reported with sigma ligands, notably at the central level. For review see Walker et al.[33] and Su et al.[9] Several effects on the digestive tract have been reported either in vitro[34–36] or in vivo[26,37–39,40] on digestive motility and secretory processes.

Effects on Stress-Induced Digestive Motility Abnormalities

Sigma ligands have no or mild effects on GI motility. However, recent findings indicate that sigma receptors may influence disturbed GI motility under stress conditions. We have developed[41] a model of emotionel stress (ES) in rat that induces colonic motor alteration. Rats with electrodes implanted on the colon are conditioned to receive an electric footshock via the cage floor. On the day of the experiments, the rats are placed in the same cage, no footshock is delivered, and colonic motility is recorded during 30 minutes. Such conditions produce an increase in the frequency of colonic spike bursts. CRF injected intracerebroventricularly (i.c.v.) increases also the frequency of colonic spike bursts, reproducing the effect of ES. A CRF antagonist, α-helical CRF_{9-41}, prevents the colonic response to stress. These findings suggest that CRF mediates the effect of ES on colonic myoelectric activity. Furthermore, CRF appears to act directly on central structures regulating colonic motility and not through the stimulation of the hypothalamic-pituitary adrenal axis (HPA) because ES induces the same motility changes in hypophysecto-mized rats as it does in intact ones.

NPY[42] and sigma ligands[43] can block the excitatory effects of stress and CRF on colonic motility. This effect is centrally mediated because it occurs at doses at least ten times lower than those required after systemic administration. Injection i.c.v. of the sigma ligand JO 1784 30 minutes before stress almost totally prevents stress-induced hyperkinesia[42] (FIG. 2). Previous treatment with a single dose of pertussis toxin given i.c.v. prevents the effect of both NPY and JO 1784, indicating a GI protein-mediated pathway as reported in other studies for both compounds.[44,45,28] The effects of NPY and JO 1784 are blocked by preadministration of the putative sigma ligand antagonist, BMY 14802.[46] These results again indicate that both compounds act through a possible common sigma receptor. Another interesting feature is that both JO 1784 and NPY effects are blocked by the cholecystokinin A (CCKA) receptor antagonist devazepide administered i.c.v. The CCKB antagonist L-365718 was less active. Gué et al.[46] have also reported that CCK8s and analogs injected i.c.v. also reverse the stress and CRF-induced colonic hypermotility. These data suggest that sigma ligands, as well as NPY, interact with the CRF pathway through CCK and/or CCKA receptors.

The observation that CCK8s and other substances such as NPY and sigma ligands, which appear to act through CCK pathways, are able to inhibit the digestive motor effects related to fear equated with an acute form of anxiety is surprising because of the existing knowledge of the proposed anxiogenic effects of CCK tetrapeptides (CCK4). Recent studies have shown that CCK4 and pentagastrin elicit panic-like attacks in patients suffering from panic disorders[47,48] and also induce

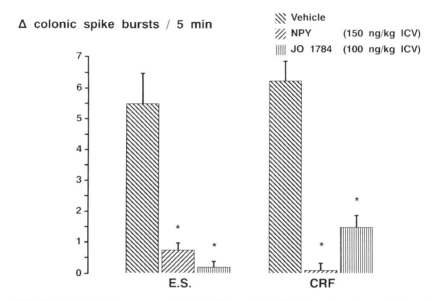

FIGURE 2. Blockade by neuropeptide Y (NPY) and JO 1784 of emotional stress (ES) and corticotropin-releasing factor (CRF) induced changes in colonic myoelectrical activity of rats. *Values significantly different ($p < 0.05$) from corresponding control values. Fasted rats were placed in a test cage where they had previously received electric footshock (ES) or were injected i.c.v. with CRF. NPY and JO 1784 were administered i.c.v. 30 minutes before stress or CRF.[43]

short-lasting panic-like attacks in healthy volunteers.[49] In contrast, peripheral administration of CCK8s does not produce any anxiety or panic-like attacks in volunteers but does induce gastrointestinal disturbances.[49] These differences could be explained either by a low penetration of the peptide into the brain or the involvement of two different CCK receptor subtypes. Indeed, the CCKA receptor has a high affinity for CCK8s but a low affinity for nonsulphated CCK8, CCK4, and pentagastrin,[50] whereas the CCKB receptor has high affinity for both of them. Several data suggest that CCKB receptors may be involved in anxiety. Antianxiety effects have been reported with the more selective CCKB antagonists, L-365260 and PD 134308.[51] In stress-induced colonic motility disorders the specific CCKA antagonist devazepide was 10 to 100 times more active than the CCKB antagonist L-365260. These results suggest that JO 1784 and NPY act specifically through CCKA receptors and that such activation is not anxiogenic because neither JO 1784 nor NPY has such an effect. NPY has even been reported to have an anxiolytic effect in the Vogel conflict test.[52,53] These results either indicate that sigma ligands interact with CCK receptors in a region not related to CCK-induced behavioral changes or that CCKA receptors are not anxiogenic.

Whether the effects of JO 1784 on CRF are due to an interaction with the psychotropic effects of this neuropeptide needs to be investigated. A possibility is that JO 1784 and other sigma ligands act on descending pathways activated by CRF at the level of the paraventricular nucleus (PVN) of the hypothalamus or the dorsal vagal complex (DVC). NPY, CCK, and sigma sites are present at the hypothalamic level in the same areas as CRF neurones. Neurones in the PVN project to the DVC from where parasympathetic fibers emerge to the periphery. CCKB receptors are widely distributed in the brain, though only a few areas have a high density of CCKA receptors, the NTS being one of the richest regions.[54] The identification of the precise localization of NPY/sigma/CCKA receptor interaction is necessary to understand the mechanisms involved and why sigma and CCKA receptors are so closely linked in various regions.

Effects of Sigma Ligands on CRF-Induced GI-Mediated Effects

To further study the interaction between sigma ligands/NPY and CRF mediated effects, Gué et al.[55] investigated the effects of JO 1784 and NPY and various fragments on the CRF inhibition of the pentagastrin-induced gastric acid response. CRF injected into the cerebrospinal fluid or selective brain nuclei alters gastric acid secretion and motor function as previously reported.[56–59,41,42] Intracisternal (i.c.) injection of CRF prior to injection of pentagastrin inhibits by 70% the plateau of acid response to pentagastrin in urethane-anesthetized rats. This inhibition is completely prevented by NPY and JO 1784 injected i.c. These effects are dose-related and occur at doses that do not influence basal or pentagastrin-stimulated gastric acid secretion. At higher doses, NPY administered i.c. or i.c.v. increases basal or pentagastrin-stimulated gastric acid secretion.[60,61] The interaction between NPY and JO 1784 with CRF is peptide-specific because i.c. injection of NPY or JO 1784 does not influence the antisecretory action of bombesin and interleukin 1β in the same experimental model (FIG. 3). These data and those reported before indicate that NPY and JO

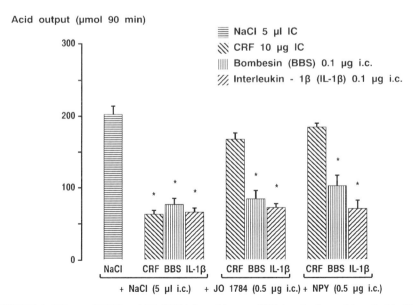

FIGURE 3. Effects of NPY and JO 1784 injected i.c. on CRF, bombesin, and interleukin-1β (hIL-1β) induced inhibition of gastric acid secretion in urethane-anesthetized rats. Fasted rats were injected i.c. with saline, NPY or JO 1784 10 minutes prior to the peptides. Ten minutes later pentagastrin (10 μg kg^{-1} h^{-1}) was infused. $p < 0.05$.[55]

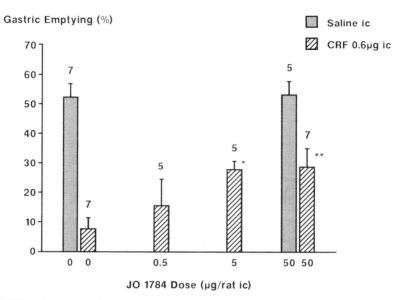

FIGURE 4. Dose-related antagonism of i.c. CRF-induced inhibition of gastric emptying by JO 1784 in conscious rats. Rats received i.c. injection of saline or JO 1784 at various doses followed by another i.c. injection of saline or CRF. $*p < 0.05$; $**p < 0.01$.[71]

1784 antagonize the alterations of gastrointestinal secretory and motor function induced by exogenous or endogenous CRF.

The central CRF-sensitive elements involved in the inhibition of gastric acid secretion have been previously localized in the PVN and lateral hypothalamus.[62] Gué et al.[55] have further investigated the anatomical sites of the functional interaction between NPY, JO 1784, and CRF. Unilateral microinjection of CRF into the PVN or lateral hypothalamus inhibits pentagastrin-stimulated acid secretion. NPY microinjected into these nuclei has no effect on gastric acid secretion by itself but inhibits the antisecretory action of CRF when microinjected into the PVN and not into the LH. Anatomical studies indicate that the PVN, including the parvicellular part which regulates autonomic function,[63] is densely innervated with NPY-immunoreactive fibers and terminals[64] and has a high density of NPY[65] and sigma receptors.[3] Briefly, the PVN may be one site where the NPY and CRF interaction takes place.

In addition to the PVN, NPY/sigma/CRF interaction may occur in other sites such as the brainstem nuclei that regulate gastric acid secretion. This is supported by the fact that i.c. injection of NPY or JO 1784 also completely prevents the CRF antisecretory effect and that drugs delivered into the cisterna magna do not enter the cerebral ventricle and act mainly in the brain stem and/or upper cervical cord. NPY immunoreactivity and receptors have also been located in brain medullary nuclei regulating autonomic outflow,[66,67] and CRF has been shown to act in the DVC to influence gastric function.[68]

Gué et al.[69] tested a series of NPY and PYY fragments in the same model. NPY1-36 and PYY1-36 were almost equally active, whereas (Leu 31, Pro 34) NPY was less active. NPY 13-36 was weakly active. They also found that PYY3-36, a peptide recently characterized in the human GI tract,[70] was as active as native NPY. Based on the relative activity of these fragments or NPY receptor subtypes, this again raises the probability that NPY effects reported here are mediated through a non-Y1Y2 receptor although dose-response curves would be necessary to definitely assess the respective potency of the peptides. This also raises the question of the exact nature of the endogenous ligand acting on the sigma receptor.

More recently Yoneda et al.[71] reported that the sigma ligand JO 1784 is also able to reduce CRF-induced inhibition of gastric emptying in conscious rats as well as its effect on gastric acid secretion. Injection of CRF i.c. in conscious pylorus-ligated rats reduces gastric output by 95%. Intracisternal injections of JO 1784 immediately before that of CRF reduces dose-dependently CRF-induced inhibition of gastric acid secretion. Administration of JO 1784 i.v. did not modify CRF antisecretory action, showing the centrally mediated effect of the compound. The rate of gastric emptying of non-nutrient liquid meal is strongly inhibited by CRF in conscious rats. JO 1784 reverses by almost 50% the 83% decrease induced by CRF (FIG. 4). JO 1784 has no effect by itself either on acid secretion or gastric emptying at the doses tested.

CONCLUSIONS

Sigma sites or receptors are widely distributed in the organism and many functional effects of sigma ligands have been described. At least two different sigma subtypes exist based on their binding characteristics. However, the exact relationship between these subtypes and the functional effects of various ligands remain to be established clearly. Evidence exists that some effects of the ligands do not fit well with this classification, and further binding data and studies on the effector system(s) are needed to clarify the various characteristics of sigma receptors.

Some studies indicate that one sigma receptor that has high affinity for haloperidol-like substances, (+)-benzomorphans and JO 1784 mediates effects on the GI tract through peripheral and brain receptors. Interestingly, some of the ligands behave as agonists whereas haloperidol-like substances are antagonists. Of particular interest is the antagonist effect exerted by some of these ligands, such as JO1784 as well as NPY peptides, on profound modifications induced by stress and CRF on GI functions. How and where this interaction occurs remain to be further characterized. NPY peptides and sigma sites seem closely linked. However, the nature of this interaction at the cellular level is not elucidated nor is the role of CCK and CCKA receptors. PVN may be one site where NPY, sigma, and CRF interaction takes place as reported above, but other possibilities should be investigated which could be of therapeutic importance. In summary, these data support an interaction between sigma receptor ligand and CRF at brain sites regulating gut function which opens new interesting therapeutic avenues.

REFERENCES

1. MARTIN, W. R., C. G. EADES, J. A. THOMPSON, R. E. HUPPLER & P. E. GILBERT. 1976. J. Pharmacol. Exp. Ther. **197:** 517–532.
2. ZUKIN, S. R., A. TEMPEL, E. L. GARDNER & R. S. ZUKIN. 1984. Brain Res. **294:** 174–177.
3. LARGENT, B. L., A. L. GUNDLACH & S. H. SNYDER. 1986. J. Pharmacol. Exp. Ther. **238(2):** 739–748.
4. HEROUX, J. A., S. W. TAM & E. B. DE SOUZA. 1991. Abstract 133.11. 21st Annual meeting of the Society for Neuroscience, New Orleans, Louisiana. Nov. 10–15.
5. ROMAN, F., X. PASCAUD, D. VAUCHÉ & J. L. JUNIEN. 1988. Life Sci. **42(22):** 2217–2222.
6. SAMILOVA, N. N., L. V. NAGORNAYA & V. A. VINOGRADOV. 1988. Eur. J. Pharmacol. **147:** 259–264.

7. WOLFE, S. A., C. KULSAKDINUM & E. B. DE SOUZA. 1987. Soc. Neurosci. **13:** 1437.
8. BOWEN, W. D., S. B. HELLEWELL & K. A. McGARRY. 1989. Eur. J. Pharmacol. **163:** 309–318.
9. SU, T. P., X. Z. WU, C. E. SPIVAK, E. D. LONDON & J. A. BELL. 1991. *In* NMDA Receptor Related Agents: Biochemistry, Pharmacology and Behavior. T. Kamenyama, T. Nabeshima & E. F. Domino, Eds: 227–233. NPP Books. Ann Arbor, MI.
10. ITZHAK, Y. & M. KHOURI. 1988. Neurosci. Lett. **85:** 147–152.
11. QUIRION, R., W. BOWEN, Y. ITZHAK, J. L. JUNIEN, J. M. MUSACCHIO, R. B. ROTHMAN, T. P. SU, S. W. TAM & D. P. TAYLOR. 1992. Trends Pharmacol. Sci. **13:** 85–86.
12. ROMAN, F. J., X. PASCAUD, G. CHOMETTE, L. BUENO & J. L. JUNIEN. 1989. Gastroenterology **97:** 76–82.
13. ROMAN, F. J., X. PASCAUD, R. SALMON, G. CHOMETTE & J. L. JUNIEN. 1991. Gastroenterology **100:** A662.
14. QUIRION, R., D. A. DI MAGGIO, E. D. FRENCH, P. C. CONTRERAS, J. SHILOACH, C. B. PERT, H. EVERIST, A. PERT & T. L. O'DONOHUE. 1984. Peptides **5:** 967–973.
15. CONTRERAS, P. C., P. A. DI MAGGIO & T. L. O'DONAHUE. 1987. Synapse **1:** 57–61.
16. SU, T. P. & D. B. VAUPEL. 1988. Soc. Neurosci. Abstr. **14:** 218–222.
17. CONNOR, M. A. & C. CHAVKIN. 1990. FASEB Abstr. A330.
18. ROMAN, F. J., X. PASCAUD, O. DUFFY, D. VAUCHÉ, B. MARTIN & J. L. JUNIEN. 1989. Eur. J. Pharmacol. **174:** 301–302.
19. TAM, S. W. & K. N. MITCHELL. 1991. Eur. J. Pharmacol. **193:** 121–122.
20. BOUCHARD, P., Y. DUMONT, A. FOURNIER, S. ST-PIERRE & R. QUIRION. Submitted to J. Neurosci.
21. ROMAN, F. J., X. PASCAUD, O. DUFFY, D. VAUCHÉ & J. L. JUNIEN. 1991. *In* NMDA Receptor Related Agents: Biochemistry, Pharmacology and Behavior. T. Kamenyama, T. Nabeshima & E. F. Domino, Eds.: 211–218. NPP Books. Ann Arbor, MI.
22. FERRIS, C. D., D. J. HIRSCH, B. P. BROOKS & S. H. SNYDER. 1991. J. Neurochem. **57:** 729–737.
23. MONNET, F. P., A. FOURNIER, G. DEBONNEL & C. DE MONTIGNY. 1992. J. Pharmacol. Exp. Ther. **263(3):** 1212–1218.
24. MONNET, F. P., G. DEBONNEL, A. FOURNIER & C. DE MONTIGNY. 1992. J. Pharmacol. Exp. Ther. **263(3):** 1219–1225.
25. RIVIÈRE, P. J. M., X. PASCAUD, J. L. JUNIEN & F. PORRECA. 1990. Eur. J. Pharmacol. **187:** 557–559.
26. PASCAUD, X., M. CHOVET, C. ROZÉ & J. L. JUNIEN. Eur. J. Pharmacol. 1993. In press.
27. KARBON, E. W., K. NAPER & M. J. PONTECORVO. 1991. Eur. J. Pharmacol. **193:** 21–27.
28. MONNET, F. P., P. BLIER, G. DEBONNEL & C. DE MONTIGNY. 1992. Naunyn-Schmiedebergs Arch. Pharmacol. **346(1):** 32–39.
29. BOWEN, W. D., B. N. KIRSCHNER, A. H. NEWMAN & K. C. RICE. 1988. Eur. J. Pharmacol. **149:** 399–400.
30. RAO, T. S., S. J. MICK, J. A. CLER, M. R. EMMETTE, V. M. DILWORTH, P. C. CONTRERAS, N. M. GRAY, P. L. WOOD & S. IYENGAR. 1991. Brain Res. **561:** 43–50.
31. BELL, J. A., C. E. SPIVAK, T. P. SU & E. D. LONDON. 1988. Soc. Neurosci. Abstr. **14:** 1155.
32. ROTHMAN, R. B., A. REID, A. MAHBOUKI, C. H. KIM, B. R. DE COSTA, A. E. JACOBSON & K. C. RICE. 1991. Abstract 133.9. 21st Annual Meeting of the Society for Neuroscience, New Orleans, Louisiana.
33. WALKER, J. M., W. D. BOWEN, F. O. WALKER, R. R. MATSUMOTO, B. DE COSTA & K. C. RICE. 1990. Pharmacol. Rev. **42(4):** 355–402.
34. SU, T. P., T. H. CLEMENS & C. W. GORODETZKY. 1981. Life Sci. **28:** 2519–2528.
35. CAMPBELL, B. G., M. W. SCHERZ, J. F. W. KEANA & E. WEBER. J. Neurosci. **9(10):** 3380–3391.
36. COCCINI, T., L. G. COSTA, L. MANZO, S. M. CANDURA, N. IAPADRE, B. BALESTRA & M. TONINI. 1991. Eur. J. Pharmacol. **198:** 105–108.
37. JUNIEN, J. L., M. GUÉ, X. PASCAUD, J. FIORAMONTI, L. BUENO. 1990. Gastroenterology **99(3):** 684–689.
38. PASCAUD, X., J. P. DEFAUX, C. ROZÉ & J. L. JUNIEN. 1990. J. Pharmacol. Exp. Ther. **255(3):** 1354–1359.

39. PASCAUD, X., M. CHOVET, P. SOULARD, A. CHEVALIER, C. ROZÉ & J. L. JUNIEN. 1993. Gastroenterology. **104:** 427–434.
40. BUENO, L., M. GUÉ, C. DEL RIO, J. L. JUNIEN & J. FIORAMONTI. 1992. Gastroenterology. **102(4/2):** A432.
41. GUÉ, M., J. L. JUNIEN & L. BUENO. 1991. Gastroenterology **100(10):** 964–970.
42. JIMENEZ, M. & L. BUENO. 1990. Life Sci. **47:** 205–212.
43. JUNIEN, J. L., M. GUÉ & L. BUENO. 1991. Neuropharmacology **30(10):** 1119–1124.
44. CHANCE, W. T., S. SHERIFF, T. FOLEY-NELSON, J. E. FISCHER & A. BALASUBRAMANIAM. 1989. Peptides **10:** 1283–1286.
45. ITZHAK, Y. 1989. Mol. Pharmacol. **36:** 512–517.
46. GUÉ, M., J. L. JUNIEN, C. DEL RIO & L. BUENO. 1992. J. Pharmacol. Exp. Ther. **261(3):** 850–855.
47. BRADWEJN, J., D. KOSZYCKI, C. SHRIQUI & G. METERISSIAN. 1990. Can. J. Psychiatry **35:** 83–85.
48. ABELSON, J. L. & R. NESSE. 1990. Arch. Gen. Psychiatry **47:** 395.
49. DE MONTIGNY, C. 1989. Arch. Gen. Psychiatry **46:** 511–517.
50. INNIS, R. B. & S. H. SNYDER. 1980. Proc. Natl. Acad. Sci. USA **77:** 6917–6921.
51. RAVARD, S. & C. T. DOURISH. 1990. Trends Pharamacol. Sci. **11:** 271–273.
52. HEILIG, M., C. WAHLESTEDT & E. WIDERLÖV. 1988. Eur. J. Pharmacol. **157:** 205–213.
53. WIDERLOV, E., M. HEILIG, R. EKMAN & C. WAHLESTEDT. 1989. In Neuropeptide Y. V. Mutt, K. Fuxe, T. Hokfelt & J. M. Lundberg, Eds.: 331–342. Raven Press. New York, NY.
54. HILL, D., N. J. CAMPBELL, T. M. SHAW & G. N. WOODRUFF. 1987. J. Neurosci. **7:** 2967–2976.
55. GUÉ, M., M. YONEDA, H. MONNIKES, J. L. JUNIEN & Y. TACHÉ. 1992. Br. J. Pharmacol. **107:** 642–647.
56. STEPHENS, R. L., H. YANG, J. RIVIER & Y. TACHÉ. 1988. Peptides **9:** 1067–1070.
57. TACHÉ, Y., M. MAEDA-HAGIWARA & C. M. TURKELSON. 1987. Am. J. Physiol. **253:** G241.
58. LENZ, H. J., A. RAEDLER, H. GRETEN, W. W. VALE & J. E. RIVIER. 1988. Gastroenterology **95:** 1510–1517.
59. GUNION, M. W., G. L. KAUFFMAN & Y. TACHÉ. 1990. Am. J. Physiol. **258:** G152–G157.
60. MATSUDA, M., M. AONO, M. MORIGA & M. OKUMA. 1991. Regul. Pept. **35:** 31–41.
61. GEOGHEGAN, J. G., D. C. LAWSON, C. A. CHENG, E. OPARA, I. L. TAYLOR & T. N. PAPPAS. 1992. In press.
62. GUNION, M. W. & Y. TACHÉ. 1987. Brain Res. **411:** 156–161.
63. SAWCHENKO, P. E. & L. W. SWANSON. 1982. J. Comp. Neurol. **205:** 260–272.
64. SAWCHENKO, P. E. & S. W. PFEIFFER. 1988. Brain Res. **474:** 231–245.
65. MARTEL, J. C., S. ST. PIERRE & R. QUIRION. 1986. Peptides **55:** 60.
66. NAKAJIMA, N., Y. YASHIMA & K. NAKAMURA. 1986. Brain Res. **380:** 144–150.
67. DUMONT, Y., J. C. MARTEL, A. FOURNIER, S. ST. PIERRE & R. QUIRION. 1992. Prog. Neurobiol. **38:** 125–167.
68. HEYMANN-MONNIKES, I., Y. TACHÉ, M. TRAUNER, H. WEINER & T. GARRICK. 1991. Brain Res. **554:** 139.
69. GUÉ, M., V. EYSSELEIN, J. REEVE, J. RIVIER, J. L. JUNIEN & Y. TACHÉ. 1992. Gastroenterology **102(4/2):** 454.
70. EBERLEIN, G. A., V. E. EYSSELEIN, M. SHAEFFER, P. LAYER, D. GRANDT, H. GOEBELL, W. NIEBEL, M. DAVIS, T. D. LEE, J. E. SHIVELY & J. R. REEVE. 1989. Peptides **10:** 797–803.
71. YONEDA, M., J. L. JUNIEN & Y. TACHÉ. 1992. Eur. J. Pharmacol.

Regulation of Small Intestinal and Pancreaticobiliary Functions by CRF

H. JÜRGEN LENZ

Division of Gastroenterology, Department of Medicine
University of California, San Diego, School of Medicine
9500 Gilman Drive
La Jolla, California 92093-0671

Stress responses of the gastrointestinal tract are commonly thought of as changes in gastric acid secretion and intestinal motility. These two gut functions have been studied most thoroughly both in humans and in animals. Furthermore, stress-induced alterations in acid secretion and gastrointestinal motility have been implicated to play a role in the pathogenesis of peptic ulcer disease and the irritable bowel syndrome which are felt to be secretory and motor disorders, respectively. Several studies have indicated that corticotropin-releasing factor (CRF) appears to be an endogenous central nervous system (CNS) transmitter mediating stress-induced inhibition of gastric acid secretion, gastric emptying, and small bowel transit as well as stress-induced stimulation of large bowel transit.[1]

The small intestine, the pancreas, and the gallbladder are innervated by both the sympathetic and parasympathetic systems. Evidence for cephalic phases of exocrine pancreatic secretion and gallbladder contraction indicates that the pancreas as well as the gallbladder are controlled by neuronal efferents originating in the CNS whereas the small bowel can function rather independently. Until recently, the effects of stress and of CRF on small intestinal and pancreaticobiliary functions were completely unknown. Here we summarize our findings in animals as they relate to the effects of stress and CRF on duodenal, pancreatic, and ileal secretions and gallbladder motor function.

ANIMAL MODELS

To examine the effects of stress and exogenous CRF, studies were carried out in awake, nonanesthetized animals. Gallbladder contraction was measured in male Beagle dogs equipped with chronic, third cerebroventricular cannulae and gastric, Thomas-type, fistulae. Gallbladder volume was determined in the fasting state at basal levels, in response to cholecystokinin-8 (CCK, 20 pmol/kg.h), a mixed intragastric meal, stress, and exogenous CRF by real-time ultrasonography using a 5-mHz transducer.[2] Duodenal, ileal, and pancreatic studies were carried out in male Sprague-Dawley rats fitted with lateral cerebroventricular cannulae, internalized 2-cm duodenal loops, internalized 15-cm ileal loops or an internal pancreatic catheter after surgical biliary diversion to obtain pure pancreatic juice. Intestinal loops were perfused, and the perfusates and the pancreatic juice were drained through catheters which were exteriorized to exit at the interscapular region of the animal's neck.[2] Vagotomy, adrenalectomy, and hypophysectomy were performed by standard techniques and pharmacologic means were used to block neuronal transmission at autonomic ganglia, adrenergic, cholinergic, and opiate receptors as previously reported.[2] Plasma levels of catecholamines, β-endorphin, ACTH, cortisol, and glucose were also determined in response to stress, exogenous cerebral CRF, and intravenous infusions of norepinephrine and β-endorphin.

Two different stressors were applied. Dogs were fitted with headphones and exposed for one hour to "pop" music (70–80 dB) that was prerecorded at different speeds (17, 33, and 45 rpm in random order, 1 min each). In control experiments, dogs were equipped with headphones only, to which they were accustomed. Rats were subjected to physical restraint at room temperature using three metal clamps which allowed them to move their head, tail, and limbs but not their trunk. In control experiments, rats were freely moving in 15-L buckets to which they were accustomed. Both acoustic and restraint stress (stressor) produced plasma concentrations of ACTH, β-endorphin, epinephrine, norepinephrine, and glucose that were observed in response to cerebral administration of exogenous CRF.[2]

CRF AS MEDIATOR OF ILEAL WATER TRANSPORT

Cerebral but not intravenous administration of CRF (0.1–1.0 nmol) significantly stimulated ileal water absorption in freely moving rats for 45–60 minutes. Similarly, restraint stress stimulated ileal water absorption for 60 minutes.[3] Increased water absorption was associated with increased absorption of sodium and chloride. Both CRF- and stress-induced stimulated water absorption were abolished dose-dependently by cerebral but not by intravenous administration of the CRF receptor antagonist, α-helical CRF$_{9-41}$ (1–10 nmol). The CNS effects of CRF were abolished by ganglionic blockade with intravenously administered chlorisondamine, noradrenergic blockade with bretylium tosylate, and the α-adrenergic antagonist phentolamine.[3] In contrast, vagotomy, adrenalectomy, hypophysectomy, vasopressin, and opiate receptor blockade did not significantly alter the response produced by cerebral CRF.[3] Intravenous infusion of norepinephrine produced plasma concentrations similar to those observed in response to stress and cerebral CRF and also stimulated ileal water absorption.[3] The absorptive effect produced by norepinephrine was attenuated dose-dependently by phentolamine.[3] These results indicate that exogenous CRF administered to the CNS and endogenously released CRF during stress stimulate ileal water absorption in conscious rats. The absorptive effects produced by CRF are mediated by increased sympathetic, noradrenergic outflow to the gut. Release of norepinephrine acting on α-adrenergic receptors appears to be the final peripheral transmitter mediating the absorptive effects produced by CRF (FIG. 1).

CRF AS MEDIATOR OF PANCREATICOBILIARY FUNCTION

Acoustic stress in dogs and restraint stress in rats produced characteristic neuroendocrine stress responses: elevations in plasma concentrations of epinephrine, norepinephrine, ACTH, β-endorphin, and glucose. Acoustic stress significantly prevented CCK- and meal-induced gallbladder contraction, and restraint stress significantly inhibited pancreatic volume, protein and bicarbonate secretions. Cerebral but not intravenous CRF (0.05–0.5 nmol/kg) mimicked these stress responses in a dose-related manner. The effects of acoustic stress, restraint stress, and exogenous CRF were prevented by cerebral injection of the CRF receptor antagonist, α-helical CRF$_{9-41}$ (0.1–10.0 nmol/kg). The effects of acoustic stress, restraint stress and exogenous CRF on both CCK-induced gallbladder contraction and resting and

CCK/secretin-stimulated pancreatic secretions were prevented by intravenous injection of the ganglionic blocking agent chlorisondamine and the noradrenergic blocking agent bretylium, but not by vagotomy or adrenalectomy. Intravenous infusion of norepinephrine (10 μmol/kg.h) produced norepinephrine plasma levels that were similar to those observed in response to acoustic stress, restraint stress, and CRF.[4] The effects of acoustic stress, restraint stress, intravenous norepinephrine, and cerebroventricularly administered CRF on CCK-induced gallbladder contraction and exocrine pancreatic secretions were abolished dose-dependently by intravenous administration of phentolamine.[4] These results indicate that stress, exogenous CRF, and norepinephrine inhibit canine gallbladder contraction and murine exocrine pancreatic secretion. Different stressors (acoustic and restraint stress) in distinct species (dogs and rats) release CRF that acts on specific receptors within the brain.

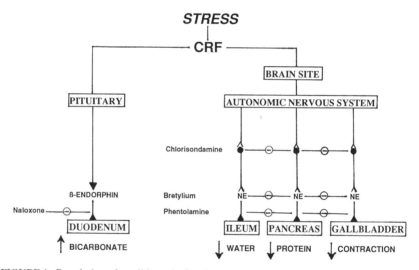

FIGURE 1. Regulation of small intestinal and pancreaticobiliary function by CRF: a working model. CRF released in response to stress *stimulates* duodenal bicarbonate secretion by release of β-endorphin from the pituitary which acts on opiate receptors. In contrast, CRF released in response to stress *inhibits* ileal water and electrolyte secretion, exocrine pancreatic secretion, and gallbladder contraction by activating sympathetic, noradrenergic efferents releasing norepinephrine that acts on α-adrenergic receptors. NE, norepinephrine; $\ominus$, inhibited by.

Stress and CRF stimulate sympathetic, noradrenergic outflow to the gut. Release of norepinephrine appears to be the final common pathways resulting in inhibition of gallbladder contraction and exocrine pancreatic secretion during stress mediated by endogenous CRF (FIG. 1).

CRF AS MEDIATOR OF DUODENAL BICARBONATE SECRETION

Proximal duodenal mucosal bicarbonate secretion is an important factor in the pathogenesis of duodenal ulcer disease. Patients with duodenal ulcer disease have decreased proximal duodenal mucosal bicarbonate production at rest and in response to intraluminal hydrochloric acid. An animal model was developed that allowed cerebroventricular and intravenous injections as well as collection of duodenal perfusates in awake, freely moving rats.[5] In contrast to the observations on ileal, pancreatic, and biliary functions, cerebral as well as intravenous injections of CRF (0.01–1.0 nmol) produced similar effects, that is, significant stimulation of proximal duodenal bicarbonate secretion. These responses were reversed dose-dependently by cerebral and intravenous infusion of α-helical CRF_{9-41} (0.1–10.0 nmol).[5] Restraint stress stimulated duodenal bicarbonate secretion to a similar degree as did the highest dose of CRF (1.0 nmol) studied. In contrast to all previous observations, blockade of autonomic nervous system efferents using chlorisondamine, bretylium, adrenalectomy or vagotomy did not affect the bicarbonate responses produced by stress or CRF.[5]

Hypophysectomy and pretreatment with naloxone completely abolished duodenal bicarbonate secretion in response to stress and CRF. Furthermore, intravenous infusion of β-endorphin that mimicked plasma concentrations of β-endorphin observed after either stress or exogenous CRF stimulated duodenal bicarbonate secretion similarly compared with stress and exogenous CRF. Finally, the effects of exogenous β-endorphin on duodenal bicarbonate secretion were also abolished by naloxone.[5] These results indicate that endogenous CRF released during stress and exogenously administered CRF stimulate duodenal bicarbonate secretion by release of β-endorphin from the pituitary, thus demonstrating a functional hypothalamus-pituitary-gut axis (FIG. 1).

PHYSIOLOGIC AND PATHOPHYSIOLOGIC IMPLICATIONS

Stress is usually not implicated as the sole cause for any disease in man, but numerous reports indicate that stress may aggravate, exacerbate, and modify the illness itself and the associated symptoms. It is a myth, for example, that ordinary life stresses (physical, mental, conflict, work- or family-related) cause gastric or duodenal ulcers, yet different stressors may accentuate symptoms such as abdominal pain, fullness, bloating, diarrhea, and constipation. Similarly, stress is unlikely the only cause for the irritable bowel syndrome, but, clearly, stressful life events may exacerbate and have been associated with cramping abdominal pain and a change in bowel habits.

Are the gastrointestinal effects of CRF of any physiologic or pathophysiologic significance? The answer to this question is based solely on observations made in experimental animals. Nevertheless, some cautious extrapolations may be made. (1) CRF, in general, inhibits visceral and digestive functions; this enhances availability of oxygen and energy sources in other organ systems such as the cardiovascular and musculoskeletal systems. (2) During stress, such as hemorrhagic shock, CRF contributes to the maintenance of blood pressure not only by increasing cardiac output but also by inhibiting small bowel secretions, that is, enhancing water and electrolyte absorption. (3) During some forms of stress, CRF may prevent formation of gastric and duodenal ulcers by inhibiting gastric acid secretion and stimulating duodenal bicarbonate production. (4) Although pancreatic digestive enzyme inhibition mediated by CRF during stress may be beneficial to the organism, inhibition of gallbladder emptying during stress (such as in a patient in an intensive-care unit) may facilitate formation of biliary crystals (sludge) and subsequent acalculous cholecystitis. (5) The irritable bowel syndrome is characterized by various gastrointestinal motility patterns. It is possible that *some* of the motility disturbances are mediated by CRF.

UNRESOLVED QUESTIONS

CRF exerts its central nervous system effects via both sympathetic and parasympathetic efferents and via different peripheral transmitters at the end organ. For example, CRF-induced inhibition of gastric acid secretion may be mediated by sympathetic, noradrenergic efferents, noncholinergic vagal efferents, vasopressin- and opiate-sensitive pathways (at least in the dog) and "substance(s)" (not epinephrine) from the adrenal gland.[6] Although redundancy in neuronal circuits is a frequently seen phenomenon, it is unclear, at this time, how much each of these pathways contributes to mediation of acid inhibition. The inhibitory effects of CRF on gastric emptying appear to be mediated via sympathetic, noradrenergic or vagal efferents whereas the stimulatory effects of CRF on colonic motility are mediated by vagal efferents only. The mechanisms underlying this pattern of control are unclear. One could hypothesize that different CNS sites stimulated (or inhibited) by CRF are operative in the control of gastric and colonic motility or that peripheral or spinal control mechanisms alter the central (CRF-sensitive) common pathway. Finally, at least in the dog, CRF increases plasma vasopressin concentrations, and peripheral vasopressin inhibits duodenal bicarbonate secretion; yet, duodenal bicarbonate secretion is increased by stress and CRF. It is possible that the stimulatory effect of β-endorphin released by CRF overrides the inhibitory effect of vasopressin. Finally, adrenalectomy abolishes the inhibitory effects of CRF on gastric acid secretion via a pathway that does not appear to depend on epinephrine. However, other inhibitors of gastric acid secretion derived from the adrenal cortex or medulla have not been identified. "Desensitization of the system" after adrenalectomy has been implicated; however, adrenalectomy does not abolish other effects of CRF on gastrointestinal functions. Additional comparative and confirmative studies as well as different strategies to block autonomic efferents may be needed to resolve some of these discrepancies.

FUTURE CHALLENGES

Because the site of action of CRF, as it relates to changes in gastrointestinal function, appears to be primarily the central nervous system, the physiologic and pathophysiologic significance of CRF in humans is not likely to be elucidated any time soon. Further insight may be gained from studies utilizing techniques such as immunoneutralization, chronic administration of a CRF receptor antagonist or from animals either deficient in the CRF gene (if viable) or from animals with impaired expression of the gene (ideally, animals in which the expression of the CRF gene can be controlled in a restricted fashion). Further direct evidence for a (patho)physiologic importance of CRF in humans may be gained once technology has advanced so that agonist and antagonist may be delivered to the central nervous system after peripheral, intravenous or oral administration.

REFERENCES

1. LENZ, H. J. 1990. Mediation of gastrointestinal stress responses by corticotropin-releasing factor. Ann. N.Y. Acad. Sci. **597:** 81 91.
2. LENZ, H. J. 1991. Stress-induced alteration of gastrointestinal function: Role of corticotropin-releasing factor. *In* Brain-Gut Interactions. Y. Taché & D. Wingate, Eds.: 285–295. CRC Press. Boca Raton, FL.

3. LENZ, H. J. & T. M. SILVERMAN. 1993. Stimulation of ileal water absorption in conscious rats by exogenous and endogenous corticotropin-releasing factor. Gastroenterology. In press.

4. LENZ, H. J., B. MESSMER & F. G. ZIMMERMAN. 1992. Noradrenergic inhibition of canine gallbladder contraction and murine pancreatic secretion during stress by corticotropin-releasing factor. J. Clin. Invest. **89:** 437–443.

5. LENZ, H. J. 1989. Regulation of duodenal bicarbonate secretion during stress corticotropin-releasing factor and β-endorphin. Proc. Natl. Acad. Sci. USA **86:** 1417–1420.

6. LENZ, H. J. 1991. Stress-induced alteration in gastrointestinal function. *In* Encyclopedia of Human Biology. R. Dulbecco, Ed. Vol. **7:** 285–292. Academic Press. San Diego, CA.

Immunopathology of Ulcer Disease[a]

AKIRA UEHARA[b] AND MASAYOSHI NAMIKI

Department of Internal Medicine (III)
Asahikawa Medical College
4-5 Nishikagura
Asahikawa, Hokkaido 078, Japan

Recent advances of genetic engineering have made it possible to produce many kinds of recombinant cytokines in large amounts. The greater availability of cytokines mass-produced by the recombinant technique has paved the way to the comprehensive investigation of various biological actions of these cytokines, particularly nonimmunological actions. Interleukin-1 (IL-1), a cytokine released mainly from activated monocytes and macrophages, is a typical example of these cytokines investigated from various points of view. For example, we have reported that IL-1 activates the hypothalamic-pituitary-adrenal axis,[1-3] the principal neuroendocrine regulatory mechanism of stress responses, and furthermore that IL-1 suppresses feeding behavior via hypothalamic corticotropin-releasing factor (CRF).[4-5] Thus, this recent surge of interest in numerous bilateral interactions between the immune and neuroendocrine systems has established a rapidly expanding interdisciplinary field, which is called immunoneuroendocrinology or psychoneuroimmunology.

In extending our immunoneuroendocrine studies on IL-1, we found that the intraperitoneal injection of IL-1 inhibited the secretion of gastric acid and output of pepsin in pylorus-ligated rats.[6-7] Since then, we have been conducting a series of studies in which we have demonstrated that IL-1 acts centrally in the brain to inhibit gastric secretion and also to exert potent mucosal protective actions against various ulcerogenic stimuli.[8-10] Other investigators have confirmed these findings and have also found these novel biological effects of IL-1 on the stomach; as a result, the investigation of the effects of IL-1 on the gastrointestinal tract seems to have become one of the primary topics in gastroenterology today. On the basis of these findings, we have proposed the possible existence of an "immune-brain-gut" axis, which may be involved in the physiology and pathophysiology of digestive diseases, especially of peptic ulcer.[10] Reflecting these current trends in the field of gastroenterology, we discuss in this paper the immunopathological aspects of ulcer disease by reviewing reports produced from our group as well as those from other research groups.

EFFECTS OF INTERLEUKIN-1 ON GASTRIC FUNCTIONS

Gastric Secretion

What prompted us to speculate that IL-1 might have gastric antisecretory actions was based upon the following two lines of scientific evidence. First, it has been shown

[a]This study was supported by Grant (12-A) from the National Center of Neurology and Psychiatry (NCNP) of the Ministry of Health and Welfare of Japan, and by grants from the Meiji Welfare Foundation, the Uehara Memorial Foundation, and the Nanba Memorial Foundation in Japan.
[b]Corresponding author.

that the transmission of immune signals carried by blood-borne IL-1 across the blood-brain barrier is mediated by the prostaglandin (PG) system in the brain[11] and that central PGs inhibit gastric acid secretion.[12] Second, IL-1 stimulates the secretion of CRF,[2,13,14] a neuropeptide that centrally inhibits acid secretion.[15] We therefore speculated that IL-1 might suppress gastric acid secretion via a mechanism involving the central PG system or central CRF, or both. As expected, the intraperitoneal injection of IL-1 resulted in a dose-related and long-lasting inhibition of gastric acid in pylorus-ligated rats, and this gastric antisecretory action of IL-1 was completely abolished by pretreatment with indomethacin, a blocker of PG biosynthesis.[6] This was the very first report that suggested that a cytokine produced by the immune system is ever involved in the regulation of gastric acid secretion. The possibility of CRF involvement in this IL-1 action was excluded by the observation that the CRF antagonist α-helical CRF$_{9-41}$ failed to affect the IL-1-induced suppression of acid secretion.

Next, we decided to determine if this antisecretory action of IL-1 was mediated by the central nervous system, by comparing the effects of intraperitoneally (i.p.) injected IL-1 and intracerebroventricularly (i.c.v.) injected IL-1 on gastric acid output.[9] The i.c.v. administration of IL-1 led to the dose-dependent inhibition of gastric secretion, as did the i.p. injection of IL-1. In addition, it was found that i.c.v. IL-1 was about a hundred times more potent in its suppressive action than i.p. IL-1. These results strongly indicate that IL-1 inhibits gastric acid secretion via a mechanism which is mediated by the central nervous system.

Besides gastric acid, pepsin is another important component in the physiology of gastric secretion. We therefore examined the effects of IL-1 on pepsin secretion. IL-1, either i.c.v. or i.p. injected, inhibited pepsin secretion with i.c.v. IL-1 being far more powerful than i.p. IL-1, in a similar manner to acid inhibition by IL-1.[7] Taken together, IL-1 seemed likely to participate in the mechanism by which gastric secretion of both acid and pepsin is regulated, particularly under certain pathophysiological conditions that can stimulate the immune system to secrete cytokines including IL-1.

To determine whether endogenously released IL-1 as well as exogenously administered IL-1 will exert a similar effect, we examined the effects of lipopolysaccharide (LPS), a potent stimulant of the secretion and production of endogenous IL-1, on gastric secretion. The i.c.v. injection of LPS dose-dependently suppressed the secretion of gastric acid[6,16] and pepsin,[17] and this biological activity of LPS was a reversible and PG-dependent reaction.[18,19] These results indicate that IL-1 has indeed a physiological relevance in terms of the regulatory mechanism of gastric secretion.

It should be noted here that the antisecretory actions of IL-1 were reported independently and almost simultaneously by other research groups as well.[20-21] All these reports, including ours, are in good agreement with the finding that IL-1 acts centrally in the brain to potently inhibit gastric acid secretion and that this IL-1 action is PG-dependent. They also demonstrated, by examining the influence of the CRF antagonist α-helical CRF$_{9-41}$, bilateral adrenalectomy and noradrenergic blockade, that neither CRF nor the noradrenergic system was involved in the antisecretory effect of IL-1.[20-21] Furthermore, Saperas et al.[22] have very recently reported that the microinjection of IL-1 into the medial preoptic area, anterior hypothalamus, and paraventricular nucleus inhibited gastric acid secretion, thereby indicating that these areas in the hypothalamus are brain sites of action of IL-1 to exert its antisecretory effect.

Although it seems to be well accepted that IL-1 inhibits gastric acid secretion in a PG-dependent manner via the central nervous system, a number of unsolved problems or disputes still remain regarding IL-1 and acid secretion. First, where is the site of action of this IL-1 effect—Is it located centrally in the brain or peripherally in the stomach? A great dose differential between centrally injected IL-1 and peripherally injected IL-1 strongly suggests that this is mediated by the central nervous system. It is true, however, that peripheral IL-1 results in a dose-related and long-lasting inhibition of gastric secretion.[6,7,21,23] It is possible, therefore, that IL-1 may act both at peripheral and central sites through different mechanisms. In this respect, Robert et al.[23] went so far as to speculate that the stomach may possess IL-1 receptors possibly located on parietal cells or other cells, including as yet unidentified cells. Second, how is the IL-1 signal of inhibiting acid secretion transmitted to the local effector organ stomach? One may readily consider that the vagal system mediates the IL-1-induced suppression of acid output. Saperas et al.[21] demonstrated that intracisternal injection (i.c.) of IL-1 inhibited the gastric acid secretion stimulated by thyrotropin-releasing hormone, which acts by increasing vagal efferent activity, suggesting that central IL-1 decreases acid output through modification of the parasympathetic outflow to the stomach. By contrast, peripheral IL-1-induced antisecretory action is not influenced by bilateral vagotomy.[24] Third, most investigators have agreed that the integrity of PG pathways is required for acid inhibition by IL-1;[6,20–23] however, there is a paper that shows that the inhibitory effect of IL-1 on acid secretion was not blocked by pretreatment with indomethacin.[24] Taken together, these data indicate that IL-1 can be now added to the list of many neuropeptides that are involved in the central nervous system regulation of gastric acid secretion (see ref. 25, for review).

Gastric Emptying

Compared with the effects of IL-1 on gastric acid secretion, much less information is available concerning the effects of IL-1 on gastric motility, an important function of the gut. Robert et al.[23] first reported that IL-1 retarded gastric emptying in rats.[23] They demonstrated that i.p. IL-1 dose-dependently suppressed the gastric emptying of solid meals. Of great intrigue was the observation that this inhibitory action of IL-1 on gastric motility was not abolished by pretreatment with indomethacin;[23] this is in sharp contrast with the antisecretory action of IL-1 which is PG-dependent. We have also confirmed these findings that either i.p. or i.c.v. IL-1 inhibit gastric emptying in a dose-related and PG-independent manner (unpublished data). These results suggest that IL-1 affects gastric function, that is, secretion and motility, through at least two different mechanisms: PG-dependent and -independent pathways. However, many more studies should be performed to further clarify the characteristics of this IL-1 action on gastric motility. For example, it would be of interest to test the effects of IL-1 on the gastric emptying of liquid meals as well as solid meals, or to see the effects of IL-1 on the contractile activity of stomach. Another important aspect of this inhibitory effect of IL-1 on gastric motility is that this property of IL-1 may contribute to the mucosal protective actions of IL-1. There is increasing evidence that hypermotility is an important factor in the pathogenesis of gastric ulcer formation.[26–28] Detailed discussion of this follows.

EFFECTS OF INTERLEUKIN-1 ON EXPERIMENTAL ULCERS

Mucosal Protective Actions

The novel findings that IL-1 inhibited both gastric secretion and motility, two major pathogenetic factors of gastric ulceration, promptly led us to hypothesize that pretreatment with IL-1 might reduce the severity of gastric mucosal lesions induced by various ulcerogenic manipulations.[8-11] These mucosal protective effects of IL-1 have been reported by several different research teams as well.[23,29-32]

First, we examined[8] the effects of IL-1 in the water-immersion restraint stress ulcer model, a well-established stress maneuver to produce gastric mucosal lesions in rats.[32] Overnight fasted rats were preinjected with i.c.v. IL-1 60 minutes prior to being placed in individual restraint cages. Then they were immersed and kept into cold water (23 °C) up to the xiphoid process for 5 hours. The severity of gastric mucosal lesions was assessed by the total length of all lesions observed. Pretreatment with IL-1 dose-dependently prevented the development of gastric mucosal lesions induced by the stress manipulations. A similar mucosal protective action of IL-1 was also observed against the i.c.v. injection of an ulcerogenic dose of thyrotropin-releasing hormone (TRH),[9] which produces gastric lesions by increasing acid secretion through stimulation of vagal efferent activity.[33]

Wallace et al.[29] reported that pretreatment with i.p. IL-1 decreased the severity of ethanol- or indomethacin-induced gastric damage or cyteamine-induced duodenal injury, suggesting that IL-1 has protective actions in three different experimental models of gastroduodenal ulceration. Robert et al.[30] also found that i.c. IL-1 protects the gastric mucosa against the oral administration of absolute ethanol.[30] Likewise, it has been shown that i.p. IL-1 exerts a gastroprotective effect against the gastric damage by aspirin, another nonsteroidal anti-inflammatory drug (NSAID).[31]

Although the route of administration of IL-1 differs among these studies, that is, centrally injected or peripherally injected, all these findings clearly suggest that IL-1 possesses powerful mucosal protective effects against a wide variety of ulcerogenic challenges such as stress, TRH, NSAID, cysteamine, and ethanol, which have different pathogenetic properties to some extent. It is amazing, at least to us, that a cytokine produced by the immune system can influence the gastric mucosal defensive mechanism, because heretofore there had been no report which suggested that the immune system is associated with the pathogenesis and pathophysiology of ulcer disease.

Underlying Mechanisms

As to underlying mechanisms by which IL-1 exhibits its protective actions in the gastroduodenal tract, it appears likely to conclude at the present time that IL-1 can protect the gastric mucosa through several different underlying mechanisms, the contribution of each of which varies from ulcer model to model.

Considering that gastric acid and motility are major aggressive factors for ulceration, it may be easily assumed that the inhibitory actions of IL-1 on acid and motility significantly contribute to its anti-ulcer actions. To examine this assumption, we conducted a series of experiments (unpublished data). As described above, the antisecretory action of IL-1 is PG-dependent whereas the inhibitory action of IL-1 on motility is PG-independent. One may therefore speculate that when you preinject a PG-blocking dose, but not ulcerogenic dose, of indomethacin (5 mg/kg) and then block PG synthesis, the next injection of IL-1 would result in an inhibition of gastric motility but not an inhibition of gastric and secretion. By utilizing these pharmacological manipulations, we examined the effects of IL-1 in the two experimental ulcer models: stress ulceration and NSAID gastropathy. Pretreatment with indomethacin abolished the anti-ulcer effect of IL-1 against water-immersion restraint stress. On the other hand, indomethacin pretreatment failed to block the mucosal protective action of IL-1 against NSAID. These results suggest that the antisecretory effect of IL-1 is essential for its mucosal protective action in the stress ulcer model, whereas this is not the case for NSAID gastropathy, in which on the other hand the inhibitory effect of IL-1 on gastric motility is required for its protective action. In other words, the underlying main mechanism by which IL-1 exhibits its protective actions differs among experimental models of ulceration. In this respect, it should be stressed that Wallace et al.[34] also recently reported that the ability of IL-1 to protect the gastric mucosa against NSAID challenge was not completely attributable to the antisecretory action of IL-1; this is in accordance with our data that IL-1 can exert its protective actions in NSAID gastropathy in spite of the absence of its antisecretory action. Rather, the same group presented experimental data which suggested that the inhibitory effects of IL-1 on neutrophil function possibly through endogenous corticosteroids might contribute to its protective actions.[31]

As to the cytoprotective actions of IL-1 against absolute ethanol, the PG system in the stomach may play a crucial role. In fact, Mugridge et al.[35] first reported that IL-1 stimulated the biosynthesis of PGs in the stomach; this was later confirmed by Robert et al.[23] It is therefore possible that IL-1 increases PG production locally in the stomach, which in turn exerts cytoprotective actions against the necrotizing agent ethanol. This possibility has also been indirectly supported by the observation that the cytoprotective action of IL-1 was blocked by indomethacin pretreatment.[23,30] Mugridge and his colleagues, however, demonstrated in their recent papers[32,34] that IL-1 does not affect gastric PG synthesis, excluding the possible involvement of the gastric PG system in the protective actions of IL-1, at least in NSAID-induced gastric damage. It is not immediately known whether this apparent discrepancy may have derived from the differences in the experimental ulcer models employed, or from as yet unidentified causes. This problem warrants future experiments.

Although a number of unsolved problems remain with regard to underlying mechanisms for the mucosal protective actions of IL-1, it appears to be true that IL-1 activates several mechanisms to exhibit its protective effects. The comprehensive investigation of these as yet unknown mechanisms will certainly provide fruitful and significant information in the near future.

EFFECTS OF OTHER CYTOKINES

Comparison of Interleukin-1α and Interleukin-1β

There are the two different molecules of IL-1: IL-1α and IL-1β. It was previously considered that both forms of IL-1 shared the common spectrum of biological activities and bound to the common IL-1 receptor despite their limited homology (less than 30%) in amino acid sequences. Ample evidence now exists, however, that, depending on the cell type or animal species, the two forms of IL-1 likely have distinctly different binding sites on the IL-1 receptor, and accordingly demonstrate marked differences in biological activities (see ref. 36, for review). For example, we found that IL-1β was much more potent in its ability to release ACTH from the pituitary gland than IL-1α.[3] Since then, we have been exclusively using the β-form in our immunoneuroendocrine studies on IL-1. However, it would be of interest to see possible differences between the α- and β-forms of IL-1 in their antisecretory and anti-ulcer actions. It seems generally accepted that IL-1β is more powerful than IL-1α in both its inhibitory effect on gastric acid secretion[20,21,24] and its mucosal protective effects.[34] Inasmuch as IL-1α binds best to the type I receptor and IL-1β to the type II,[36] it is possible that the type II receptor is predominantly involved in the induction of IL-1 effects on the gut function. This may be a critical factor in interpreting the effects of an IL-1 receptor antagonist[37] on these biological activities of IL-1 in the gastrointestinal tract.

Tumor Necrosis Factor and Interleukin-6

The biological properties of tumor necrosis factor (TNF) share remarkable similarities to those of IL-1, particularly the nonimmunological effects of IL-1. Is this also true for the effects of IL-1 on the stomach? Wallace *et al.* have addressed this question. According to their results, TNF is nearly without effect in inhibiting acid secretion[24] and protecting the mucosa from NSAID gastropathy.[34] It is well known, however, that when IL-1 and TNF are used together in experimental studies, the net effect often exceeds the additive effect of each cytokine. It is possible, therefore, that this type of potentiation or synergism between these two molecules may occur in the stomach as well; this has not yet been investigated.

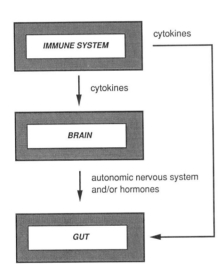

FIGURE 1. A hypothetical model of an "immune-brain-gut" axis, which may be involved in the pathogenesis and pathophysiology of various diseases in the gastrointestinal tract, particularly ulcer disease. In this organ axis, it is speculated that cytokines including IL-1 affect the central nervous system, which in turn influences the gut function through autonomic nervous pathways or neuropeptides, or both. It is possible that cytokines exert direct effects on the gastrointestinal tract through specific receptors that may be present locally. (Uehara *et al.*[10] Reproduced, with permission, from *Journal of Clinical Gastroenterology.*)

Because the production of IL-6 appears to be under the control of IL-1 in some models and both cytokines possess many biological activities in common, one may assume that the effects of IL-1 on the gut function may be mediated by IL-6 produced in response to IL-1 stimulation. This possibility would be worth investigating in the future.

IS GASTRIC ULCER AN IMMUNE DISEASE?

Gastric ulcer is a multifaceted disease with a complex, pluricausal etiology that is not fully understood.[38] A hypothesis used frequently to account for gastric mucosal injury or resistance to injury is that of an interaction or balance between aggressive factors and defensive factors in the gut. Aggressive factors include various mechanisms, from the long-held clinical dictum "no acid—no ulcer" to *Helicobacter pylori*, recently implicated as a causal factor in antral gastritis and possibly also in gastric and duodenal ulcerogenesis. Defensive mechanisms are represented by classic factors such as mucus and biocarbonate secretion, as well as by PGs, sulfhydryls, polyamines, and the more recently characterized gastroprotectants including endothelium-derived relaxing factor/nitric oxide and dopamine. These discussions have generally included only physicochemical events or agents which occur locally in the stomach. But is gastric ulcer a local disease in the gut alone?

As has been described in this paper, accumulating evidence strongly suggests that IL-1, a cytokine produced by the immune system, has potent mucosal protective actions against various ulcerogenic stimuli through different mechanisms. These observations indicate that the immune system may be also involved in the pathogenesis or pathophysiology of ulcer formation. On the basis of all these findings, we have proposed the presence of an immune-brain-gut axis (FIG. 1), which may play an important role in ulcerogenesis. In our view, gastric ulcer should be considered as not simply a local disease in the stomach, but as a general disease involving even the immune system as well as the brain.

Finally, we end this paper by asking a rather provocative question: Is gastric ulcer an immune disease? Most readers likely would immediately answer in the negative, but future advances in immunoneuroendocrine studies on the pathogenesis of ulcer disease may lead to an answer in the affirmative.

ACKNOWLEDGMENTS

The authors wish to thank Y. Yoshida for her excellent technical assistance.

REFERENCES

1. UEHARA, A., S. GILLIS & A. ARIMURA. 1987. Effects of interleukin-1 on hormone release from normal pituitary cells in primary culture. Neuroendocrinology 45: 343–347.
2. UEHARA, A., P. E. GOTTSCHALL, R. R. DAHL & A. ARIMURA. 1987. Interleukin-1 stimulates ACTH release by an indirect action which requires endogenous corticotropin-releasing factor. Endocrinology 121: 1580–1582.
3. UEHARA, A., P. E. GOTTSCHALL, R. R. DAHL & A. ARIMURA. 1987. Stimulation of ACTH release by human interleukin-1 beta, but not by interleukin-1 alpha, in conscious, freely-moving rats. Biochem. Biophys. Res. Commun. 146: 1286–1290.
4. UEHARA, A., C. SEKIYA, Y. TAKASUGI, M. NAMIKI & A. ARIMURA. 1989. Anorexia induced by interleukin-1: Involvement of corticotropin-releasing factor. Am. J. Physiol. 257: R613–R617.
5. UEHARA, A., Y. ISHIKAWA, T. OKUMURA, K. OKAMURA, C. SEKIYA, Y. TAKASUGI & M. NAMIKI. 1989. Indomethacin blocks the anorexic action of interleukin-1. Eur. J. Pharmacol. 170: 257–260.
6. UEHARA, A., T. OKUMURA, C. SEKIYA, K. OKAMURA, Y. TAKASUGI & M. NAMIKI. 1989. Interleukin-1 inhibits the secretion of gastric acid in rats: Possible involvement of prostaglandin. Biochem. Biophys. Res. Commun. 162: 1578–1584.
7. OKUMURA, T., A. UEHARA, K. OKAMURA, Y. TAKASUGI & M. NAMIKI. 1990. Inhibition of gastric pepsin secretion by peripherally or centrally injected interleukin-1 in rats. Biochem. Biophys. Res. Commun. 167: 956–961.
8. UEHARA, A., T. OKUMURA, S. KITAMORI, Y. TAKASUGI & M. NAMIKI. 1990. Interleukin-1: A cytokine that has potent gastric antisecretory and anti-ulcer actions via the central nervous system. Biochem. Biophys. Res. Commun. 173: 585–590.
9. OKUMURA, T., A. UEHARA, S. KITAMORI, Y. TAKASUGI & M. NAMIKI. 1990. Prevention by interleukin-1 of thyrotropin-releasing hormone (TRH)-induced gastric mucosal lesions in rats. Neurosci. Lett. 125: 31–33.

10. Uehara, A., T. Okumura, S. Kitamori, Y. Shibata, K. Harada, K. Okamura, Y. Takasugi & M. Namiki. 1992. Gastric antisecretory and anti-ulcer actions of interleukin-1: Evidence for the presence of an "immune-brain-gut" axis. J. Clin. Gastroenterol. 14: S149–S155.

11. Katsuura, G., P. E. Gottschall, R. R. Dahl & A. Arimura. 1989. Interleukin-1 beta increases prostaglandin E_2 in rat astrocyte cultures: Modulatory effect of neuropeptides. Endocrinology 124: 3125–3127.

12. Puurunen, J. 1983. Central inhibitory action of prostaglandin E_2 on gastric secretion in the rat. Eur. J. Pharmacol. 91: 245–249.

13. Berkenbosch, F., J. van Oers, A. del Rey, F. Tilders & H. Besedovsky. 1987. Corticotropin-releasing factor–producing neurons in the rat activated by interleukin-1. Science 238: 524–526.

14. Sapolsky, S., C. Rivier, G. Yamamoto, P. Plotsky & W. Vale. 1987. Interleukin-1 stimulates the secretion of hypothalamic corticotropin-releasing factor. Science 238: 522–524.

15. Taché, Y., Y. Goto, M. W. Gunion, W. Vale, J. Rivier & M. Brown. 1983. Inhibition of gastric acid secretion in rats by intracerebral injection of corticotropin-releasing factor. Science 222: 935–937.

16. Impicciatore, M., D. G. Hansen, D. Rachmilewitz, S. K. Maitra, G. Lugaro & M. I. Grossman. 1980. Comparison of human urine gastric inhibitor (HUGI) and bacterial endotoxin as inhibitors of acid secretion. Eur. J. Pharmacol. 65: 365–368.

17. Uehara, A., T. Okumura, K. Okamura, Y. Takasugi & M. Namiki. 1990. Lipopolysaccharide-induced inhibition of gastric acid and pepsin secretion in rats. Eur. J. Pharmacol. 181: 141–145.

18. Uehara, A., T. Okumura, K. Tsuji, Y. Taniguchi, S. Kitamori, Y. Takasugi & M. Namiki. 1992. Evidence that gastric antisecretory action of lipopolysaccharide is not due to a toxic effect on gastric parietal cells. Dig. Dis. Sci. 37: 1039–1044.

19. Tsuji, K., A. Uehara, T. Okumura, Y. Taniguchi, S. Kitamori, Y. Takasugi & M. Namiki. 1992. The gastric antisecretory action of lipopolysaccharide is blocked by indomethacin. Eur. J. Pharmacol. 210: 213–215.

20. Ishikawa, T., S. Nagata, Y. Ago, K. Takahashi & M. Karibe. 1990. The central inhibitory effect of interleukin-1 on gastric acid secretion. Neurosci. Lett. 119: 114–117.

21. Saperas, E. S., H. Yang, C. Rivier & Y. Taché. 1990. Central action of recombinant interleukin-1 to inhibit acid secretion in rats. Gastroenterology 99: 1599–1606.

22. Saperas, E., H. Yang & Y. Taché. 1992. Interleukin-1β acts at hypothalamic sites to inhibit gastric secretion in rats. Am. J. Physiol. 263: G414–G418.

23. Robert, A., A. S. Olafsson, C. Lancaster & W. Zhang. 1991. Interleukin-1 is cytoprotective, antisecretory, stimulates PGE_2 synthesis by the stomach, and retards gastric emptying. Life Sci. 48: 123–134.

24. Wallace, J. L., M. Cucala, K. Mugridge & L. Parente. 1991. Secretagogue-specific effects of interleukin-1 on gastric acid secretion. Am. J. Physiol. 261: G559–G564.

25. Taché, Y. 1987. Central nervous system regulation of gastric acid secretion. In Physiology of the Gastrointestinal Tract. L. R. Johnson, Ed.: 911–930. Raven Press. New York, NY.

26. Yano, S., M. Akahane & M. Harada. 1978. Role of gastric motility in development of stress-induced gastric lesions of rats. Jpn. J. Pharmacol. 28: 607–615.

27. Garrick, T., S. Buack & P. Bass. 1986. Gastric motility is a major factor in cold restraint-induced lesion formation in rats. Am. J. Physiol. 250: G191–G199.

28. Takeuchi, K., S. Ueki & S. Okabe. 1986. Importance of gastric motility in the pathogenesis of indomethacin-induced gastric lesions in rats. Dig. Dis. Sci. 31: 1114–1121.

29. Wallace, J. L., C. M. Keenan, K. G. Mugridge & L. Parente. 1990. Reduction of the severity of experimental gastric and duodenal ulceration by interleukin-1β. Eur. J. Pharmacol. 186: 279–284.

30. Robert, A., E. Saperas, W. Zhang, A. S. Olafsson, C. Lancaster, D. E. Tracey, J. G. Chosay & Y. Taché. 1991. Gastric cytoprotection by intracisternal interleukin-1β in the rat. Biochem. Biophys. Res. Commun. 174: 1117–1124.

31. Perretti, M., K. G. Mugridge, J. L. Wallace & L. Parente. 1992. Reduction of

aspirin-induced gastric damage in rats by interleukin-1β: Possible involvement of endogenous corticosteroids. J. Pharmacol. Exp. Ther. **261:** 1238–1247.

32. TAKAGI, K., Y. KASUYA & K. WATANABE. 1964. Studies on the drugs for peptic ulcer. A reliable method for producing stress ulcer. Chem. Pharm. Bull. **12:** 465–472.

33. GOTO, Y. & Y. TACHÉ. 1985. Gastric erosions induced by intracisternal thyrotropin-releasing hormone (TRH) in rats. Peptides **6:** 153–156.

34. WALLACE, J. L., C. M. KEENAN, M. CUCALA, K. G. MUGRIDGE & L. PARENTE. 1992. Mechanisms underlying the protective effects of interleukin 1 in experimental nonsteroidal anti-inflammatory drug gastropathy. Gastroenterology **102:** 1176–1185.

35. MUGRIDGE, K. G., D. DONATI, S. SILVESTRI & L. PARENTE. 1989. Arachidonic acid lipoxygenation may be involved in interleukin-1 induction of prostaglandin biosynthesis. J. Pharmacol. Exp. Ther. **250:** 714–720.

36. DINARELLO, C. A. 1991. Interleukin-1 and interleukin-1 antagonism. Blood **77:** 1627–1652.

37. HANNUM, C. H., C. J. WILCOX, W. P. AREND, F. G. JOSLIN, D. J. DRIPPS, P. L. HEIMDAL, L. G. ARMES, A. SOMMER, S. P. EISENBERG & R. C. THOMPSON. 1990. Interleukin-1 receptor antagonist activity of a human interleukin-1 inhibitor. Nature **343:** 336–340.

38. GLAVIN, G. B. & S. SZABO. 1992. Experimental gastric mucosal injury: Laboratory models reveal mechanisms of pathogenesis and new therapeutic strategies. FASEB J. **6:** 825–831.

Stress and Behavior in Domestic Animals

Temperament as a Predisposing Factor to Stereotypies

ANDRÉ DALLAIRE

Faculté de Médecine Vétérinaire
C.P. 5000, St-Hyacinthe
Québec J2S 7C6, Canada

The objective of this paper is to relate the concept of abnormal stereotyped behaviors observed in domestic animals that were kept in inappropriate environment to a predisposition that seems linked to temperament and that is dependent upon the way each animal reacts to stress according to its behavioral profile. The data sources come mainly from published studies in animal sciences and from personal observation of domestic animal behavior. Research in fundamentals of stress, neuroendocrinology, pharmacology, and brain disorders in humans has provided veterinary medicine with new insights into these abnormal behaviors in animals, from which new therapeutics and preventive strategies begin to emerge.[1]

STEREOTYPIES IN DOMESTIC ANIMALS

A stereotypy is defined as a behavior pattern which is repetitive, invariant, and without any apparent goal or function.[2-4] This definition is useful for identification of and discussion about abnormal stereotyped behaviors. However, careful analysis of behavioral characteristics of a given stereotypy in one particular animal may reveal some degree of variation. In fact, repetitiveness and invariability should be considered as dependent both upon the nature of the stereotypy and the species concerned.[5]

Cribbing or wind sucking in horses, whereby the horse applies upper incisive teeth onto a protruding object in order to contract neck muscles and to swallow air, appears as ritualistic both in form and timing of sequential gestures. On the other hand, flank sucking in Dobermans, which consists of repetitive actions of biting and licking mainly at the abdomen, is quite variable in its behavioral manifestations and eliciting situations. Accordingly, stereotypies must be regarded as relatively invariable rather than absolutely invariable;[5] some of them are like fixed action patterns recognized by ethologists, whereas others seem closer to learned or acquired behaviors.

In veterinary medicine, the same criteria used in human medicine for diagnosis of stereotypies are now applied to animals. At present, stereotyped abnormal behaviors are considered as obsessive-compulsive disorders (OCD). The essential diagnostic features of OCDs are the clinical manifestations of a recurrent compulsion severe enough to cause physical injury or to interfere with normal activities or to become a nuisance to others. Thus, for the clinical diagnosis of an OCD, a criterion of severity is involved.

Mild wood chewing by a horse may not be regarded as an OCD, but persistent and recurrent wood chewing that interferes with the normal activity of the animal and causes physical injury or damage to its surroundings would be considered as a stereotyped abnormal behavior. Deciding which cases are of a sufficient degree of

TABLE 1. Obsessive-Compulsive Disorders (OCDs) in Domestic Animals

Nature of OCD	Species		
	A. In Food-Producing Animals		
	Pig	*Hen*	*Cattle*
Oral	Bar chewing	Feather pecking	Tongue rolling
	Snout rubbing		Head rubbing
Locomotor	Head weaving	Head flicking	
		Pacing	
Social	Tail biting	Hysteria	Destructive behavior
	B. In Companion Animals		
	Dog	*Cat*	*Horse*
Oral	Flank sucking	Self-licking	Crib biting
	Lick granuloma	Lick granuloma	Wood chewing
	Self-scratching	Hair chewing	
Locomotor	Circling	Head shaking	Head nodding
	Pacing	Pacing	Pacing
	Digging		Pawing
	Freezing	Freezing	
	Staring		Weaving
Social	Rhythmic barking		
	Unpredictable aggression	Periodic aggression	Self-mutilation
	Destructive behavior		

severity to confirm the diagnosis may be difficult at times, mainly in the early stages of development.

A significant number of OCDs are known to occur in domestic species. TABLE 1 is a summary of the most important of them in food-producing and companion animals.

STEREOTYPIES AND WELFARE

Stereotyped behavioral anomalies have been regarded for a long time as the result of an individual being placed in a suboptimal environment. Inadequate or improper environmental conditions such as social isolation, overfeeding, lack of a sufficient level of kinetic activities, and overcrowding are regarded usually as causative factors.[3] These factors are of concern to food-producing animals as well as to companion animals.

Frustration or boredom occurs in situations in which an animal is motivated to perform a behavior but is unable to do it because of physical or social limitations. Resultant stress or anxiety may initiate the search for a displacement or a redirected activity. For example, in a horse kept in a loose box but restricted to the barn most of the time, stereotyped pacing is recognized as "stall walking." The horse constantly circles around its box. This OCD is thought to appear under conditions of exercise deprivation and restriction to a small area. This behavior is also well known in polar bears kept at zoos.[6] Head rubbing in cattle confined to stalls for long periods during winter is also regarded as a behavioral anomaly that results from lack of movement and from overfeeding.[4] In dogs, a number of erratic behavioral manifestations occur in relation to separation anxiety. Many dogs suffer from the social isolation resulting from being left alone at home during working hours. Displacement activities such as destructive behavior or constant or rhythmic barking may develop in such a situation.[7]

Most of the OCDs recognized in domestic species have been associated with a barren environment or with restrictive conditions which are thought to generate frustration, boredom, anxiety or fear. This is the reason why these behavioral anomalies are regarded as signs of poor welfare, that is, the animal is suffering from a welfare condition that produces some form of stress. If this stress is chronic or intense enough, it may initiate a disorder that is subsequently recognized as a clinical sign of a behavioral disease.

INCIDENCE OF OBSESSIVE-COMPULSIVE DISORDERS

Although OCDs have been considered for many years as evidence of poor management or poor animal keeping practices, we do not have many statistics on their incidence. They are regarded as important and frequent problems, but we do not know exactly how frequently they occur. In food-producing animals, we have no statistics. When we consider data obtained from small animal veterinary clinics which offer behavioral services to their clients, we find a partial answer to the question about incidence of these anomalies. That is, from all dogs that presented with abnormal behaviors, we found that a significant percentage of these behaviors could be considered as OCDs (TABLE 2).

These statistics, however, do not provide us with a measure of incidence of stereotypies in an unbiased population. More useful indications have been obtained on the incidence of OCDs in horses. Figures from three independent studies[9-11] conducted in the United Kingdom, Italy, and Canada show that 8 to 20% of the horses kept permanently in stables have one or more OCDs. TABLE 3 summarizes these observations. When we consider most of the OCDs that can occur in this species, we find that nearly 20% of horses kept permanently at stables may develop a stereotypy during their life. In comparison to the incidence of OCDs in humans, which is considered to be less than 3%,[12] the frequency of OCDs among captive domestic animals seems very high. This could be related to generalizations about management conditions or attitudes in regard to domestic animals as well as to intensive breeding.

TABLE 2. Incidence of Abnormal Behaviors in a Clinical Population of Dogs (expressed in percentages)[a]

Aggression (all forms)[b]	58
Submission	2
Inappropriate elimination	18
Excitability[b]	6
Barking[b]	5
Destructive behavior[b]	14
Fear and phobias[b]	6
Stereotypies (tail biting, lick granuloma)[c]	2

[a]Adapted from Landsberg.[8]

[b]OCDs were included in these classifications. [c]Although only two abnormal behaviors were considered as stereotypies, their total incidence should be between 15 and 20%.

CAUSES OF OBSESSIVE-COMPULSIVE DISORDERS

The question one should ask at this point is why all animals in a given species kept in the same situation of confinement or in the same barren or improper environment do not develop abnormal behaviors in the form of OCDs. Why, for instance, in a given stable, do *only* two horses out of ten develop a stereotypy to cope with environmental constraints, whereas the others do not? Why do some develop an oral stereotypy, like wood chewing, whereas others develop a locomotor stereotypy, like stall walking?

Until very recently, we considered improper management practices as the cause of OCDs.[3,4] It now appears that environment should not be regarded as the sole cause of abnormal behaviors. Individuality of behavioral responses to environmental constraint should also be considered and probably regarded as a primary cause.

Certain stereotypies are more frequent in certain breeds of dogs, for example, flank sucking in Doberman and fly chasing in miniature schnauzer. In horses, it has been observed that individuals from some thoroughbred bloodlines are more likely to develop stereotyped behaviors.[10] If there is an increased probability for individuals

TABLE 3. Incidence of OCDs in Horses Kept Mostly in Barns. Results of Three Studies (expressed in percentages)[a]

OCD	A	B	C	X̄
Wood chewing	—	8.9	7.8	—
Crib biting	2.4	4.2	5.3	4.0
Aggression	—	—	6.4	—
Weaving	2.5	2.8	0.9	2.1
Head nodding	—	—	1.4	—
Pacing (stall walking)	2.5	1.1	2.5	2.0
Pawing	—	—	3.6	—
Total incidence	7.4	17.0	28.5	17.5

[a]Data in column **A** are from Vecchiotti and Galanti;[10] **B,** from Prince;[9] and **C,** from Dallaire.[11]

from one particular breed or from some bloodlines to present the clinical sign of an OCD, then we have to consider that genetics has something to do with stereotypies. Some individuals may inherit a predisposition to develop abnormal behaviors under stressful situations. Thus the cause of OCDs is not only an improper environment but also a predisposition to develop coping mechanisms to resist stress that involve a substitutive behavior.

Barren or improper environment is responsible for emotional perturbations that trigger physiological and behavioral processes to enable an individual to cope with these emotional perturbations. Individuality of reactions should be considered both at the level of emotional perturbations and of coping mechanisms. Because of individual differences in physiological processes and in behavioral strategies, the threshold between normal and abnormal probably varies among individuals.

Barrey[13] suggested that pathological behaviors emerge in horses when an animal has explored all possible behavioral strategies to cope with environmental pressure without finding an appropriate outcome. This exploration occurs according to a priority ranking, with those functions related to fighting or fleeing and to feeding as first-order homeostatic behaviors and functions related to rest, body care, motion, exploration, and territorialism as second-order homeostatic behaviors.[4] When an animal is unable to find a solution in its natural repertoire of behaviors, then a substitutive abnormal behavior may serve as the solution. When this outcome is no longer possible, inhibition of action or helplessness becomes the last resort;[14] this may ultimately help avoid further destructive effects from the environment. OCDs may be regarded as an inappropriate release of fixed action patterns or the release of an instrumental motor pattern which may delay the evolution of the pathological outcome toward an insoluble situation.

PREVENTION OF OBSESSIVE-COMPULSIVE DISORDERS

The neurobiological mechanisms underlying emotions and behaviors are not thoroughly understood. However, with respect to stereotypies, enough evidence exists that modifications in serotonin and/or dopamine metabolism are involved.[12] Recent research in the neurobiology of OCDs has led to new pharmacological approaches to these behavioral diseases. Antianxiety drugs seem useful, as well as narcotic antagonists, to modify stereotyped behavioral anomalies.[11,15] However, some stereotypies in animals are difficult to cure; some even seem intractable.

As useful as neuropharmacology in animals may be, we also have the opportunity to address the genetic component of OCDs. Significant data have been obtained on the heritability of many traits of temperament in dogs. Scott and Fuller[16] initiated this search in the late 1950s. It has been extended recently, using different approaches, by Hart and Hart[17] in California and Tortora[18] in New York. For instance, dimensions of temperament like nervousness and touch shyness seem to have a significant degree of inheritance.[19] If we consider that some animals may inherit a predisposition to develop an OCD, probably this predisposition is linked to one or more dimensions of their temperament. If we accept that a genetic predisposition seems to be linked to stereotypies—at least in dogs and in horses—even if we do not know the exact interaction between environment and temperament which is responsible for the development of an OCD, we have to consider that it may be possible to reduce the incidence of these anomalies by a twofold intervention: careful genetic selection based on behavior in addition to use of the sound management practices that are presently being promoted.

In conclusion, temperament must be regarded as a predisposing factor in relation to behavioral diseases that occur in most domestic species. We cannot ignore the influence of suboptimal environment in relation to stereotypies, but we must also address the issue of selecting for behavioral soundness in animals intended for use by humans.

REFERENCES

1. MARDER, A. R. & V. VOITH, Eds. 1991. Advances in companion animal behavior. Vet. Clin. North Am. **21(2):** 203–418.
2. FOX, M. 1968. Abnormal Behavior in Animals. W. B. Saunders Co. Philadelphia, PA.
3. KILEY-WORTHINGTON, M. 1977. Behavioral Problems of Farm Animals. Oriel Press. London.
4. FRASER, A. F. & D. M. BROOM. 1990. Farm Animal Behaviour and Welfare. Baillieres Tindall. London.
5. MASON, G. J. 1991. Stereotypies: A Critical Review. Anim. Behav. **41:** 1015–1037.
6. WECHSLER, B. 1992. Stereotypies and Attentiveness to Novel Stimuli: A Test in Polar Bears. Appl. Anim. Behav. Sci. **33:** 381–388.

7. O'FARRELL, V. 1991. Problem Dogs. London.
8. LANDSBERG, C. M. 1991. The distribution of canine behavior cases at three behavior referral practices. Vet. Med. **11:** 1011–1018.
9. PRINCE, D. 1987. Stable vices. *In* Behaviour Problems in Horses. S. McBane, Ed. David and Charles. London.
10. VECCHIOTTI, G. G. & R. GALANTI. 1986. Evidence of heredity of cribbing, weaving and stall-walking in thoroughbred horses. Livest. Prod. Sci. **14:** 91–95.
11. DALLAIRE, A. 1991. Problèmes de comportement chez les chevaux. lère Conférence vétérinaire de Gramat, France.
12. RAPPAPORT, J. L. 1989. The neuro-biology of obsessive-compulsive disorders. JAMA **260(19):** 2888–2890.
13. BARREY, J. C. 1990. Hiérarchie des comportements et comportements d'appétence. CEREOPA, 16ième Journée d'étude: 184–190. Paris.
14. LABORIT, H. 1986. L'inhibition de l'action: biologie comportementale et physiopathologie. 2nd edit. Masson. Paris.
15. DODMAN, N. H., L. SHUSTER, S. D. WHITE, M. H. COURT, D. PARKER & R. DIXO. Use of narcotic antagonists to modify stereotypic self-licking, self-chewing and scratching Behavior in Dogs. JAVMA **193(7):** 815–819.
16. SCOTT, J. P. & J. G. FULLER. 1965. Dog Behavior: The Genetic Basis. The University of Chicago Press. Chicago, IL.
17. HART, B. & L. A. HART. 1988. The Perfect Puppy. Freeman. New York, NY.
18. TORTORA, D. F. 1980. Choosing the right dog for you. Simon and Schuster. New York, NY.
19. MACKENZIE, S. A., E. A. B. OLTENACU & K. A. HOUPT. 1986. Canine behavioral genetics—A review. Appl. Anim. Behav. Sci. **15:** 365–393.

Stress and Reproduction in Domestic Animals

ROBERT M. LIPTRAP

Department of Biomedical Sciences
University of Guelph
Guelph, Ontario N1G 2W1, Canada

Severe stress of a chronic or intermittent duration can have detrimental effects on reproductive processes in animals. These effects are important because of their potential economic implications and because of concerns for animal welfare. The types of stressful situations encountered by farm animals include transportation, overcrowding, poor housing, fighting, and social rank. Oliverio[1] has emphasized the integrated response of the hypothalamo-adenohypophyseal-adrenocortical and the sympatho-adrenomedullary systems by farm animals in their adaptation to stressful situations. The role of the adrenocortical system in regard to the stress-mediated influence on reproduction has been the most studied. Little attention has been given to ultradian and circadian variations in adrenocortical hormone secretion and to possible alterations in the rate of clearance of hormones from the circulation during stress.[2] This brief review will be centered upon the hypothalamo-adenohypophyseal-adrenocortical axis and its potential impact on the hypothalamo-adenohypophyseal-gonadal axis in cattle, sheep, pig, and horse.

INFLUENCE OF STRESS ON THE ESTROUS CYCLE

Reproductive processes in the nonpregnant female depend upon a carefully synchronized sequence of endocrine events. Disruption in the timing and occurrence of these events probably makes the female more vulnerable to the effects of stress than her male counterpart.[3] The estrous cycle is more sensitive to the influence of stress than gestation. The length of the estrous cycle in the cow, sow, and mare is about 21 days, whereas that of the ewe is 16 days. The predominant structure on the ovary for most of the estrous cycle is the progesterone-secreting corpus luteum or the corpora lutea. Two major events in the estrous cycle must occur for reproductive success: (1) luteolysis or regression of the corpus luteum and (2) follicular growth and ovulatory release of the oocyte.

FIGURE 1 depicts an idealized scheme of the hormonal events leading up to the surge in luteinizing hormone (LH) and ovulation. The box on the left presents the plasma hormone changes during luteolysis. In several species, concomitant pulses of prostaglandin $F_{2\alpha}$ ($PGF_{2\alpha}$) and oxytocin are present. Prostaglandin $F_{2\alpha}$ has been confirmed as the principal luteolytic factor secreted by the uterus in the cow, ewe, sow, and mare.[4] It is secreted as a series of pulses into the utero-ovarian vein that reach the ovary by countercurrent transfer,[5] although other vascular pathways including the lymphatics may also be involved. Prostaglandin suppresses cholesterol synthesis and its conversion to progesterone, antagonizes LH binding, and reduces blood flow.

Oxytocin involved in luteal regression is primarily of luteal origin in ruminants.[6] Although somewhat of an oversimplification, it can be said that progesterone seems

275

to favor $PGF_{2\alpha}$ synthesis whereas estrogens favor $PGF_{2\alpha}$ release.[7] In contrast, for nonruminants such as the sow and mare, the neurohypophysis is suspected as an important oxytocin source. The sow[8] and mare[9] also differ from ruminants in that estrogens encourage continued luteal function. A positive feedback relationship exists between the secretion of $PGF_{2\alpha}$ and oxytocin. This prostaglandin-oxytocin interplay is thought to shorten the time required for luteolysis and to ensure a rapid drop in progesterone concentrations.

With the decline in progesterone levels, ovulatory follicle selection and growth can proceed. In FIGURE 1 the box on the right depicts the hormonal changes in plasma that occur at estrus and ovulation. During this follicular growth, estrogen production by the granulosa cells predominates. The aromatase system for estrogen synthesis is under follicle-stimulating hormone (FSH) regulation and is dependent upon a supply of androgen precursors (androstenedione and testosterone), which

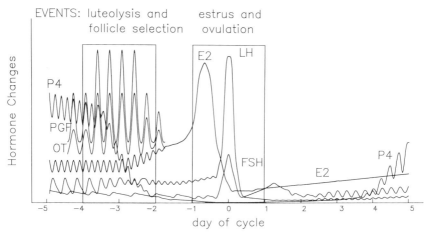

FIGURE 1. Idealized scheme of plasma hormone changes associated with luteolysis and with ovulation during the estrous cycle in a typical farm mammal. Hormone concentrations are not proportional to each other, and the exact timing of events varies somewhat between species. P4, progesterone; PGF, prostaglandin $F_{2\alpha}$; OT, oxytocin; E2, estradiol; LH, luteinizing hormone; FSH, follicle-stimulating hormone. See text for details.

are produced by the theca cells under LH control.[10] A positive feedback action by rising estrogen levels involves both an increase in hypothalamic gonadotropin-releasing hormone (GnRH) secretion,[11] as well as an increased pituitary sensitivity to GnRH. As a result, a dramatic increase in plasma LH concentrations occurs to initiate the biochemical events associated with ovulation. Ovulation with release of the oocyte has been compared to processes associated with the inflammatory response.[12]

In farm animals the dynamic changes associated with luteolysis and with ovulation share three characteristics that may make them reproductive events of particular vulnerability to stress: (1) Both events, at least in the cow and ewe, are controlled by positive feedback processes—oxytocin and $PGF_{2\alpha}$ for luteolysis and estrogen and luteinizing hormone for ovulation; (2) both events are accompanied by dramatic shifts in hormone values, that is, a progesterone decline, pulsatile $PGF_{2\alpha}$ secretion, and commencement of estrogen dominance around luteolysis, and marked increases in estrogen secretion and the LH surge around ovulation; and (3) morphological changes on the ovary, that is, from corpora lutea to follicles with luteolysis and from follicles to corpora lutea with ovulation. If these are truly periods of vulnerability then one would expect to observe disturbances of the estrous cycle involving a high incidence of prolonged cycle length or poor follicular development and a high incidence of failure in ovulation.

Effect of Stress on the Luteolysis Period

The stress of pen confinement on beef heifers removed from pasture extends the estrous cycle and maintains progesterone concentrations an additional two days.[13] Persistence of the corpus luteum with elevated progesterone concentrations has been observed also in ewes.[14,15] Measurement of $PGF_{2\alpha}$[16] or its metabolite[17] at the expected time of luteolysis reveals a decrease in the critical pulse frequency but not in the pulse amplitude.

Similar extensions of the estrous cycle can be mimicked by the injection of adrenocorticotrophic hormone (ACTH) or glucocorticoids. When the synthetic glucocorticoid, dexamethasone (DXM), is given to cows before luteal regression (days 16 through 20) an extended luteal life span is seen.[18] Although single injections of glucocorticoid are ineffective,[19] injections from days 10 to 19 can extend luteal function by an average of 10 days.[20] Plasma progesterone concentrations remain elevated, and the expected increase in prostaglandin metabolite is not seen.[21] Adrenocorticotropin treatment on days 12 to 16 extends the estrous cycle in ewes, depresses prostaglandin metabolite values, and delays the decline in progesterone values.[22] Because ACTH treatment also inhibits the ability of oxytocin to elicit $PGF_{2\alpha}$ secretion, the uterine component of the positive feedback relationship seems to be affected. Elevated glucocorticoid concentrations may depress the synthesis of uterine prostaglandin by suppressing phospholipase A_2 activity, thereby reducing the availability of the precursor, arachidonic acid.[23] Glucocorticoids could exert an indirect effect also in ruminants to cause a prolonged cycle. Estrogens from the small follicles present late in the luteal phase facilitate uterine prostaglandin release and enhance its action on the corpus luteum. When glucocorticoids are administered in the late luteal phase,[21] less LH is secreted in response to injection of GnRH. Glucocorticoid administration from days 13 to 17 reduces pulsatile LH secretion, and the dependent estrogen values are diminished significantly.[24] Hence, the facilitating action of estrogens on uterine prostaglandin release would be diminished, causing an extended cycle and delayed estrus.

In contrast to the cow and ewe, injection of sows with glucocorticoids from days 9 to 14 of the cycle[25] does not inhibit luteal regression nor the pulsatile secretion of LH and FSH. However, on the fifth day of the next expected cycle, follicular structures of small diameter (<5 mm), instead of corpora lutea, can be seen in numbers that exceed the expected ovulatory cohort.[25,26] This has been interpreted as a direct effect of increased glucocorticoid concentrations on preselection follicles. The retardation in follicular development appears to be associated with decreases in follicular fluid concentrations of androstenedione precursor and estradiol. The decrease in estradiol is accompanied by a morphological disorganization of the follicle[26] and degenerative changes in the oocyte-cumulus complex.[27] In mares, although most instances of persistent corpus luteum are due to early embryonic death, about 10% of cases occur in the unbred animal.[28] Inasmuch as these cases are accompanied by continuously elevated plasma progesterone values from a corpus luteum that is responsive to exogenously administered prostaglandin $F_{2\alpha}$,[29] the problem may be due to an inability of the uterus to synthesize adequate amounts of $PGF_{2\alpha}$. Unlike ruminants, dexamethasone injection of mares from day 10 for the next 20 days does not result in persistent corpora lutea.[30] Like the sow, estrogens extend luteal activity in the mare. It is, therefore, of interest to note that mares developing persistent corpora lutea possess greater urinary estrogen values on days 5 to 10 of the cycle than do mares with normal corpora lutea.[31] Some experimental evidence indicates that an adrenal origin of estrogens is possible.[32]

Effect of Stress on the Estrous Period

The stress of severe handling increases cortisol values in cattle to a greater extent relative to changes in catecholamine values.[33] This response is distinctly different from that of a brief transport stress where changes in catecholamines are much greater than those of cortisol. The degree to which the adrenal medulla or adrenal cortex responds varies with the type of stress. Transportation for prolonged periods, however, does increase cortisol levels such that a reduction in the ovulation rate occurs when beef heifers are administered a superovulation treatment.[34] With time, crowding and social disruption result in adrenal enlargement and increased production of glucocorticoids.[35] In ewes, prolonged stressful situations such as exposure to severely cold winds and rain[36,37] or to the application of a simulated rainfall throughout the estrous cycle[38] cause a delay or suppression of overt estrous behavior and a depression in the mean ovulatory rate. The rise in cortisol concentrations is due to an increased cortisol secretion and not an alteration in clearance rate.[39] Injection of ACTH during the follicular phase of the bovine estrous cycle results in ovulatory delay or anovulation.[40–42] Treatment with ACTH fails to alter the LH response to GnRH injection in adrenalectomized heifers but repeated cortisol administration is successful.[43] The lack of ovulation is attributable to a deficiency in the LH surge as shown by decreased plasma values in animals subjected to restraint stress, or hormone treatment.[42,44] Continuous infusion of cortisol or twice daily injections of ACTH[45] or betamethasone[21] result in reduced peaks in plasma LH concentrations following GnRH stimulation. A pituitary site of action was demonstrated by the suppression of GnRH-stimulated LH release in the presence of glucocorticoids in pituitary cell culture.[46,47]

The ability of an estradiol injection to elicit an ovulatory release of LH is impaired or delayed as a result of transportation stress.[48] More cows are affected early in the postpartum period compared to later. The difference found between early and late postpartum cows may be due to the greater numbers of opioid receptors present in the former.[49] Because opioids are secreted also during stress and are able to suppress LH secretion,[50] they may act with glucocorticoids to inhibit reproductive processes. The stress-mediated alterations in estrous behavior, ovulation rate, and LH values in the ewe can be mimicked also by injection of ACTH[51] but not by cortisone or cortisol. Other products of the adrenal cortex in sheep such as progesterone are believed to mediate these effects of ACTH treatment.

It has been known for 40 years that early weaning or removal of piglets immediately after parturition (zero weaning) can result in a high incidence of anovulation and cystic follicles in lactating sows.[52,53] Elevated cortisol levels accompany the absence of LH and ovulation in 50% of zero-weaned sows.[54] Other stressful circumstances such as stall tethering,[55] surgery or illness,[56] and transportation[57,58] can increase the duration of the estrous cycle, decrease the expression of estrous behavior, and reduce the proportion of successful matings. The behavioral signs of estrus seen when estradiol benzoate is injected into ovariectomized and intact gilts are reduced when glucocorticoids are administered concomitantly.[59,60] Administration of ACTH, twice daily injections of cortisol or potent synthetic glucocorticoids during the follicular phase of the estrous cycle delays the onset of estrus and blocks the ovulatory surge in LH with subsequent cystic follicle formation.[61,62] A suppressive action of cortisol on LH release in response to GnRH has been demonstrated in porcine pituitary cell culture.[63] The surge of LH expected after injection of estradiol can be blocked by glucocorticoids.[64] The possibility exists that glucocorticoid hormones also influence the ovary directly. Specific cortisol-binding globulin exists in porcine follicular fluid,[65,66] and glucocorticoid receptors have been noted in the rat ovary.[67] Treatment of sows with ACTH results in significantly higher concentrations of cortisol, but lower values of estradiol and its precursor, androstenedione, in follicular fluid compared to control sows.[68,69] The cystic ovarian follicle condition as seen in the cow, ewe, and sow does not truly occur in the mare. Nevertheless, injection of DXM can limit the size of the largest developing follicle, reduces maximum LH concentrations, and suppresses estrous behavior and ovulation.[30]

In summary, considerable evidence exists to suggest that both the time around luteolysis and the time around ovulation are vulnerable to the effects of stress and increased adrenal glucocorticoids. In ruminants, glucocorticoids can suppress $PGF_{2\alpha}$ levels prolonging the estrous cycle, whereas in the sow it is the emergence of the ovulatory cohort of follicles that is affected. In the cow, ewe, and sow, stressful situations with elevated glucocorticoid hormone concentrations near the onset of estrus can block the ovulatory surge in LH and ovarian steroidogenesis. The possible effects of elevated temperature stress are likely to be physical because environmental heat stress only raises cortisol values on the first day of exposure; by the third or fourth day, they are depressed.[70] With seasonal changes in ambient temperature, no suppression of the ovulatory LH release in dairy cattle[71] is seen in the hot summer months.

INFLUENCE OF STRESS ON PREGNANCY

Heat stress applied to cows immediately after breeding results in a significant increase in both abnormal and poorly developed embryos and in increased embryo mortality.[72,73] Ambient heat stress also affects early pregnancy in the ewe. A body temperature increase in ewes of 1 to 1.5 °C can cause a mortality rate as high as 75%, although breed differences exist.[74] Young ewes are more affected than older ewes.[75] The effect of ambient heat stress has been examined in the pregnant sow, and has revealed that a brief exposure of two hours at 40 °C between days 2 and 13 can increase embryonic death.[76,77] This does not occur if exposure occurs between days 14 and 25. Embryo transfer in ewes has been used to more precisely define the time during the first two weeks of pregnancy that is most sensitive to heat stress.[78] The initial three days after the onset of estrus exhibited the greatest reduction in embryo survival. Morphological examination of zygotes in the ewe confirmed that the heat stress effect involved alterations in the initial stages of embryo cleavage while in the oviduct.[79] Survival rates tended to increase with time after conception.[70] Embryo mortality in cows may result, in part, from an alteration in embryo growth so that development is insufficient to inhibit the luteolytic mechanism.

Other types of stresses can affect embryo survival also. In ewes during the 20-day period after mating, daily transportation, rough herding by dogs or handling by strangers may significantly increase embryonic mortality.[80] Young sows stressed by boar harassment at the time of mating exhibit higher levels of embryo mortality.[81]

The potential for stress to disrupt pregnancy in the mare has been studied less. Transport of mares in early pregnancy does not affect embryo survival.[82] Pain, infectious disease, the emotional disturbance of early weaning[83] or the stress of a drastic reduction in dietary protein for 10 days in the second or third month of gestation[84] can result in equine embryonic death.

The detrimental effects resulting from prolonged heat stress in pregnancy are probably physical in nature, but adrenal cortical hormones could mediate some effects of other stress including the initial exposure to high ambient temperatures. Injection of ACTH[80] or up to 225 mg/day of cortisol,[85] but not lower doses of cortisol (60 mg/day),[86] reduces embryo survival in the early stages of sheep pregnancy. Similarly in sows, injection of repository ACTH from days 11 to 15 after breeding doubles the plasma values of glucocorticoids and results in an embryo survival rate of 48% compared to the 70% survival usually seen.[87]

Reproductive steroid levels have been measured during stress in pregnancy. Progesterone levels tend to be greater in stressed gilts than control animals during heat stress from the day of estrus to day 8,[88] whereas estradiol concentrations are lower. Whether these changes alter conception rate or embryonic survival is unknown, but it should be noted that tubal transport of gametes and uterine secretion are important steroid-dependent processes in early pregnancy. Exposure of sows to elevated temperatures from days 8 to 16 results in lower saphenous vein levels of estradiol than those present in control sows.[89] It is at this time that dynamic embryo and uterine changes occur related to pregnancy recognition. In the pregnant mare injection of prednisolone[83] is associated with a decline in progesterone concentrations. Exposure of dams to stress later in pregnancy does not influence fetal mortality although offspring may be born with a reduced body weight.

INFLUENCE OF STRESS ON MALE REPRODUCTION

Reproductive function in male farm animals is regulated by the more familiar negative feedback system between the testes and the hypothalamic-adenohypophyseal axis. As pointed out by Moberg,[3] the continuing process of spermatogenesis is less likely to be affected by stress than the more discrete event of ovulation. Sexual behavior is probably more sensitive to the effects of stress.

The effect of elevated ambient temperature has been extensively studied in male farm species. In the bull[72,90] and ram,[91] heat stress brings about a significant reduction in semen quality with a decline in both percent motility and numbers of morphologically normal sperm. Ambient heat stress probably exerts a physical effect. During induced heat stress only a temporary lowering of testosterone values accompanied by elevated cortisol values was seen in bulls[92] and in boars.[93] Single injections of ACTH are ineffective but repeated administration of the long-acting form to bulls can suppress the episodic secretion of LH and testosterone.[94] Injections of DXM also lower LH and testosterone values.[95] Imposition of restraint stress or pretreatment of rams with ACTH reduces the degree of increase in LH secreted in response to GnRH injection.[96] As in the ewe, ACTH injection but not cortisol infusion is able to depress the ability of GnRH to elicit LH secretion,[97] suggesting the involvement of other adrenal steroids.

In boars, long-acting ACTH depresses LH and urinary androgen levels.[98] Glucocorticoids appear to be involved inasmuch as cortisol, but not ACTH treatment, was effective in the adrenalectomized animal. Treatment with DXM decreases the number of episodic LH secretory pulses but not their individual size.[99] Fewer studies of the effect of stress hormones on reproductive parameters have been explored in the stallion. Injection of a long-acting form of ACTH or injection of cortisol is able to suppress testosterone concentrations.[100] Less well explored is the possibility that glucocorticoids can directly decrease androgen production by the testes of farm mammals. Glucocorticoids have been shown to lower LH receptor numbers and testosterone production in a dose-dependent manner in rat[101] and porcine[102] testicular tissue.

POSITIVE EFFECTS OF STRESS ON REPRODUCTION

Do stress and the glucocorticoids have any positive effects on reproductive activity? Certainly, Selye[103] believed that some stress was beneficial and necessary. Two examples may illustrate the point.

Boar contact is the most potent factor stimulating precocious puberty in gilts, and olfactory cues involving pheromones are particularly important.[104] Transportation is also a well-known stimulator of advanced puberty,[105] but is only effective near the time of puberty and is dependent upon exposure to the boar within 10 days of movement. As indicated above, prolonged stress, repeated injections of ACTH or long acting glucocorticoids can suppress fertility. In contrast, administration of short-acting glucocorticoids to gilts indicates that although the adrenal cortex is not solely responsible for the advancement in puberty,[106] briefly stressful events may actually enhance other known stimuli such as boar pheromones and physical contact.[107]

How might the adrenal cortex facilitate the onset of puberty? As in many species, plasma cortisol values in pigs display a circadian rhythm with high levels present early in the morning and low levels present in the afternoon. This rhythm is disrupted for several days when sows come into estrus.[57,108] The authors[108] suggest that the occurrence of estrus itself can increase cortisol levels and does not require the presence of the boar. *In vitro* experiments have indicated that brief exposure to cortisol can enhance estrogen production by ovarian granulosa cells[109] and thecal cell production of the estrogen precursor, androstenedione.[110] By facilitating an increase in estrogen secretion under gonadotropic stimulation, behavioral estrus may be more evident.

Positive effects of glucocorticoid secretion can occur also in the male. Mating behavior is associated with a sharp increase in cortisol, as well as testosterone concentrations, in bulls,[111] boars,[112,113] and stallions.[114] A brief increase in plasma testosterone concentrations in bulls is seen after treatment with DXM before the eventual suppression previously described occurs.[95] Similarly, in the boar[115,116] and stallion,[117] administration of a rapid-acting form of ACTH increases plasma testosterone concentrations as well as those of cortisol. Experimentally, the increase in testosterone in boars after ACTH injection is not accompanied by an increase in LH concentrations,[118] and the absence of a response in the castrated animal[113,114] suggests a direct action of glucocorticoids on the testes. However, glucocorticoids may enhance LH secretion also because intracarotid infusion of cortisol can facilitate the pituitary response to GnRH injection.[119] This could be significant at the time of mating because limiting glucocorticoid synthesis with metyrapone limits the normal increase in secretion of testosterone to about half of that seen in control animals, although the testes are still responsive to gonadotropic stimulation.[112,113]

In summary, glucocorticoids do not directly induce puberty and male sexual behavior. However, they can play a facilitating role by enhancing the secretion or action of other hormones of the reproductive system. The rapidity of the rise in cortisol values and the brief time of the increase may be significant. Brief increases exert a positive influence, whereas a sustained increase in activity by the hypothalamic-adenohypophyseal-adrenal cortical system has the potential to suppress activity of the hypothalamic-adenohypophyseal-gonadal axis.

REFERENCES

1. OLIVERIO, A. 1987. *In* Biology of Stress in Farm Animals: An Integrative Approach. P. R. Wiepkema & P. W. M. van Adrichem, Eds.: 3–12. Martinus Nijhoff Publishers. Boston, MA.
2. LADEWIG, J. 1987. *In* Biology of Stress in Farm Animals: An Integrative Approach. P. R. Wiepkema & P. W. M. van Adrichem, Eds.: 13–25. Martinus Nijhoff, Publishers. Boston, MA.
3. MOBERG, G. P. 1985. *In* Animal Stress. G. P. Moberg, Ed.: 245–267. American Physiological Society. Bethesda, MD.
4. HAFEZ, E. S. E. *In* Reproduction in Farm Animals. 5th edit. E. S. E. Hafez, Ed.: 107–129. Lea and Febiger. Philadelphia, PA.
5. MCCRACKEN, J. A., M. E. GLEW & R. J. SCARAMUZZI. 1970. J. Clin. Endocrinol. Metab. **30:** 544–546.
6. FLINT, A. P. F., E. L. SHELDRICK, T. J. MCCANN & D. S. C. JONES. 1990. Domest. Anim. Endocrinol. **7:** 111–124.
7. SILVIA, W. J., G. S. LEWIS, J. A. MCCRACKEN, W. W. THATCHER & L. WILSON, JR. 1991. Biol. Reprod. **45:** 655–663.
8. BAZER, F. W., J. L. VALLET, R. M. ROBERTS, D. C. SHARP & W. W. THATCHER. 1986. J. Reprod. Fertil. **76:** 841–850.
9. BERG, S. L. & O. J. GINTHER. 1987. J. Anim. Sci. **47:** 203–208.
10. GORE-LANGTON, R. E. & D. T. ARMSTRONG. 1988. *In* The Physiology of Reproduction. E. Knobil & J. D. Neill, Eds.: 331–385. Raven Press. New York, NY.
11. CLARKE, I. J. & J. T. CUMMINS. 1985. Endocrinology **116:** 2376–2383.
12. ESPEY, L. L. 1980. Biol. Reprod. **22:** 73–106.
13. POOL, S. H., R. H. INGRAHAM & R. A. GODKE. 1983. Theriogenology **20:** 257–265.
14. QUIRKE, J. F. & J. P. GOSLING. 1979. Anim. Prod. **28:** 1–12.
15. YENIKOYE, A., J. PELLETIER, D. ANDRE & J. C. MARIANA. 1982. Theriogenology **17:** 355–364.
16. HOOPER, S. B. & G. D. THORBURN. 1987. Acta Endocrinol. **115:** 469–477.
17. ZARCO, L., G. H. STABENFELDT, H. KINDAHL, J. F. QUIRKE & E. GRANSTRÖM. 1984. Anim. Reprod. Sci. **7:** 245–267.
18. INGRAHAM, R. H., S. H. POOL & R. A. GODKE. 1984. Theriogenology **21:** 875–886.
19. GIMÉNEZ, T., M. L. ENDER & B. HOFFMANN. 1974. Dtsch. Tierärztl. Wochenschr. **81:** 29–52.
20. KANCHEV, L. N., H. DOBSON, W. R. WARD & R. J. FITZPATRICK. 1976. J. Reprod. Fertil. **48:** 341–345.
21. DOBSON, H., M. G. S. ALAM & L. N. KANCHEV. 1987. J. Reprod. Fertil. **80:** 25–30.
22. COOKE, R. G. & K. M. BENHAJ. 1989. Anim. Reprod. Sci. **20:** 201–211.
23. DEY, S. K., R. C. HOVERSLAND & D. C. JOHNSON. 1982. Prostaglandins **23:** 619–630.
24. VIGHIO, G. H. & R. M. LIPTRAP. 1990. Am. J. Vet. Res. **51:** 1711–1714.
25. FRAUTSCHY, S. A. & R. M. LIPTRAP. 1988. Am. J. Vet. Res. **49:** 1270–1275.
26. GEE, C. M., H. D. GEISSINGER & R. M. LIPTRAP. 1991. Can. J. Vet. Res. **55:** 206–211.
27. CASTRO, L., R. M. LIPTRAP & P. K. BASRUR. 1991. Proceedings of the 24th World Veterinary Congress, Rio de Janeiro. Abstract 07.
28. GINTHER, O. J. 1979. Reproductive Biology of the Mare: Basic and Applied Aspects. Equiservices. Cross Plains, WI.
29. STABENFELDT, G. H., J. P. HUGHES, J. W. EVANS & D. P. NEELY. 1974. Equine Vet. J. **6:** 158–162.
30. ASA, C. S. & O. J. GINTHER. 1982. J. Reprod. Fertil. **32:** 247–251.
31. PALMER, E. & B. JOUSSET. 1975. J. Reprod. Fertil. **(Suppl. 23):** 213–221.

32. ASA, C. S., D. A. GOLDFOOT, M. C. GARCIA & O. J. GINTHER. 1980. Horm. Behav. **14:** 55–64.
33. MITCHELL, G., J. HATTINGH & M. GANHAO. 1988. Vet. Rec. **123:** 201–205.
34. EDWARDS, L. M., C. H. RAHE, J. L. GRIFFIN, D. F. WOLFE, D. N. MARPLE, K. A. CUMMINS & J. F. PITCHETT. 1987. Theriogenology **28:** 291–299.
35. FRIEND, T. H., C. E. POLAN, F. C. GWAZDAUSKAS & C. W. HEALD. 1977. J. Dairy Sci. **60:** 1958–1963.
36. MACKENZIE, A. J., C. J. THWAITES & T. N. EDEY. 1975. Aust. J. Agric. Res. **26:** 545–551.
37. GRIFFITHS, J. G., R. G. GUNN & J. M. DONEY. 1970. J. Agric. Sci. **75:** 485–488.
38. DONEY, J. M., R. G. GUNN & J. G. GRIFFITHS. 1973. J. Reprod. Fertil. **35:** 381–384.
39. PANARETTO, B. A. & M. R. VICKERY. 1970. J. Endocrinol. **47:** 273–285.
40. LIPTRAP, R. M. & P. J. MCNALLY. 1976. Am. J. Vet. Res. **37:** 369–375.
41. DUNLAP, S. E., T. E. KISER, N. M. COX, F. N. THOMPSON, G. B. RAMPACEK, L. L. BENYSHEK & R. R. KRAELING. 1981. J. Anim. Sci. **52:** 587–593.
42. STOEBEL, D. P. & G. P. MOBERG. 1982. J. Dairy Sci. **65:** 1016–1024.
43. LI, P. S. & W. C. WAGNER. 1983. Biol. Reprod. **29:** 11–24.
44. STOEBEL, D. P. & G. P. MOBERG. 1982. J. Dairy Sci. **65:** 92–96.
45. MATTERI, R. L. & G. P. MOBERG. 1982. J. Endocrinol. **92:** 141–146.
46. LI, P. S. & W. C. WAGNER. 1983. Biol. Reprod. **29:** 25–37.
47. PADMANABHAN, V., C. KEECH & E. M. CONVEY. 1983. Endocrinology **112:** 1782–1787.
48. NANDA, A. S., H. DOBSON & W. R. WARD. 1990. Res. Vet. Sci. **49:** 25–28.
49. TROUT, W. E. & P. V. MALVEN. 1988. J. Anim. Sci. **66:** 954–960.
50. WHISNANT, C. S., T. E. KISER, F. N. THOMPSON & C. R. BARB. 1986. J. Anim. Sci. **63:** 561–564.
51. DOBSON, H., S. A. ESSAWY & M. G. S. ALAM. 1988. J. Endocrinol. **118:** 193–197.
52. BAKER, L. N., H. L. WOEHLING, L. E. CASIDA & R. H. GRUMMER. 1953. J. Anim. Sci. **12:** 33–38.
53. PETERS, J. B., R. E. SHORT, N. L. FIRST & L. E. CASIDA. 1969. J. Anim. Sci. **29:** 20–24.
54. KUNAVONGKRIT, A., L.-E. EDQVIST & S. EINARSSON. 1983. Zentralbl. Veterinaermed. A **30:** 625–636.
55. BARNETT, J. L. & P. H. HEMSWORTH. 1991. Anim. Reprod. Sci. **25:** 265–273.
56. HENNESSY, D. P. & P. WILLIAMSON. 1983. Theriogenology **20:** 13–26.
57. BECKER, B. A., J. A. NIENABER, J. A. DESHAZER & G. L. HAHN. 1985. Am. J. Vet. Res. **46:** 1457–1459.
58. DALIN, A.-M., L. NYBERG & L. ELIASSON. 1988. Acta Vet. Scand. **29:** 207–218.
59. FORD, J. J. & R. K. CHRISTENSON. 1981. Horm. Behav. **15:** 427–435.
60. ESBENSHADE, K. L., A. M. PATERSON & B. N. DAY. 1983. J. Anim. Sci. **56:** 460–465.
61. LIPTRAP, R. M. 1970. J. Endocrinol. **47:** 197–205.
62. BARB, C. R., R. R. KRAELING, G. B. RAMPACEK, E. S. FONDA & T. E. KISER. 1982. J. Reprod. Fertil. **64:** 85–92.
63. LI, P. S. 1987. Life Sci. **41:** 2493–2501.
64. PATERSON, A. M., T. C. CANTLEY, K. L. ESBENSHADE & B. N. DAY. 1983. J. Anim. Sci. **56:** 466–470.
65. COOK, B., R. H. F. HUNTER & A. S. L. KELLY. 1977. J. Reprod. Fertil. **51:** 65–71.
66. MAHAJAN, D. K., R. B. BILLIAR & A. B. LITTLE. 1980. J. Steroid Biochem. **13:** 67–71.
67. SCHREIBER, J. R., K. NAKAMURA & G. F. ERICKSON. 1982. Steroids **39:** 569–584.
68. LIPTRAP, R. M. & E. CUMMINGS. 1991. Anim. Reprod. Sci. **26:** 303–310.
69. VIVEIROS, M. M. & R. M. LIPTRAP. 1992. Biol. Reprod. **46(Suppl. 1):** 154.
70. ABILAY, T. A., H. D. JOHNSON & M. L. MADAN. 1975. J. Dairy Sci. **58:** 1836–1840.
71. VAUGHT, L. W., D. E. MONTY, JR. & W. C. FOOTE. 1977. Am. J. Vet. Res. **38:** 1027–1030.
72. VINCENT, C. K. 1972. J. Am. Vet. Med. Assoc. **161:** 1333–1338.
73. PUTNEY, D. J., M. DROST & W. W. THATCHER. 1988. Theriogenology **30:** 195–209.
74. THWAITES, C. J. 1967. J. Reprod. Fertil. **14:** 5–14.
75. SHELTON, M. 1964. J. Anim. Sci. **23:** 360–364.
76. OMTVEDT, I. T., R. E. NELSON, R. L. EDWARDS, D. F. STEPHENS & E. J. TURMAN. 1971. J. Anim. Sci. **32:** 312–317.
77. WILDT, D. E., G. D. RIEGLE & W. R. DUKELOW. 1975. Am. J. Physiol. **229:** 1471–1475.

78. ALLISTON, C. W. & L. C. ULBERG. 1961. J. Anim. Sci. **20:** 608–613.
79. DUTT, R. H. 1963. J. Anim. Sci. **22:** 713–719.
80. DONEY, J. M., W. F. SMITH & R. G. GUNN. 1976. J. Agric. Sci. **87:** 133–136.
81. RICH, T. D., E. J. TURMAN & J. C. HILLIER. 1986. J. Anim. Sci. **27:** 443–446.
82. BAUCUS, K. L., S. L. RALSTON, C. F. NOCKELS, A. O. MCKINNON & E. L. SQUIRES. 1990. J. Anim. Sci. **68:** 345–351.
83. VAN NIEKERK, C. H. & J. C. MORGENTHAL. 1982. J. Reprod. Fertil. **(Suppl. 32):** 453–457.
84. VAN NIEKERK, C. H., J. C. MORGENTHAL & C. J. STARKE. 1983. J. S. Afr. Vet. Assoc. **54:** 65–66.
85. HOWARTH, B. JR. & H. W. HAWK. 1968. J. Anim. Sci. **27:** 117–121.
86. THWAITES, C. J. 1970. J. Reprod. Fertil. **21:** 95–107.
87. ARNOLD, J. D., H. G. KATTESH, T. T. CHEN & R. L. MURPHREE. 1982. Theriogenology **17:** 475–484.
88. WETTEMANN, R. P. & F. W. BAZER. 1985. J. Reprod. Fertil. **(Suppl. 33):** 199–208.
89. HOAGLAND, T. A. & R. P. WETTEMANN. 1984. Theriogenology **22:** 15–24.
90. MYERHOEFFER, D. C., R. P. WETTEMANN, S. W. COLEMAN & M. E. WELLS. 1985. J. Anim. Sci. **60:** 352–357.
91. HOWARTH, B., JR. 1969. J. Reprod. Fertil. **19:** 179–183.
92. RHYNES, W. E. & L. L. EWING. 1973. Endocrinology **92:** 509–515.
93. LARSSON, K., S. EINARSSON, K. LUNDSTRÖM & J. HAKKARAINEN. 1983. Acta Vet. Scand. **24:** 305–314.
94. JOHNSON, B. H., T. H. WELSH, JR. & P. E. JUNIEWICZ. 1982. Biol. Reprod. **26:** 305–310.
95. THIBIER, M. & O. ROLLAND. 1976. Theriogenology **5:** 53–60.
96. MATTERI, R. L., J. G. WATSON & G. P. MOBERG. 1984. J. Reprod. Fertil. **72:** 385–393.
97. FUQUAY, J. W. & G. P. MOBERG. 1983. J. Endocrinol. **99:** 151–155.
98. LIPTRAP, R. M. & J. I. RAESIDE. 1968. J. Endocrinol. **42:** 33–43.
99. GAON, D. & R. M. LIPTRAP. 1989. Theriogenology **32:** 79–85.
100. COX, J. E. & N. M. A. JAWAD. 1979. Equine Vet. J. **11:** 195–198.
101. WELSH, T. H., JR., T. H. BAMBINO & A. J. W. HSUEH. 1982. Biol. Reprod. **27:** 1138–1146.
102. BERNIER, M., W. GIBB, R. COLLU & J. R. DUCHARME. 1984. Can. J. Physiol. Pharmacol. **62:** 1166–1169.
103. SELYE, H. 1956. The Stress of Life. McGraw-Hill Book Co. New York, NY.
104. PEARCE, G. P. & P. E. HUGHES. 1987. **44:** 293–302.
105. DU MESNIL DU BUISSON, F. & J. P. SIGNORET. 1962. Ann. Zootech. **11:** 53–59.
106. ESBENSHADE, K. L. & B. N. DAY. 1980. J. Anim. Sci. **51:** 153–157.
107. EASTHAM, P. R. & D. J. A. COLE. 1987. Anim. Prod. **44:** 435–441.
108. BECKER, B. A., J. J. FORD, R. K. CHRISTENSON, R. C. MANAK, G. L. HAHN & J. A. DESHAZER. 1985. J. Anim. Sci. **60:** 264–270.
109. RYAN, P. L., G. J. KING & J. I. RAESIDE. 1990. Anim. Reprod. Sci. **23:** 75–86.
110. RAESIDE, J. I. & H.-C. XUN. 1986. Anim. Reprod. Sci. **12:** 39–46.
111. BORG, K. E., K. L. ESBENSHADE & B. H. JOHNSON. 1991. J. Anim. Sci. **69:** 3230–3240.
112. LIPTRAP, R. M. & J. I. RAESIDE. 1978. J. Endocrinol. **76:** 75–85.
113. WANG, L. X., P. HUETHER, E. DOBLE & R. M. LIPTRAP. 1986. Can. J. Vet. Res. **50:** 540–542.
114. TAMANINI, C., N. GIORDANO, F. CHIESA & E. SEREN. 1983. Acta Endocrinol. **102:** 447–450.
115. LIPTRAP, R. M. & J. I. RAESIDE. 1975. J. Endocrinol. **66:** 123–131.
116. JUNIEWICZ, P. E. & B. H. JOHNSON. 1981. Biol. Reprod. **25:** 725–733.
117. COX, J. E. & J. H. WILLIAMS. 1975. J. Reprod. Fertil. **(Suppl. 23):** 75–79.
118. PITZEL, L., A. HARTIG, W. HOLTZ & A. KÖNIG. 1980. Acta Endocrinol. **94(Suppl. 234):** 35–36.
119. LIPTRAP, R. M. & J. I. RAESIDE. 1983. J. Endocrinol. **97:** 75–81.

Stress and Disease in Domestic Animals

LASZLO DeROTH

Faculté de Médecine Vétérinaire
Université de Montréal
3200, rue Sicotte
Saint-Hyacinthe, Québec J3H 3W3, Canada

It is rare for any animal not to be confronted with stressful situations, whether they be found in the wild, on the family farm, or in an industrial setting. In general, physiological responses, immunological mechanisms, and behavioral adaptations allow animals to adapt to these stressful events. However, these events can act as causal factors leading to specific pathological conditions.

In 1976 Hans Selye[1] reviewed the various stress-related conditions of importance in veterinary medicine. He noted that "the numerous reviews dealing with this subject in different languages have generally led to the conclusion that stress can cause essentially the same diseases in animals as in men." Since then, several other reviews have been published in order to crystallize the concept of stress in veterinary medicine.[2-6]

The present review is not exhaustive, but rather is a conceptual view of stress-related diseases in the various domestic animal species. The approach is rather generalist and was inspired by Selye's "Letter to John" in the introduction to his book *From Dream to Discovery*: "The specialist loses perspective, and by now I am sure that there will always be a need for integrators, for naturalists who keep trying to survey the broad fields."[7] The objective of this paper is to present stress through disease models in which it is a recognized entity and through models of stressful management practices. The conditions presented include a genetic model, the porcine stress syndrome; an environmental model, bovine shipping fever; an exercise model, equine paroxysmal atrial fibrillation; a housing model, confinement stress in chickens; a handling-related stress model, sheep shearing stress; and finally a psychosocial model, the human–animal interaction related stress in dogs.

MODELS OF STRESS IN DOMESTIC ANIMALS

Genetic Model

In recent decades, growth rate and meat to body weight ratio of fattening pigs have been steadily increasing. Efficient genetic selection programs resulted in rapid weight gain and lean meat in large-scale swine productions. At the same time, the percentage of pigs that die when subjected to stressful situations, such as routine handling and transportation, has also increased.

In the 1950s, the pig was already considered as an animal predisposed to heart disease.[8] In a study on systole to diastole ratios in different domestic animals, it was established that at a resting heart rate the horse had the lowest systole to diastole ratio and the pig had the highest. A parallel was drawn between the length of diastole and bodily ability, and it was concluded that this could explain the apparent predisposition of pigs to "heart death" (literal translation of the German term *Herztod*).[9] Furthermore, genetic selection produced an animal which, even in his basic characteristics, is evidently quite different from its ancestors. In relation to body mass the modern Landrace pig has a relatively small heart (0.21% of total body weight) as compared to the much smaller European wild boar (0.38% of total body weight). It is speculated that the smaller heart is overstrained during locomotion in order to provide sufficient blood supply to the muscular periphery. In the Mangalitza breed, in which the heart weight to body weight ratio and total body mass are similar to that of the Landrace pig, the heart is not affected because the periphery contains much fatty tissue with a significantly lower blood supply.[10]

As the genetic selection was giving tangible results on the profitability and on the healthy growth of pig muscle, it was also observed that some of these lean pigs, shortly after slaughter, had a discolored and watery muscle. Ludvigsen[11] provided the first substantial report on these observations, and the condition is now known as pale, soft, exudative muscle (PSE). In 1966, Hall et al.[12] reported the deaths of three pigs undergoing halothane and suxamethonium anesthesia, and two years later another group reported the occurrence of acute hyperthermia in pigs given halothane alone.[13] The descriptions provided by these groups tallied well with descriptions of the human malignant hyperthermia (MH) syndrome, and consequently the pig became the animal model of choice for the condition.

Concurrently, extreme stress susceptibility of pigs was also described as a syndrome rather than a single disease entity and was identified as porcine stress syndrome (PSS).[14] When stress-susceptible animals are subjected to stressful events such as transport, fighting, parturition, and pre-slaughter rough handling, a cascade of physiological events develop, and in the final stages of the syndrome, marked muscle rigidity and hyperthermia occur, resulting in sudden death in a shocklike state.

Because of the economic consequences of PSE and PSS in pigs and MH syndrome in human anesthesia, the various aspects of porcine biochemistry, physiology, and pathology have been extensively studied to elucidate this trilogy of syndromes. The relationships that exist between the three expressions of the same disease are now better understood (FIG. 1).

Susceptibility to these syndromes is of genetic origin and is related to an autosomal recessive gene with variable penetrance.[15] The halothane-screening method was used to identify susceptibility of individual animals to PSS, PSE, and MH.[16] The ultimate objective was to identify genetic carriers in order to better control their frequency in a given population. However, the halothane test was costly and only homozygote-susceptible pigs (genotype $Hal^n Hal^n$) could be identified. Homozygote-resistant (genotype $Hal^N Hal^N$) and heterozygote ($Hal^N Hal^n$) pigs are not sensitive to halothane. However, because of incomplete penetrance of the gene, some susceptible animals ($Hal^n Hal^n$) do not respond to halothane, and some carriers ($Hal^N Hal^n$) do react positively.[17] Because the Hal gene belongs to a linkage group including blood group loci S and H, erythrocyte enzyme loci phosphohexose isomerase (Phi), 6-phosphogluconate dehydrogenase (Pgd), and plasma postalbumin 2 (Po2), erythrocyte typing has been used in many countries.[18]

Most recently, a noninvasive, simple, and accurate test to identify stress-susceptible animals was developed, based on the identification of an arginine to cysteine mutation in porcine ryanodine receptor. It is suggested that Arg^{615} is located on the surface of the Ca^{2+}-release channel and that its alteration leads to hypersensitive channel gating. It is postulated that endocrine responses to stress raise the intracellular concentration of physiological channel-gating agents to a level that could trigger the opening of the hypersensitive Ca^{2+}-release channels. The high level of intracellular Ca^{2+} would render these same channels unresponsive to the Ca^{2+}- and Mg^{2+}- related closing mechanisms, thereby inducing muscle contracture, hypermetabolism, and hyperthermia.[19]

Environmental Model

Transportation of animals is considered a major stress-inducing event because it comprises several perturbing factors such as exposition to a novel environment, confrontation with unfamiliar animals, lack of space, noise, movement, hunger, and thirst. The major cause of mortality in the American feedlot cattle industry is a stress-related disease known as transit fever (shipping fever, pasteurellosis).

Although *Pasteurella haemolytica* is often quoted as the principal causal organism in association with various viral agents, transit fever is mainly considered to be stress induced; thus the etiology of the condition is still open to disagreement. *P. haemo-*

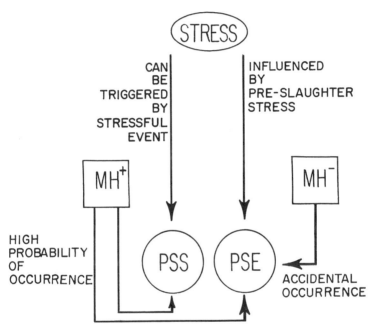

FIGURE 1. Interrelationships of the porcine stress syndromes (PSS). PSE: Pale, soft, exudative muscle syndrome; MH+: Animal with symptoms of malignant hyperthermia reacts to halothane; MH−: Animal with symptoms of malignant hyperthermia does not react to halothane.

lytica can be isolated from the respiratory passages in clinically healthy animals, but as the calves are transported, the number of biotype AI increases in the nasotracheal tract and the lungs, where bronchopneumonia results.[20] The effects of stress are very difficult to quantify and have not been successfully used to produce transit fever experimentally.[21] Transportation, however, results in a rise in plasma fibrinogen levels in cattle, which is considered as an indicator of stress.[22]

Parainfluenza-3 (PI3) and infectious bovine rhinotracheitis (IBR) viruses have long been known to interfere with alveolar macrophage function. They inhibit phagosome-lysosome fusion and thus pave the way for secondary infections with *Pasteurella* in stressed calves.[23] In addition, the PI3 virus is excreted in nasal mucus, ocular secretion, and in droplets, and is very stable in aerosols of nasal secretion, particularly where temperatures are low.[24]

In cattle, the role of stress-associated corticosteroids remains unclear because, on the one hand, the mode of action of their immunosuppressive effect has not yet been elucidated, and, on the other hand, there are corticosteroid-sensitive and -resistant animal species. For example, laboratory rodents and humans are much more sensitive to the immunosuppressive effect of corticosteroids than are common domestic animals. Consequently, laboratory animal data should not be directly extrapolated to the domestic species.[25]

In many outbreaks of transit fever, it is likely that the combined stress of movement plus mixing with other animals, the introduction to an unknown environment, and a new diet are contributing factors. Virus, bacteria, and stress function are in synergy to provoke this disease in cattle.

Handling Model

Relatively transient or routine handling is another potential source of stress in domestic animals. Handling is especially stressful in the ovine, because sheep is defined as "a defenceless, vigilant, tight-flocking, visual, wool-covered ruminant evolved within a mountain grassland habitat, displaying a 'follower-type' dam-offspring relationship with strong imitation occurring between young and old with regard to habits."[26] Because of the very nature of this species, isolation from the group and introduction to a novel environment are the principal variables that could increase plasma cortisol levels. Shearing increases adrenaline and noradrenaline levels right at the outset, and plasma glucocorticoids increase steadily and reach peak levels after 30 minutes after the beginning of handling for shearing.[2] The development of automated systems for shearing to replace traditional methods may increase the severity of stressors to which sheep are routinely exposed.[27]

Housing Model

Social interactions among chickens can be a serious source of stress. Although not always evident in the hormonal profile, aggressive behavior in chickens results from stress related to housing, and, in particular, to that of confinement. Social instability in a group of animals is a stress factor that is manifested in high levels of plasma corticosterone. In addition, a high concentration of chickens in a confined environment results not only in physiological changes, but will provoke various manifestations of abnormal aggressive behavior. When two animals are in the same cage, they show eight types of aggressive behavior during a 20-minute period. This aggressive behavior will increase if the animals are presented food in an inaccessible container.[28] In some studies of laying hens, confinement and crowding were found to increase plasma corticosterone levels; in other reports they remained unchanged,[29] but crowding had a significant effect on adrenal response to adrenocorticotropic (ACTH) challenge.[30]

Exercise Model

The champion runner of the 1500-meter race at the 1932 Olympics finished the race in a time of 3:51.2 minutes. In 1980, the same distance was run in 3:38.4 minutes, an improvement of 12.8 seconds in 50 years. During that same period the performance of a Thoroughbred horse on a distance of 2.4 kilometers improved only one second. This could be explained by the fact that Thoroughbreds for a long time were selected based on their physical performance.[31] If the horse, because of proper selection, did not improve significantly its performance in its natural pace, then in its artificial pace (pacers and trotters) the improvement is more significant.

With regard to heart rate, domestic species have been classified in parasympathetic and sympathetic dominant groups. The horse has a significantly lower resting heart rate than its intrinsic heart rate because of overwhelming parasympathetic control (FIG. 2). This dominance by the parasympathetic nervous system manifests itself in frequent second degree atrioventricular blocks, considered as physiological at normal heart rate and at a low incidence per unit of time. Hogs and chickens are at the other end of the spectrum with a sympathetic dominance.[32,33]

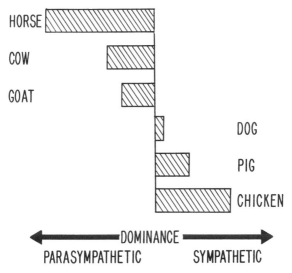

FIGURE 2. Comparative autonomic tone relative to heart rate in different domestic species (based on data from refs. 32, 33, and 40).

In the horse, from a baseline of 35 beats per minute, the heart rate increases during racing, to its peak, in the last straight, to 220 beats per minute, over six times of its baseline rate.[34] In spite of such cardiovascular performance, this athletic animal par excellence suffers from cardiac arrhythmias induced by the stress of the sporting event.[35] Paroxysmal atrial fibrillation is a reoccurring arrhythmia induced by the stress of racing. It probably appears in the last straight of the race which results in a significant slowdown in the speed of the animal. The atrial fibrillation will disappear shortly after the end of the race, but it can reoccur at the next event and eventually could result in a sustained atrial fibrillation.[36]

Psychosocial Model

From time immemorial the dog has been the "most" domestic of all animals. Some scientists suggest that the dog was not domesticated by man, but he was smart enough to become domestic by choice. Its scientific name, *Canis familiaris,* goes one step further and calls it the "dog relating to a family." Our ancestors quickly recognized the advantages of the human–canine partnership, and the co-habitant dog became the co-hunter, the co-traveler, then the companion animal, and finally the co-therapist.

In the last decade animals, especially dogs, have been used more and more for therapeutic visits to homes, hospices, and hospitals. These animals are taken to unfamiliar places, and these visits are filled with unpredictable events. Both the unknown and the unpredictable are considered major stress factors.[37] Although no specific studies have been done on the effect of therapy visits on the working dogs themselves, there are some data scattered in the literature that warrant more attention to this particular aspect of stress.[38]

Heart rate is often used as a basic clinical parameter in evaluating stress.[39] Incorporated in the classification of the different species of domestic animals relative to sympathetic and parasympathetic dominance, the dog is situated between the goat and the pig.[40] The importance of the psychosocial aspects in the human–animal interaction is not a recent concern. Pavlov in considering this wrote: "Finally, we have come across in our dogs a definite social reflex, operative under the influence of an agent of the social surroundings." Although heart rate is always affected by the presence of a person in the vicinity of a dog, the amplitude and the duration is influenced by the various characteristics of the surroundings. The presence of a person induces a significant tachycardia, but if that same person is also petting the dog, the heart rate increases only slightly and declines back to the baseline much more rapidly.[41] On the other hand, whereas a normal dog will react to the presence of a person with increased heart rate, a nervous dog will respond with a significant bradycardia. This pattern is already present at three months of age and becomes more evident at six months and nine months. Although the normal resting heart rate is not significantly different between the two types of dogs, it decreases with age.[42]

Discussing the results of a study made on the effect of a person on coronary blood flow in dogs, the authors remark that "whatever the ultimate answers to these questions, it is worth noting that man, an old friend of the dog, makes striking impression on the dog's heart, on the blood supply as well as the overall output."[43] More and more evidence is accumulating on the beneficial effects of animal ownership in dealing with everyday stress[44] and also in the successes of animal-assisted therapy.[45] The assessment quoted above is even more pertinent today than it was in 1969.

CONCLUSION

It is generally recognized that everything is potentially stressing for the animal, but because the phenomenon itself is not self-evident, the topic of stress in domestic animals is a controversial one. Stress can be viewed as the result of an imposed factor, but it can also be considered as the consequence of a loss of control. The models discussed in this paper seem to fit the latter: loss of natural selection, loss of free movement, loss of self-determined speed, loss of company, loss of vital space, and loss of free interaction.

Furthermore, the concern about stress in the animals is now beyond its economic consequence and even welfare, and is now at the point where the very well-being of the animals is being examined. This is one of the many reasons why stress research should be encouraged. Through communication and interaction between the scientists of the various specialty areas of stress research, the exchange of information will result in cross-fertilization of knowledge to the benefit of all. It is hoped, therefore, that a session on stress in domestic animals will become an integral part of future Hans Selye Symposia.

REFERENCES

1. SELYE, H. 1976. Stress in Health and Disease. Butterworth. Boston, MA.
2. DANZER, R. & P. MORMÈDE. 1979. Le stress en élevage intensif. Masson. Paris.
3. MOBERG, G. P. 1985. Animal Stress. American Physiological Society. Bethesda, MD.
4. YOUSEF, M. 1985. Stress Physiology in Livestock. (3 vols.). CRC Press. Boca Raton, FL.
5. BRUGÈRE, H. & P. MORMÈDE. 1988. Le stress. Rec. Med. Vet. **164:** 703–873.
6. FRASER, A. F. 1988. Proceedings of an International Symposium on Animal Bio-Ethics and Applied Ethology. Appl. Anim. Behav. Sci. **20:** 1–207.
7. SELYE, H. 1964. From Dream to Discovery. McGraw-Hill. Toronto.
8. SPÖRRI, H. 1954. Warum ist das Schwein für den Herztod prädisponiert? Zentralbl. Veterinaermed. **1:** 799–604.
9. SPÖRRI, H. 1954. Untersuchungen über die Systolen- und Diastolendauer des Herzens bei den vershiedenen Haustierarten und ihre Bedentung für die Klinik und Beurteilungslehre. Schweiz. Arch. Tierheilkd. **96:** 593–604.
10. MICHEL, G. 1963. Zum Bau der Herzmuskulatur bei Haus- und Wildschweinen. Zentralbl. Veterinaermed. A **10:** 381–396.
11. LUDVIGSEN, J. 1953. "Muscular degeneration" in hogs (Preliminary report). Proceedings of the 25th International Veterinary Congress **1:** 62.
12. HALL, L. W., N. WOOLF, J. W. P. BRADLEY & D. W. JOLLY. 1966. Unusual reaction to suxamethonium chloride. Br. Med. J. **2:** 1305.
13. HARRISON, G. G., J. F. BIEBUYCK, J. TERBLANCHE, D. M. DENT, P. HICKMAN & J. SAUNDERS. 1968. Hyperpyrexia during anaesthesia. Br. Med. J. **3:** 594–595.
14. TOPEL, D. G., E. J. BICKNELL, K. S. PRESTON, L. L. CHRISTIAN & C. Y. MATSUSHIMA. 1968. Porcine stress syndrome. Mod. Vet. Pract. **49:** 40–41, 59–60.
15. CHRISTIAN, L. L. 1972. A review of the role of genetics in animal stress susceptibility and meat quality. Proceedings of the Pork Quality Symposium. University of Wisconsin, Madison, WI.
16. DeROTH, L., S. D'ALLAIRE S. & M. BÉLANGER. 1981. Épreuve de susceptibilité au syndrome de stress du porc. Med. Vet. Que. **11:** 16–19.
17. DOIZÉ, F., I. ROUX, B. MARTINEAU-DOIZÉ & L. DeROTH. 1990. Prediction of the halothane (Hal) genotypes by means of linker marker loci (Phi, Po2, Pgd) in Quebec Landrace pigs. Can. J. Vet. Res. **54:** 397–399.
18. CHRISTIAN, L. I. & K. LUNDSTROM. 1992. Porcine Stress Syndrome. *In* Diseases of Swine. A. D. Leman, B. E. Straw, W. L. Mengeling, S. D'Allaire & D. L. Talor, Eds. Iowa State University Press. Ames, IA.
19. FUJII, J., K. OTSU, F. ZORZATO, S. DE LEON, V. K. KHANNA, J. E. WEILER, P. J. O'BRIAN & D. H. MACLENNAN. 1992. Identification of a mutation in porcine ryanodine receptor associated with malignant hyperthermia. Science **253:** 448–451.
20. FRANK, G. H. & P. C. SMITH. 1983. Prevalence of Pasteurella haemolytica in transport calves. Am. J. Vet. Res. **45:** 2622–2624.
21. ANDREWS, A. H. 1992. Respiratory disease. *In* Bovine Medicine; Diseases and Husbandry of Cattle. A. H. Andrews, R. W. Blowey, H. Boyd & R. G. Eddy, Eds. Blackwell Scientific Publications. London.
22. PHILLIPS, W. A. 1984. The effects of assembling and transit stresses on plasma fibrinogen concentration of beef cattle. Can. J. Comp. Med. **48:** 35–41.
23. BRYSON, D. G. 1990. Parainfluenza-3 virus in cattle. *In* Virus Infections of Ruminants. Z. Dinter & B. Morein, Eds. Elsevier. New York, NY.
24. ELHAZARY, M. A. S. Y. & J. B. DERBYSHIRE. 1979. Aerosol stability of bovine parainfluenza type-3 virus. Can. J. Comp. Med. **43:** 295–305.
25. TIZARD, I. 1992. Veterinary Immunology. 4th edit. Saunders. Montreal.
26. KILGOUR, R. 1976. Sheep behaviour: Its importance in farming systems, handling trans-

port and pre-slaughter treatment. Proceedings of the Western Australia Department of Agriculture Workshop on Sheep Assembly and Transport: 9–12. Perth.

27. RUSHEN, J. 1986. Aversion of sheep for handling treatments: Paired choice study. Appl. Anim. Behav. Sci. **16:** 363–370.
28. DUNCAN, I. J. H. & D. G. M. WOOD-GUSH. 1971. Frustration and agression in the domestic fowl. Anim. Behav. **19:** 496–500.
29. FAURE, J. M., H. LAGADIC & A. D. MILLS. 1988. Le stress chez la poule. Rec. Med. Vet. **164:** 857–861.
30. KOELKEBECK, K. W., J. R. CAIN & M. S. AMOSS. 1986. Use of adrenocorticotropin challenges to indicate chronic stress responses of laying hens in several housing alternatives. Domest. Anim. Endocrinol. **3:** 301–305.
31. CUNNINGHAM, P. 1991. The genetics of thoroughbred horses. Sci. Am. May: 92–98.
32. MATSUI, K. & S. SUGANO. 1987. Species differences in the changes in heart rate and T wave amplitude after autonomic blockade in Thoroughbred horses, ponies, cows, pigs, goats and chickens. Jpn. J. Vet. Res. **49:** 637–644.
33. MALO, D. & L. DEROTH. 1986. Effects of bolus injection of epinephrine and norepinephrine on systolic time intervals in normal and stress susceptible pigs. Am. J. Vet. Res. **47:** 1565–1568.
34. PHYSICK-SHEARD, P. W. 1983. The physiology of equine performance: An overview. Guelph Task Group on Horse Research. Guelph, Ontario, Canada.
35. PHYSICK-SHEARD, P. W. 1991. Diseases of the cardiovascular system. *In* P. T. Colahan, I. G. Meyhee, A. M. Merritt & J. N. Moore. Equine Medicine and Surgery. American Veterinary Publications. Goleta, CA.
36. DEROTH, L., A. VRINS & M. MARCOUX. 1980. Fibrillation auriculaire chez le cheval. Med. Vet. Que. **10:** 67–68.
37. LEVINE, S. 1985. A definition of stress. *In* Animal Stress. G. P. Moberg, Ed. American Physiological Society. Bethesda, MD.
38. DEROTH, L. 1992. Approche conceptuelle au stressindexe animal dans le contexte d'interaction humain-animale (Abstracts). 6th International Conference: Animals & Us. Human-Animal Bond Association of Canada. Montreal.
39. PORGES, S. W. 1985. Spontaneous oscillations in heart rate: Potential index of stress. *In* Animal Stress. G. P. Moberg, Ed. American Physiological Society. Bethesda, MD.
40. GABRIEL, A., T. ART & P. LEKEUX. 1989. Effets physiologiques de différents types de stress chez le chien avant et après blocage β-adrénergique par le carazol. Ann. Med. Vet. **133:** 229–244.
41. LYNCH, J. J. & J. F. MCCARTHY. 1969. Social responding in dogs: Heart rate changes to a person. Psychophysiology **5:** 389–393.
42. NEWTON, J. E. O. & L. A. LUCAS. 1982. Differential heart-rate responses to person in nervous and normal pointer dogs. Behav. Genet. **12:** 379–393.
43. NEWTON, J. E. O. & W. EHRLICH. 1969. Coronary blood flow in dogs: Effect of person. Cond. Reflex. **4:** 81–88.
44. BERGLER, R. 1988. Man and Dog. Blackwell Scientific Publications. Boston, MA.
45. THE 6TH INTERNATIONAL CONFERENCE: ANIMALS & US. 1992. Abstracts. Human-Animal Bond Association of Canada. Montreal.

Subject Index

Index of Contributors